Photo credits

Gerdi Orterer: page 331 left and right.

Weleda archive, Schwäbisch Gmünd: page 20, 148, 229 right.

The following photos are taken from the free encyclopaedia Wikipedia (www. wikipedia.de): Alvesgaspar: page 276 right; birdy: page 333 left; Curtis Clark: page 187 left; LucaLuca: page 150; Nova: page 276 left; Peter Presslein: page 333 right; Peter Schmidt: page 248; Waugsberg: page 246; Stefan Wernli: page 178; Yikrazuul: page 125.

All remaining photographs are from the author or his wife Anne Sommer-Solheim.

Notes

Preface

1. Translated by William Riggins from Eichendorff, *Werke*, Vol. 1, p. 132. Original German is:
   Wünschelrute
   Schläft ein Lied in allen Dingen,
   Die da träumen fort und fort,
   Und die Welt hebt an zu singen,
   Triffst du nur das Zauberwort.
2. From: Schimmel, A., *Rumi. Ich bin Wind und du bist Feuer.* p. 43.
3. For example, in Steiner's basic work *An Outline of Esoteric Science.*
4. Buber, *Die Erzählungen der Chassidim*, p.187.

Chapter 1: Our Inner Garden

1. Livingstone, *Narrative of an Expedition.*
2. Verbal communication to Dr Karl Köller.
3. Schoner W., Scheiner-Bobis G.: Endogenous cardiac glycosides and ther mechanisms of action. *Am J Cardiovasc Drugs* 2007; 7:173–93.

Chapter 2: Bulbs

1. It would not create a great deal of enthusiasm if the patient were to come to the doctor's surgery with an onion bag, because it is not only the patient who is affected by the side effects of the penetrating smell.
2. Benavides, G.A., Squadito, G.L., Mills, R.W. et al., Hydrogen sulfide mediates the vasoactivity of garlic, *Proc Natl. Acad. Sci.* USA 104 (2007) 17977–82.
3. An overview of the effects of hydrogen sulphide which is created in the body from substances in the plants described, is given in Rui Wang, Giftgas mit Heilkraft, *Spektrum der Wissenschaft* 3 (2011) 22–27.

Chapter 3: Yarrow

1. Leeser, Lehrbuch der Homöopathie, Vol. B/II Pflanzliche Arzneistoffe.
2. Khan, A.U., Gilani, A.H., Blood pressure lowering, cardiovascular inhibitory and bronchodilatory effects of Achillea millefolium, Phytother. Res. 25 (2010) 577–83.
3. Weisser, S., Effekt von Leberwickeln auf die exkretorische Leberfunktion – eine randomisierte Cross-over-Studie. Dissertation Freiburg University 2006.

Chapter 4: Dandelion

1. Science daily Oct. 28 2013: Fraunhofer-Gesellschaft: Making rubber from dandalion juice. www.sciencedaily.com/releases/2013/10/131028114547.httm
2. Steiner, *Agriculture,* lecture of June 13, 1924.

3. Diederich, K., Taraxacum officinale, *Merkurstab* 60 (2007) 566–71; Paepke, D., Taraxacum off. in der Behandlung des Ovarialkarzinoms, (lecture of May 8, 2010 at second congress Ganzheitliche Medizin in Perinatalmedizin und Gynäkologie, at University Hospital Klinikum rechts der Isar, Munich).
4. Diederich, K., Taraxacum officinale, *Merkurstab* 60 (2007) 566–71.
5. Paepke, D., Taraxacum off. in der Behandlung des Ovarialkarzinoms, (lecture of May 8, 2010 at second congress Ganzheitliche Medizin in Perinatalmedizin und Gynäkologie, at University Hospital Klinikum rechts der Isar, Munich).
6. Jachens also wrote several descriptions of the remedy, such as in *Dermatologie*, and in his article 'Die Behandlung von Hautkrankheiten über die Leber' *Merkurstab,* 2004; 57 (4): 248–59.

Chapter 5: Peppermint

1. There is a large number of species of mint which can only be distinguished by an expert. The real peppermint does not occur in nature but is a cultivated form produced by crossing several mint species.
2. For details see www.jungebad.com
3. Madish A., Heydenreich C-J, Wieland V, Hufnagl R, Hotz J., Treatment of functional dyspepsia with a fixed peppermint oil and caraway oil combination preparation as compared to cisapride. A multicenter, reference-controlled double-blind equivalence study. *Arzneim*

Forsch/Drug Research 49 (II) 11, 925–32 (1999); Hoffmann G, Gschossmann J, Bunger L., Wieland V., Heydenreich C.-J., Effects of afixed peppermint oil caraway oil combination (FPCO) on symptoms of functional dyspepsia accentuated by pain or discomfort, *Gastroenterology* 122 (Suppl 1) A-471.

Chapter 6: Daisy

1. See Mommsen, J., Das ausdauernde Gänseblümchen: ein heilkräftiger Immerblüher, *Merkurstab* 61 (2008) 270–83.
2. This is tyrosinase, which is an important enzyme in the process of producing the dark skin pigment melanin.

Chapter 7: Birch

1. Major, H., Untersuchungen zur Wirkungsweise von Birkenblättern *(Betula folium)* und phenolischen Verbindungen, unter besonderer Berücksichtigung der Beeinflussung von Metallopeptidasen, Dissertation, Berlin 2002.
2. Further information is available at www.imlan.de.

Chapter 8: Cowslip

1. A detailed description of this remedy is given in Sommer, M., Plantago Primula cum Hyoscyamo – ein fast vergessenes Arzneimittel gegen Muskelerkrankungen, *Merkurstab* 61 (2009) 65–72.

Chapter 9: Pasque Flower

1. Vithoulkas, *Essenzen Homöopathischer Arzneimittel*, p. 134.

Chapter 10: Wild Strawberry

1. Steiner, *Introducing Anthroposophical Medicine*, lecture of March 30, 1920.
2. Olsson M E, Andersson C S, Oredson S, Beglund R H, Gustavsson K E, Antioxidant levels and inhibition of cancer cell proliferation in vitro by extracts from organically and conventionally cultivated strawberries, *J Agric Food Chem* 2006, 54:1248–55.
3. Mudnic I, Modun D, Brizic I, Vokovic J, Generalic I, et al, Cardiovascular effects of aqueous extracts of wild strawberry (Fragaria vesca L.) leaves, *Phytomecicine* 2009, 16:462–69.

Chapter 11: Greater Celandine

1. Teschke, R., Frenzel, C., Glass, X., Eichhoff, A., 'Greater Celandine hepatotoxicity: a clinical review', *Annals of Hepatology* 2012, 11, 838–48.
2. A detailed study on the issue of potential adverse reactions to medicines was published on Wala remedies containing Chelidonium and came to very reassuring results. Stahnke, G., Mörbt, N., Jäckel, B., Sobeck, U., Meyer, U., Sicherheit und Unbedenklichkeit von Chelidonium ferm-Urtinktur enthaltenden Arzneimitteln *Merkurstab* 2012; 65 (2) 136–42. Undesirable effects appear to be very rare events which, in any case, seem to occur in the case of very

concentrated preparations.
3. Servan-Schreiber, *Das Antikrebs-Buch.*
4. This led to the development of Ukrain, a medicine made from a combination of Chelidonium extract and a cytostatic agent for treating cancers. This remedy is highly controversial. On the one hand there is a series of reports on amazing effects in some cancer sufferers, on the other there are no clear research results which substantiate its efficacy but significant misgivings, particularly because of the cytostatic Thiotepa which is used in its manufacture along with the greater celandine. Ukrain is not licensed anywhere in the EU. At the beginning of 2012 it was classified by the German Federal Institute for Drugs as an unsafe drug whose use is liable to prosecution. A current review is available, 'Ukrain – ein Dauerbrenner' in *Tägliche Praxis*, 53, 2012 (3) 633–35.

Chapter 12: Chamomile

1. In Chapter 3 on yarrow it was noted that when making biodynamic compost preparations, medicinal herbs are processed using particular animal organs. Physicians will notice that those plants often have a therapeutic effect on exactly the organ which is used. For instance yarrow, which is a proven remedy for bladder complaints, is filled into a stag bladder, and chamomile flowers are filled into cow intestines.
2. Breg, M., Fickler, C., Das

Kamillendampf-Sitzbad zur Prävention von Harnwegsinfekten bei Frauen. Transplant Unit of Munich University Hospital.

3. Gyllenhaal, C., Merritt, S.L., Paterson, S.D., Block, K.L., Grouchenour, T., Efficacy and safety of herbal stimulants in sleep disorders, *Sleep Med. Rev.* 4 (2000) 229–51; Viola, H., Wasowski, C., Levi de Stein, M., et al, Apigenin, a component of matricaria recutita flowers is a central benzodiazepine receptor-ligard with anxiolytic effects, *Planta Med.* 61 (1995) 251–52.

Chapter 13: Plantain

1. A detailed description of this remedy is given in Sommer, M., Plantago Primula cum Hyoscyamo – ein fast vergessenes Arzneimittel gegen Muskelerkrankungen, *Merkurstab* 61 (2009) 65–72.

Chapter 14: Horsetail

1. Husemann, *Anthroposophische Medizin.*
2. A group of pharmacists systematically examined the degree to which different preparation methods released the constituents of horsetail. See Meyer, U., Staiger, K., Seitz, A., Rechnen Sie mit der Kieselsäure: Pharmazeutische Gesichtspunkte zu einer möglichen Optimierung der Equisetum-Therapie, *Merkurstab* 65 (2012) 112–16.

Chapter 15: St John's Wort

1. Schempp, C.M., Wölfle, U., Meyer, U., Schaette, R., Johanniskraut *(Hypericum perforatum L.):* heilkräftige Lichtpflanze der Sommersonnwende, *Merkurstab* 2011; 64 (6) 596–606.
2. Lomagno, P., Lomagno, R.C., Activity of Hypericum perforatum oil in the treatment of bedsores in old people, *Fitoterapia* 1979; 50: 201–5.
3. Glaser, *Erfolgreiche Wundbehandlung.*
4. Schempp, C.M., Müller, K.A., Winghofer, B., Schöpf, E., Simon, J.C., Johanniskraut *(Hypericum perforatum L.)* eine Pflanze mit Relevanz für die Dermatologie, *Hautarzt* 2002; 53: 316–21.
5. Schempp, C.M., Pelz, K., Wittmer, A., Schöpf, E., Simon, J.C., Antibacterial activity of hyperforin from St. John's wort against multiresistant Staphylococcus aureus and grampositive bacteria, *Lancet* 353 (1999) 2129.
6. Reuter, J., Wölfle, U., Weckesser, St., Schempp, C.M., Which plant for which skin disease? *Journal of the German Society of Dermatology* 8 (2010) 788–796.

Chapter 16: Starry Elder

1. Madaus, *Lehrbuch der Homöopathischen Heilmittel,* Volume 3.
2. Schaefer, O., 'Holunder,' in *Der grüne Ton,* p. 98. German original is:
   Sitze ich im Dunkelgrün
   Träumend an der grauen Rinde
   Eingewiegt vom Sommerwinde –
   Sehe ich dein helles Blühn
   Überall im Dunkelgrün,
   Sehe still dein Wunder,
   Sterniger Holunder.

Blätter spielen über mir
Fingergleich im Licht und Schatten
Auf den zarten Phloxrabatten,
Und ich ruhe ganz im Hier,
Glut und Mittag über mir,
Lausche Deinem Wunder,
Sterniger Holunder.

Chapter 17: Lime (Linden)

1. Rispens, J.A., Die Linde: Der Baum des Menschen, *Merkurstab* 59 (2006) 423–35.
2. Further information in Sommer, M., Soldner, G., Therapeutische Erfahrungen mit der Lindenmistel, *Merkurstab* 59 (2006) 435–37.

Chapter 19: Coneflower, Echinacea

1. There has been much speculation as to whether there were in fact cases of syphilis in Europe before Columbus. As far as I understand the current state of research on this question, there are now in fact good reasons to believe that the actual strain causing the life-threatening syphilis was imported from South America at the end of the fifteenth century but that related, far less dangerous but similar diseases (which were probably not transmitted sexually) were present before this.
2. Barrett, B., Brown, R., Rakel, D., Mundt, M., et al., Echinacea for treating the common cold. A randomized trial, *Ann. Intern. Med.* 153 (2010) 769–777.
3. Jawad, M., Schoop, R., Suter, A., Klein, P., Eccles, R., Safety and efficacy of *Echinacea purpurea* to prevent common cold epsiodes: A randomized double-blind placebo-

controlled trial. *Evidence-Based Complementary and Alternative Medicine* 2012. Article ID 841315 dx.doi.org/10.1155/2012/841315.

Chapter 20: Lemon balm (Melissa)

1. See Akhondzadeh, S., Noroozian, M., Mohammadi, M., Ohadivia, S., Jamshidi, A.H., Khani, M., *Melissa officinalis* extract in the treatment of Alzheimer's disease: a double blind, randomised, placebo controlled trial, *J. Neurol. Neurosurg. Psychiatry* 74 (2003) 863–66.
2. Ballard, O.C., O'Brien, J.T., Reichelt, K., Perry, D.K., Aromatherapy as a safe treatment for the management of agitation in severe dementia: The results of a double-blind placebo-controlled trial with melissa, *J. Clin. Psychiatr.* 63 (2002) 553–58.
3. Burns, A., Perry, E., Holmes, C., Francis, P., Morris, J., Howes, M.J., Chazot, D., Lees, G., Ballard, C., A double-blind placebo-controlled randomised trial of *Melissa officinalis* oil and donepezil for the treatment of agitation in Alzheimer's disease, *Dement Geriatr Cogn Disord* 2011; 31: 158–64
4. Fung, K.M., Tsang, H.W.H., Chung, R.C.K., A systematic review of the use of aromatherapy in treatment of behavioral problems in dementia, *Geriatr Gerontol Omt* 2012; 12: 372–82.
5. Kurz, A., Psychosoziale Interventionen bei Demenz, *Nervenarzt* 2013; 84: 93–103.
6. See Akhondzadeh, S., Noroozian, M., Mohammadi, M., Ohadivia, S., Jamshidi, A.H., Khani, M., *Melissa*

officinalis extract in the treatment of
Alzheimer's disease: a double blind,
randomised, placebo controlled
trial, *J. Neurol. Neurosurg. Psychiatry*
74 (2003) 863–66.

Chapter 21: Rosemary

1. When rosemary aroma was
introduced into the rooms then
the subjects' memory improved
and their degree of wakefulness
increased, while with the aroma of
lavender they were more relaxed
but their memory declined. See
Moss, M., Cook, J., Wesnes, K.,
Kucket, P., Aromas of rosemary and
lavender essential oils differentialy
affect cognition and mood in
healthy adults, *Int. J. Neurosci.* 113
(2003) 15–38.
2. Steiner, *Introducing
Anthroposophical Medicine,* lectures
of April 3 and 4, 1920.
3. Bakirel, T., Bakirel, O.U., Selgen,
S.G., Yardibi, H., In vivo assessment
of antidiabetic and antioxidant
activities of rosemary *(Rosmarinus
officinalis)* in alloxan-diabetic
rabbits, *J. Ethnopharmacol.* 116
(2008) 64–73. In this work it says:
'*Rosmarinus officinalis* extracts exert
remarkable antidiabetic effects.'
4. Jimbo, D., Kimura, Y., Taniguchi,
M., Inoue, M., Urakami, K., Effect
of aromatherapy in patients with
Alzheimer's disease, *Psychogeriatrics*
9 (2009) 173–79.
5. Steiner, *Introducing
Anthroposophical Medicine,* lectures
of April 3 and 4, 1920.

Chapter 22: Rose

1. Translated from German by Lynda
Hepburn, from Rumi, *Ghaselen des
Dschelâleddîn Rumi.*
2. Translated from German by
Lynda Hepburn, from Atabay, *Die
schönsten Gedichte.*
3. Translated from German by Lynda
Hepburn, from Rumi, *Ghaselen des
Dschelâleddîn Rumi.*

Chapter 23: Arnica and Calendula

1. Eckermann, J.P., *Gespräche mit
Goethe,* p. 453.
2. Karow, H., Abt, H.-P., Fröhling,
M., Ackermann, H., Efficacy of
Arnica montana D4 for Healing
of Wounds after Hallux Valgus
Surgery Compared to Diclofenac,
J. Altern. Compl. Med. 14 (2008)
17–25.
3. Steiner, *Introducing
Anthroposophical Medicine*, lecture
of April 3, 1920.
4. In the study, 128 patients were
given the commonly used
Trolamin gel after each session of
radiation and 126 patients were
given Calendula ointment. The
allocation to groups was random.
Grade II and higher radiodermatitis
occurred in 41% of patients in
the Calendula group and 63% of
patients in the standard treatment
group. This means there was over
a third less radiation reactions
which exceeded a simple reddening
of the skin and involved at least
slight skin damage, weeping and
pain. The women in the Calendula
group also had significantly less pain
and were more satisfied with the

treatment. Pommier, P., Gomez, F., Sunyach, M.P., D'Hombres, A., Carrie, C., Montbaron, X., Phase III randomized trial of *Calendula officinalis* with Trolamine for the prevention of acute dermatitis during irradiation of breast cancer, *J. Clin. Oncol.* 2004: 12 (8) 1447–53.

5. A number of case studies on this are given in Sommer, M. Lokale und systemische Behandlung mit Calendula bei komplizierten Wundheilungsstörungen: eine Kasuistik, *Merkurstab* 1996; 49 (2) 127–30. An interesting description of this medicinal plant is given in the article by Diederich K, Riggers U., Die Calendula, *Merkurstab* 2005; 59 (1) 47–55.

6. See also Sommer, M., Lokale und systemische Behandlung mit Calendula bei komplizierten Wundheilungsstörungen: eine Kasuistik, *Merkurstab* 1996; 49 (2) 127–30.

Chapter 24: What Bees Tell Us

1. Günther, et al., *Urania Tierreich,* Vol. 3, p. 470.

Chapter 25: Yellow Gentian

1. Deshpande, D.A., Wang, C.H.W., McIllmoyle, E., Robinett, K.S., et al., Bitter taste receptors on airway smooth muscle bronchodilate by localized calcium signaling and reverse obstruction, *Nature Med.* 16, 1299–1304 (2010).

Chapter 26: Monkshood

1. Nilius, B., Properties of aconitine-modified Na chanels in single cells of ventricular mouse myocardium,

Gen. Physiol. Biophys. 5 (1986) 473–482; Iurievichius, I.A., Rosenstraukh, L.V., Ishmanova, A.V., Formation of ectopic stimulation in the heart under the action of aconitine, *Kardiologija* 20 (1980) 75–78.

Chapter 27: Chicory

1. Schwarz R., Alkali comp. Kurzdarmsyndrom, in *Vademecum Anthroposophische Medizin,* p. 53.

Chapter 28: Stinging Nettle

1. Singh, R., Hussain, S., Rajish, V., Sharma, P., Anti-mycobacterial screening of five Indian medicinal plants and partial purification of active extracts of *Cassia sophera* and *Urtica dioica. Asian Pacific Jnl. Trop. Med.* (2013) 366–71.

2. Steiner, *Agriculture,* lecture of June 13, 1924.

3. Dr Wolfgang Engel described the manufacture of this fertiliser and the complex background to the process in detail in Vegetabilisierte Metalle Teil I: Grundlagen des pharmazeutischen Verfahrens und Zubereitung der Metall-Dünger, *Merkurstab* 66 (2013) 4–17.

Chapter 29: Bilberries

1. Kern, P., Ammon, A., Kron, M., et al., Risk factors of alveolar echinococcosis in humans, *Emerg. Inf. Dis.* 9 (2003) 343–49.

2. Heidelbeeren, Bärlauch und Hund: Wo der Fuchsbandwurm wirklich lauert. *Bild der Wissenschaft,* May 30, 2007.

Chapter 30: Grapevines

1. Zajicek, G., Oren, R., Weinreb, M. jr., The streaming liver, *Liver* 6 (1985) 293–300.

Chapter 31: Bryophyllum

1. Hassauer, W., Schreiber, K., Von der Decken, D., Ein neuer Weg in der tokolytischen Therapie, *Erfahrungsheilkunde* 34 (1985) 683–87.
2. Daub, *Vorzeitige Wehentätigkeit*. Vilaghi, I., Decreasing the rate of premature delivery with phytotherapy: results from general practice, *Ther. Umsch.* 59 (2002) 696–701.
3. Planegger, N., Rist, L., Zimmermann, R., von Mandach, U., Intravenous tocolysis with Bryophyllum pinnatum is better tolerated than beta-agonist application, *Eur. J. Obstet. Gynecol. Reprod. Biol.* 124 (2006) 168–72.
4. It has been shown using rodents that Bryophyllum increases the length of sleep (Pal, S., Sen, T., Chadhurim, A.K., Neuropsychopharmacological profile of the methanolic fraction of Bryophyllum pinnatum leaf extract, *J. Pharm. Pharmacol.* 51 (1999) 313–18), and a calming and muscle relaxing effect has also been demonstrated experimentally (Yemitan, O.K., Salahdeen, H.M., Neurosedative and muscle relaxant activities of aqueous extract of Bryophyllum pinnatum, *Fitoterapia* 76 (2005) 187–93).

Chapter 32: Ivy

1. Mezger, *Gesichtete Homöopathische Arzneimittellehre,* Vol. 1; Stephenson, *Hahnemannian provings.*

Chapter 33: Blackthorn

1. The paper by Ulrich Meyer gives an excellent overview of the blackthorn, its effects and its many uses throughout history: Die Schlehe: Heilpflanze für Zeitgenossen, *Merkurstab* 2011, 64 (2) 100–114. In a further paper Meyer deals with hydrocyanic acid which, as has already been mentioned above, is to be found in blackthorn: 'Dem Stoff sich verschreiben, heißt Seelen zerreiben'. Zur historischen Signatur und toxikologischen Problematik reiner Blausäure, *Merkurstab* 2011, 64 (3) 123–32.

Chapter 34: Frankincense

1. An overview is given by Ammon, H.P.T., Salai-Guggal-(Indischer Weihrauch-) Gummiharz aus *Boswellia serrata, Dtsch. Ärztebl.* 95 (1998) 30–31.
2. A current review of brain tumours also recommends considering the use of incense: Schneider, T., Marri, C., Scherlach, C., et al., Die Gliome des Erwachsenen, *Dtsch. Ärztebl.* 107 (2010) 799–808.
3. Ammon, H.P.T., Salai-Guggal-(Indischer Weihrauch-) Gummiharz aus *Boswellia serrata, Dtsch. Ärztebl.* 95 (1998) 30–31; and Schneider, T., Marri, C., Scherlach, C., et al., 'Die Gliome des Erwachsenen, *Dtsch. Ärztebl.* 107 (2010) 799–808.

Chapter 35: Mistletoe

1. Göbel, Th., Dorka, R., Zur Raumgestalt und zur Zeitgestalt der Weißbeerigen Mistel (*Viscum album L.*) *Tycho de Brahe Jahrbuch für Goetheanismus* 1986, 167–94.

2. Kienle & Kiene, *Die Mistel in der Onkologie.*

3. Britsch, M., Heidecke, H., Meyer, U., Angiogenesehemmung durch Iscucine: Ergebnisse aktueller Untersuchungen, *Merkurstab* 63 (2010) 218–22.

4. See Madeleyn, R., Gesichtspunkte zur Epilepsie und deren Behandlungsmöglichkeit bei Kindern, *Merkurstab* 43 (1990) 369–84.

5. See also Soldner & Stellmann, *Individal Paediatrics.*

6. Wilkens, J., Sommer, M., Soldner, G., et al., Die Behandlung des Fibromyalgie-Syndroms mit Weidenmistel-Extrakten, *Merkurstab* 58 (2005) 264–71.

7. Simon, L., Chronisches Gelenkrheuma/Chronische Polyarthritis, in Glöckler, *Anthroposophische Arzneitherapie,* Vol. 1, 31.1–12.

8. Orange, M., Fonseca, M., Lace, A., von Laue, B., Geider, S., Durable tumour responses following primary high-dose induction with mistletoe extracts: Two case reports. *Eur. J. Integr. Med.* 2010, 1 (4) 227. Orange, M., Lace. A., Fonseca, M., von Laue H.B., Geider, S., Kienle, G.S., Durable Regression of Primary Cutaneous B-cell Lymphoma following Fever-inducing Mistletoe Treatment: Two Case Reports. *Global Adv. in Health & Med.* 2012 1(1) 16–23. Seifert, G., Tautz, C., Seeger, K., Henze, G., Laengler, A., Therapeutic use of mistletoe for CD30+ cutaneous lymphoproliferative disorder/lymphomatoid papulosis, *J. Eur. Acad. Dermatol. Venereol.* 2007 Apr, 21 (4) 558–60. Werthmann, P.G., Strater, G., Friesland, H., Kienle, G.S., Durable response of cutaneous squamous cell carcinoma following high-dose peri-lesional injections of Viscum album extracts: A case report. *Phytomedicine* 2013 Feb 15; 20 (3–4) 324–27. Mabed, M., El-Helw, L., Sharma, S., Phase II study of viscum fraxini-2 in patients with advanced hepatocellular carcinoma. *British Journal of Cancer* 2004 (90) 65–69. Mahfouz, M.M., Ghaleb, H.A., Hamza, M.R., Fares, L., Moussa, L., Moustafua, A., El-Za Wawy, A., Kourashy, L., Mobarak, L., Saed, S., Fouad, F., Tony, O., Tohamy, A., Multicenter open labeled clinical study in advanced breast cancer patients. A preliminary report. *Journal of the Egyptian Nat Cancer Inst* 1999 11 (3) 221–27.

9. Tröger, W., Galun, D., Reif, M., Schumann, A., Stankić, N,, Milićević, M., Viscum album [L.] extract therapy in patients with locally advanced or metastatic pancreatic cancer: A randomised clinical trial on overall survival. *Eur. J. Cancer* 49 (2013) 19: 3788–97.

10. Personal communication from Dr. H. Matthes, Head Physician, Gastroenterology, Havelhöhe Community Hospital, Berlin. A small retrospective study with 39 patients has shown that intratumoral application of mistletoe extracts in combination

with conventional chemotherapy in patients with advanced, unresectable pancreatic carcinoma was safe and associated with an remarkably long time of survival. The efficacy should be evaluated in a randomised controlled trial. (Schad F, Axtner J, Buchwald D, Happe A, Popp St, Kröz M, Matthes H, *Integr Cancer Ther* Dec 19, 2013 DOI: 10.1177/153735413513637)

11. Wilkens, *Mistletoe Therapy for Cancer.*
12. Werner, H., Mahfouz, M.M., Fares, L., Fouad, F., Ghaleb, H.A., Hamza, R., Kourashy, L., Mobarak, A.L., Moustafa, A., Saed, S., Zaky, O., Zawawny, A., Fischer, S., Scheer, R., Scheffler, A., Zur Therapie des malignen Pleuraergusses mit einem Mistelpräparat, *Merkurstab* 1999, 52 (5) 298–301. Salzer, G., Popp, W., Die lokale Iscadorbehandlung der Pleurakarzinose, in Jungi & Senn, *Krebs in Alternativmedizin,* Vol. 2, pp. 36–49. Girke, M., Debus, M., Kröz, M., Ascites bei Non-Hodgkin-Lymphom (V.a. splenales Lymphom) Remission nach viermaliger intraperitonealer Viscum-album-Instillation, *Merkurstab* 2012, 65 (3) 257f.
13. Schaefermeyer H., Zur Therapie des Blasenkarzinoms, *Merkurstab* 1996, 49 (3) 229–33. Simões-Wüst, A.P., Hunziker-Basler, N., Zuzak, T.J., Eggenschwiler, J., Rist, L., Viviani, A., Meyer, U., Das Mistelpräparat Iscucin Crataegi: Option für die Instillationstherapie bei Harnblasenkarzinom. *Merkurstab* 2007, 60 (3) 251–55.
14. For example, a randomized clinical study showed that patients with breast, ovarian and bronchial carcinomas tolerated chemotherapy significantly better when they were given mistletoe at the same time (Piao, B.K., Xang, Y.X., Xie, U., Mannsmann, U., Matthes, H., Beuth, J., Lin, H.S., Impact of complementary mistletoe extract treatment on quality of life in breast, ovarian and non-small cell lung cancer patients. A prospective randomized controlled clinical trial, *Anticancer Res.* 23 (2004) 303–9. In vitro studies on cell lines of breast, pancreas, lung and prostate cancer showed that mistletoe extracts which where given simultaneously with standard chemotherapeutic agents (doxorubicin, gemcitabine, docetaxel, mitoxantrone, cisplatin) did not inhibit chemotherapy induced cytostasis and cytotoxicity. In higher concentrations mistletoe extracts showed an additive inhibitory effect. (Weinstein U, Kunz M, Baumgartner St, Interactions of standardized mistletoe (Viscum album L.) extracts with chemotherapeutic drugs regarding cytostatic and cytotoxic effects in vitro. *BMC Complementary and Alternative Medicine* 2014 14:6 DOI: 10.1186/1472-6882-14-6
15. A detailed account of the scientific findings on mistletoe therapy is given in Kienle, & Kiene *Die Mistel in der Onkologie,* and in Kienle, Kiene & Albonico, *Anthroposophische Medizin in der klinischen Forschung.*
16. See also Sommer, M., Soldner, G., Die Mistel und ihre

Wirtsbäume – Differenzierung zur Optimierung der Therapie, *Merkurstab* 54 (2000) 29–48. Wilkens, J., *Misteltherapie*. Soldner, G., Sommer, M., Wilkens, J., Therapeutische Erfahrungen mit der Lindenmistel, *Merkurstab* 60 (2006) 435–37. Wilkens, J., Die Weidenmistel beim Blasenkarzinom, *Merkurstab* 60 (2007) 446–49. Wilkens, J., Die Weisstannennmistel, *Merkurstab* 62 (2008) 570–83; Wilkens, J., Die Mandelmistel, *Merkurstab* 63 (2010) 29–45.

Chapter 36: Christmas Rose

1. Mörike, 'Auf eine Christblume,' translated by Malcolm Wren, copyright © 2006, reprinted with kind permission. The German original reads:
   Tochter des Walds, du Lilienverwandte,
   So lang von mir gesuchte, unbekannte,
   Im fremden Kirchhof, öd und winterlich,
   Zum ersten Mal, o schöne, find ich dich!

   Von welcher Hand gepflegt du hier erblühtest,
   Ich weiß es nicht, noch wessen Grab du hütest;
   Ist es ein Jüngling, so geschah ihm Heil,
   Ist's eine Jungfrau, lieblich fiel ihr Teil.
   ...
   Schön bist du, Kind des Mondes, nicht der Sonne;
   Dir wäre tödlich andrer Blumen Wonne,

Dich nährt, den keuschen Leib voll Reif und Duft,
Himmlischer Kräfte balsamsüße Luft.

2. For example, Wilkens, J., *Helleborus niger*: Geschichte, Botanik und differentialtherapeutische Anwendung einer Heilpflanze, *Merkurstab* 63 (2010) 535–49.

3. Soldner, G., *Helleborus niger* in der Pädiatrie, *Merkurstab* 63 (2010) 508–17; Soldner & Stellmann, *Individual Paediatrics*.

4. Schnürer, Chr., *Helleborus niger*: Anwendung in Innerer Medizin und Psychosomatik, *Merkurstab* 63 (2010) 518–25; Soldner, G., *Helleborus niger* in der Pädiatrie, *Merkurstab* 63 (2010) 508–17.

5. Many verbal descriptions are now available as articles in a special issue on *Helleborus niger* in the journal for anthroposophical medicine, *Der Merkurstab*, 63, Vol. 6 (2010). Contributions worth noting are for example: Breitkreuz, Th., Helleborus in der Onkologie. Kasuistiken und Therapieerfahrungen aus dem Gemeinschaftskrankenhaus Herdecke 2001–2010, *Merkurstab* 63 (2010) 526–34; Debus, M., Anwendungsmöglichkeiten von *Helleborus niger* in der Onkologie, *Merkurstab* 63 (2010) 551–57 and the articles by Wilkens, Schnürer, and Soldner mentioned in Notes 2 to 4 above.

Chapter 37: Ginger and Horseradish

1. Therkleson, T., The experience of receiving ginger compresses in persons with osteoarthritis: a phenomenological study, Faculty of Nursing. Vol. PhD. Edith Cowan University. Perth, Western Australia 2009.

Chapter 38: Gold

1. This and following quotes are from Vithoulkas, G., *Essenzen Homöopathischer Arzneimittel.*

2. For example, Selawry, *Metallfunktionstypen in Psychologie und Therapie*; Selawry, *Zinn und Zinntherapie*; Selawry, *Silber und Silbertherapie*; Walter, *Die sieben Hauptmetalle.* Individual topics also appear in *Vademecum anthroposophische Arzneimittel,* and Girke, M., *Innere Medizin.*

3. More about the possibilities of anthroposophical medicine for heart disease is given in Bavastro, Fried, & Kümmell, *Herz-Kreislauf-Sprechstunde.*

Useful Organisations

UK & Ireland:
Wala & Weleda www.weleda.co.uk

USA & Canada
Weleda usa.weleda.com

Australia
Weleda www.weleda.com.au

New Zealand
Wala & Weleda www.weleda.co.nz

Weleda (international) www.weleda.com

Bibliography

Atabay, Cyrus (tr.), *Die schönsten Gedichte aus dem klassischen Persien*, Munich 2004.

Bavastro, P., Fried, A., Kümmell, H.Chr., *Herz-Kreislauf-Sprechstunde. Ein umfassender medizinischer Ratgeber*, Stuttgart 2003.

Buber, M., *Die Erzählungen der Chassidim*, Zurich 1992.

Daub, E., *Vorzeitige Wehentätigkeit. Ihre Behandlung mit pflanzlichen Substanzen*, Stuttgart 1998.

Eckermann, J.P., *Gespräche mit Goethe in den letzten Jahren seines Lebens*, Munich 1984.

Eichendorff, J. von, *Werke*, Volume 1, Munich 1981.

Girke, M., *Innere Medizin, Grundlagen und therapeutische Konzepte in der Anthroposophischen Medizin*, Berlin 2012.

Glaser H.. *Erfolgreiche Wundbehandlung: Aus der Praxis anthroposophisch erweiterter Krankenpflege*, Stuttgart 2000.

Glöckler, M. (Ed.), *Anthroposophische Arzneitherapie für Ärzte und Apotheker*, Stuttgart 2005.

Godden, Rumer, *The Story of Holly and Ivy*, London 2001.

Gunther, K., Hannemann, H.-J., Hieke, F., Konigsmann, E., Schumann, H., *Urania Tierreich*, Vol. 3, Leipzig 1994.

Hegi, Gustav, *Illustrierte Flora von Mitteleuropa*, Parey 2000.

Husemann, Friedwart, *Anthroposophische Medizin. Ein Weg zu den heilenden Kräften*, Dornach 2011.

Jachens, Lüder, *Dermatologie: Grundlagen und therapeutische Konzepte der anthroposophischen Medizin*, Berlin 2012.

Jungi, W.F., Senn, H.-J. (eds.) *Krebs in Alternativmedizin*, Berlin/Heidelberg 1990.

Kienle, G.S., Kiene, H., Albonico, H.U., *Anthroposophische Medizin in der klinischen Forschung*, Stuttgart 2006.

Kienle, G.S., Kiene, H., *Die Mistel in der Onkologie*, Stuttgart 2003.

Leeser, O., *Lehrbuch der Homöopathie*, Ulm 1973.

Livingstone, David and Charles, *Narrative of an expedition to the Zambesi and its tributaries and of the discovery of the Lakes Shirwa and Nyassa, 1856–1864*, London 1865.

Madaus, G., *Lehrbuch der Homöopathischen Heilmittel*, Vol. 3, (reprint of 1938 ed.) Hildesheim 1979.

Mezger, Julius, *Gesichtete Homöopathische Arzneimittellehre*,

Vol. 1, Heidelberg 1989.

Mörike, E., *Sämtliche Gedichte in einem Band*, (ed. B. Zeller) Frankfurt 2004.

Rumi, *Ghaselen des Dschelâleddîn Rumi*, (tr. Josef v.
Hammer-Purgstall) Stuttgart 1920.

Schaefer, O., *Der grüne Ton. Späte und frühe Gedichte*, Munich 1973.

Schimmel, A., Rumi. *Ich bin Wind und du bist Feuer. Leben
und Werk des großen Mystikers*, Cologne 1986.

Selawry, A., *Metallfunktionstypen in Psychologie und Therapie*, Ulm 1983.

—, *Silber und Silbertherapie*, Ulm 1966.

—, *Zinn und Zinntherapie*, Ulm 1963.

Servan-Schreiber, D., *Das Antikrebs-Buch. Was uns schützt: vorbeugen
und nachsorgen mit natürlichen Mitteln*, Munich 2010.

Soldner, G., Stellmann, H.M., *Individal Paediatrics: Physical Emotional and
Spiritual Aspects of Diagnosis and Counseling*, CRC Press, USA, 2014.

Steiner, Rudolf, *Agriculture*, Bio-Dynamic Farming and Gardening Ass. USA 1993.

—, *An Outline of Esoteric Science*, Anthroposophic Press, USA 1997.

—, *Introducing Anthroposophical Medicine*, Steinerbooks USA 2010.

Stephenson, J., *Hahnemannian provings: A Materia
medica and Repertory*, New Delhi, 1998.

Vademecum anthroposophische Arzneimittel, (ed. Gesellschaft
Anthroposophischer Ärzte) 3ed Stuttgart 2013.

Walter, H., *Die sieben Hauptmetalle. Ihre Beziehungen zu
Welt, Erde und Mensch*, Dornach, 2010.

Wilkens, Johannes, Misteltherapie. *Differenzierte Anwendung
der Mistel und ihrer Wirtsbäume*, Stuttgart 2006.

—, *Mistletoe Therapy for Cancer: Prevention, Treatment
and Healing*, Floris Books, 2010.

Vithoulkas, G., *Essenzen Homöopathischer Arzneimittel nach G.
Vithoulkas*, (tr. J.Faust & G. Hieronymus) Frankfurt 1986.

Plant families

Indices are not usually the most interesting parts of a book. But they unquestionably offer a good opportunity for making discoveries. Below is a list of the medicinal plants mentioned in detail in this book, arranged according to their families. A great many medicinal plants are found here as the only representative of their family (for example ivy for the *Araliaceae* and mistletoe for the *Loranthaceae*). But it is very noticeable that there is a concentration into three families: the daisy family, mint family and buttercup family. Over a quarter of all the therapeutic plants in this book belong to the daisy family (*Compositae*, also called *Asteraceae*). This is very striking, but it has to be admitted that this is also due to the fact that the *Compositae* is a very large plant family.

Plants are in principle assigned to the different families on account of the structure of their flowers. The flower of a member of the *Compositae* is actually a community made up of numerous individual flowers. This can easily be seen with the naked eye in a sunflower, which also belongs to this family. The outer flowers each have a long coloured petal, while the inner part of the flower disc is made up of inconspicuous individual tubular flowers which each have stamens and a pistil and produce their own fruits. At every point where a sunflower seed sits there was previously an individual flower of the sunflower flower community. In principle, all members of the *Compositae* family are made up of a 'composite' of individual flowers like the sunflower. A composite inflorescence like this in a way represents the ability to integrate the individual into an overall structure. Might this ability be connected to the fact that there are so many medicinal plants amongst the members of the daisy family? Ultimately, every illness can be viewed as one part of our body no longer being able to perform what is necessary for the whole (it varies from illness to illness as to whether this is a case of 'too much' organ activity – think of the increased mucus production in a cold – or 'too little' – for example in the case of a thyroid insufficiency). What is unusual is that the members of the daisy family almost never produce any poison (in contrast to those of the buttercup family, for example, which all produce substances which irritate the skin and mucus membranes). These characteristics may be a reason that plants from the daisy family are particularly suitable as 'home remedies', which can gently help to restore health when this has begun to falter.

Far fewer plants in this book come from the mint family (*Labiatae*) but they still comprise almost a tenth of the total. The members of this family are characterised by their complicated horizontally-angled flowers resembling a face, where the petals have united into a tube and often make use of a refined tilting mechanism to ensure that every insect visiting the flower gets dabbed with pollen. Many of these 'gestures' point beyond the sphere of the plant towards that of the animal realm. What is typical of plants is actually the production of surfaces, particularly those of the leaves. When plants form enclosed spaces, this goes beyond the plant nature, strictly speaking. The fast reaction of the stamens when an insect penetrates the flower in search of nectar is also an 'animal-like' gesture. The flower, in turning away from the sky into the horizontal axis, also positions itself in the same plane in which the animal lives. Like very many other flowers, the goal of the *Labiatae* is also to attract insects. Many plants make use of scent to do this. It is a characteristic of the *Labiatae* – and especially those with a medicinal effect – that there is also a large amount of scented essential oil in the leaves. It is perhaps not surprising that these plants particularly affect our mood. They can stimulate (rosemary, for example) or relax (lemon balm or lavender, for example) or they relieve organs such as the stomach that have become 'upset' due to emotional stresses (peppermint, for example).

Just as, in individual plants, we can discover gestures in their appearance that reappear in their medicinal effects, gestures typical of the family can also be found, as illustrated by these examples. An index showing the plants in this book arranged according to their families not only has a scientific purpose, but can also be the basis of our own discoveries.

Ivy family (Araliaceae)
Ivy (*Hedera helix*): page 314.

Incense tree family (Burseraceae)
Frankincense (*Boswellia serrata, Boswellia sacra*): page 330.

Birch family (Betulaceae)
Silver birch (*Betula pendula*): page 70.

Nettle family (Urticaceae)
Stinging nettle (*Urtica dioica, Urtica urens*): page 282.

Orpine family (Crassulaceae)
Bryophyllum (*Kalanchoë* (= *Bryophyllum*) *daigremontiana, Kalanchoë pinnata*): page 308.

Gentian family (Gentianaceae)
Yellow gentian (*Gentiana lutea*): page 256.

Honeysuckle family (Caprifoliaceae)
Elder (*Sambucus nigra*): page 169.

Buttercup family (Ranunculaceae)
Christmas rose (*Helleborus niger*): page 357.
Monkshood (*Aconitum napellus*): page 265.
Pasque flower (*Pulsatilla vulgaris, Pulsatilla pratensis*): page 92.

Heather family (Ericaceae)
Cranberry (*Vaccinium macrocarpon*): page 296
Bilberry (*Vaccinium myrtillus*): page 296.

Dogbane family (Apocynaceae)
Strophanthus (*Strophanthus kombé, Strophanthus gratus*): page 17.

Ginger family (Zingiberaceae)
Ginger (*Zingiber officinale*): page 365.

St John's Wort family (Hypericaceae)
St John's Wort (*Hypericum perforatum*): page 158.

Daisy family (Compositae)
Arnica (*Arnica montana*): page 228.
Artichoke (*Cynara scolymus*): page 183.
Blessed thistle or St Benedict's thistle, holy thistle (*Cnicus benedictus, formerly Carduus benedictus*): page 183.
Daisy (*Bellis perennis*): page 65.
Chamomile (*Matricaria recutita*, formerly *Matricaria chamomilla*): page 127.
Dandelion (*Taraxacum officinale*): page 42.
Milk thistle (*Silybum marianum, formerly: Carduus marianus*): page 183.
Marigold (*Calendula officinalis*): page 228.
Yarrow (*Achillea millefolium*): page 34.
Coneflower (*Echinacea angustifolia, Echinacea purpurea, Echinacea pallida*): page 192.
Chicory (*Cichorium intybus*): page 275.

Cabbage family (Brassicaceae)
Horseradish (*Cochlearia armoracia*): page 365.

Lily family (Liliaceae)
Garden onion (*Allium cepa*): page 26.

Lime family (Tiliaceae)
Lime (*Tilia cordata, Tilia platyphyllos*): page 177.

Mint family (Labiatae)
Lavender (*Lavandula officinalis*)
Melissa/Lemon balm (*Melissa officinalis*): page 201.
Peppermint (*Mentha piperita*): page 58.

Rosemary (*Rosmarinus officinalis*): page 210.
Poppy family (*Papaveraceae*)
Greater celandine (*Chelidonium majus*): page 109.

Primrose family (Primulaceae)
Cowslip/Oxlip (*Primula veris/Primula elatior*): page 82.

Mistletoe family (Loranthaceae)
Mistletoe (*Viscum album*): page 340.

Rose family (Rosaceae)
Rose (*Rosa centifolia, Rosa damascena*): page 219.
Blackthorn (*Prunus spinosa*): page 320.
Wild strawberry (*Fragaria vesca*): page 103.

Horsetail family (Equisetaceae)
Field horsetail (*Equisetum arvense*): page 146.

Plantain family (Plantaginaceae)
Ribwort plantain (*Plantago lanceolata*): page 138.

Grapevine (Vitaceae)
Grapevine (*Vitis vinifera*): page 302.

Index of Healing Plants

Index of Ailments

bowel
— diseases, inflammatory 188
— disorders 41
— irritable bowel syndrome 38, 64, 137, 142, 205, 261
brain
— tumour 333–35
— damage 254
— damage, early childhood 91, 144
— disease 359
— haemorrhages 363
— injuries 363
bronchial oversensitivity 319
bronchitis 84, 88, 198, 272, 317
—, chronic 87, 370
bruising 231, 234
burns 237, 284, 294
—, mild 167

cancer 39, 105f, 120, 156, 299, 344, 351ff, 362, 364
— chemotherapy 48, 51, 240, 242
— fatigue syndrome 353
—, ovarian 49
—, prostate 364
—, thyroid 319
candidiasis (fungal infection of the intestine) 262
carcinoma
—, bile duct 49
—, gall bladder 49
— mucilaginous adenocarcinomas 182
cardiac
— diseases 85
— infarction 229
— insufficiency 22f, 90, 327
cardiovascular, diseases 239
cataracts 73, 154
catarrh 156
cerebral palsy, spastic 144
chemotherapy 48, 51, 240, 242
— nausea caused by 367
childbirth 98
—, exhaustion post 325
cholesterol 186, 300
circulatory system
— diseases 378
— disorders 384
— problems due to infectious diseases 90
coccyx, damage to the 165

cold 52, 64, 129, 144, 156, 170, 174, 176, 179, 181, 195, 198, 259, 263, 317, 322, 324, 366
—, acute 133
—, babies with 170, 175
—, head 58
—, late phase of a 175
—, tussive irritation in 178
— with headache 368
colic 208
— in babies 130
colitis ulcerosa 279
concentration, improvement of 203
concussion 236
confusion (postoperative delirium) 383
conjunctivitis 96, 100
—, suppurating 199
constipation 142, 324f
—, persistent 171
contractions 100
convalescence 323
convulsive siezure 130
cough 28, 30, 144, 195, 198, 317
—, dry 174, 181, 319
—, persistent 370
—, persistent dry 226
cramp 39
— lower abdomen 39
—, muscle 255
—, tendency to 38
cystospasm 129

decubitus (bedsores) 325
delirium, postoperative 383
dementia 205, 359, 363
denture pressure points 132, 143, 200, 240
depression 160, 165, 188, 329, 351, 367, 383
—, mild 86, 307
depressive mental disorders 37
depressive moods 100
dermatitis 132
detox 46, 48, 51, 73, 76, 108, 287, 295, 324
diabetes 212f, 217
—, gestational 217

diarrhoea 36, 104, 277, 298, 300, 324
—, summer 107, 300

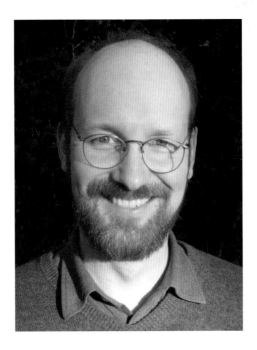

Markus Sommer, born in 1966, studied medicine in Munich and is a general physician there. His experience includes internal medicine, pediatrics, geriatry, neurology, and the practical application of homeopathic and anthroposophical medicine. He is the author of several medical books.

HEALING
PLANTS

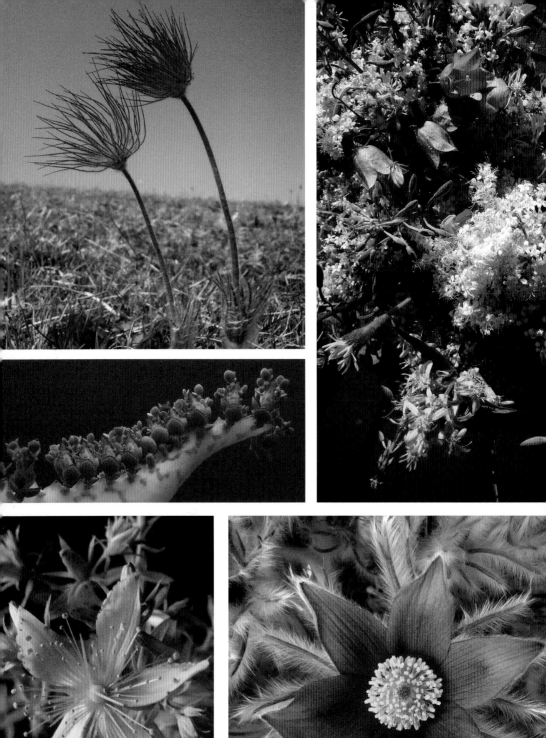
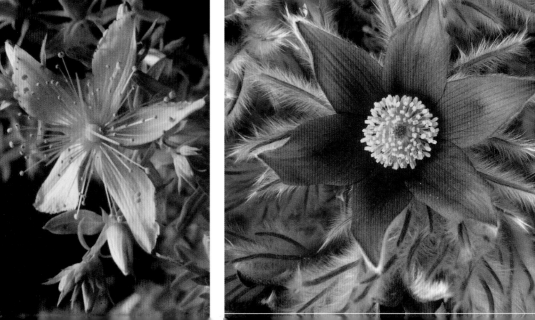

HEALING PLANTS

HERBAL REMEDIES FROM TRADITIONAL TO ANTHROPOSOPHICAL MEDICINE

MARKUS SOMMER

Floris Books

Translated by Lynda Hepburn

First published in German as *Heilpflanzen: ihr Wesen,*
ihre Wirkung, ihre Anwendung by Verlag Urachhaus in 2011
Second edition 2013
Translated from the first edition and first published in English
by Floris Books in 2014

British Library CIP Data available
ISBN 978-178250-057-5
Printed in Malaysia

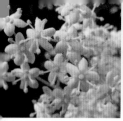
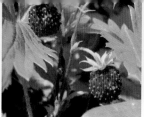
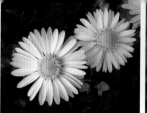
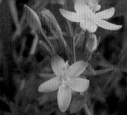

Contents

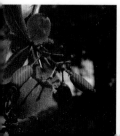
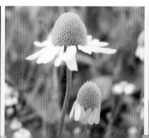
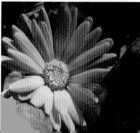
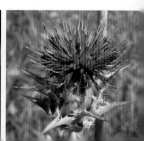

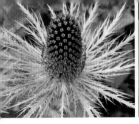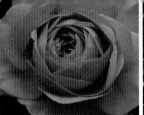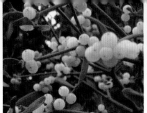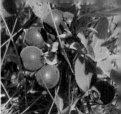

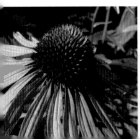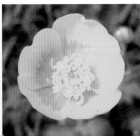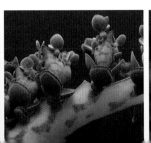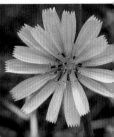

Note

Please be aware that medicines available on prescription will vary from country to country. Also names of some medicines are different in some countries. Inquire in your country about Weleda and Wala medicines (see details at back of book).

This book contains information obtained from authentic and highly regarded sources and is based on many years of clinical practice and on the current state of scientific knowledge. All reasonable efforts have been made to publish reliable data and information, but the author and the publisher cannot assume responsibility for the validity of all materials or for the consequences of their use.

Please note that anthroposophic medicine is a complementary medicine that integrates various elements of conventional medicine with anthroposophic concepts of health, illness and healing processes, homeopathy and naturopathy. It seeks to extend, not replace, mainstream medicine.

The author and the publisher disclaim any warranty of fitness for a particular purpose and warn that readers should not rely on the content herein as a substitute for conventional medical treatment. The applications and case studies described in the book cannot replace the advice and treatment of a medical specialist. For a correct diagnosis and appropriate treatment in the case of health problems, or suspected or existing disease, you should always seek the advice of your doctor/physician.

The use of general descriptive names, trade names, trademarks, etc. even if not specifically identified, does not imply that these names are not protected by the relevant laws and regulations.

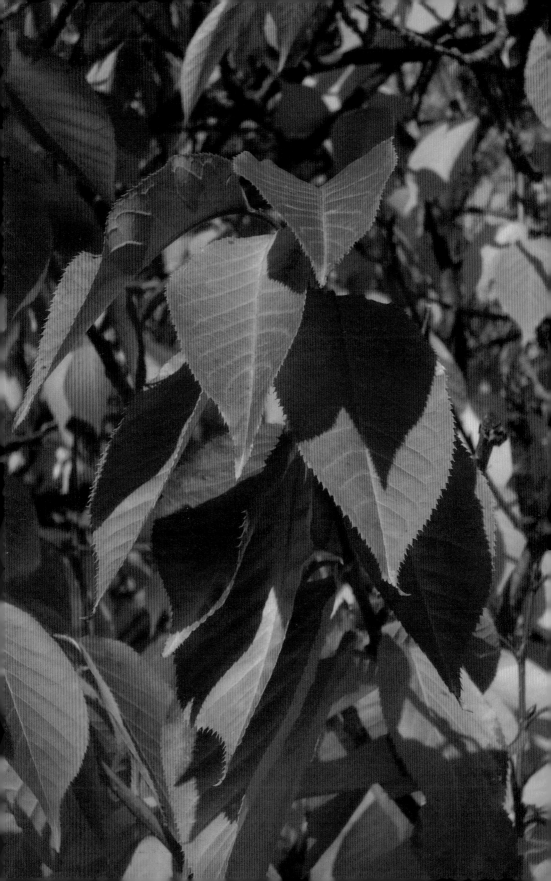

To see a world in a grain of sand
And a heaven in a wild flower,
Hold infinity in the palm of your hand
And eternity in an hour.

William Blake
(Fragments from *Auguries of Innocence*)

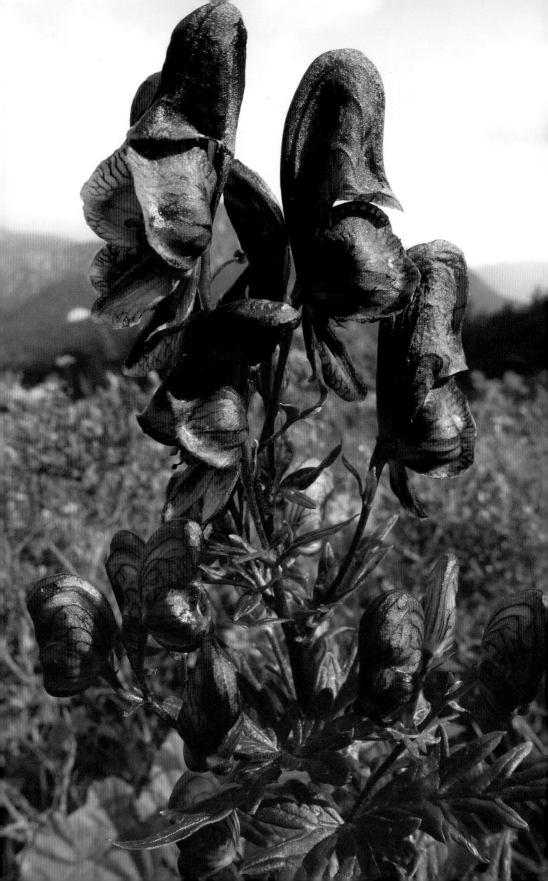

Preface

Most of us love the plants around us. Nearly everyone is moved by encountering a flowering cherry tree, and flowers like cowslips, daisies and violets likewise touch our hearts. For thousands of years we have known that some of these plants also have medicinal properties – and our knowledge of how these plants can help us continues to grow. Often, we find that current scientific findings confirm what has been known by intuitive perception of plants for hundreds of years. But even today, new aspects of plants are discovered through painstaking efforts to gain a clearer image of their inner properties, and these insights may then be confirmed in therapeutic practice at a later date. This book provides a place for both of these: the love of plants, and the knowledge of their medicinal properties. It is hoped that, by deepening both of these aspects, the reader may deepen his or her inner relationship to the plants described. This, in turn, will lead to an increased ability to use them for treating yourself both for minor and more major ailments. It can also stimulate and facilitate your discussion with a physician or other qualified therapist to discuss the possibility of your being treated with medicinal plants.

The prologue of St. John's Gospel says that everything in the world was made 'through the word' and nothing that is in the world 'came into being except through the word' (John 1:3). Thus, every thing in the world has an echo of the primordial word active within it, which is specific to that thing.

In the soul of the poet, the word is experienced as a song, which is asleep 'in all things.' We can learn to listen to and thus discover what is hidden in the world. Then things that at first seemed to be disconnected products of random chance appear full of purpose, connectedness and beauty.

The Magic Wand

There sleeps a song in every thing,
Which lies in stillness, dreams unheard.
And lo, the world begins to sing,
If you but find the magic word.

Joseph von Eichendorff [1]

When I was a small child I felt – like many children – particularly close to plants, and it seems to me that this 'singing' is still audible in the child's ear for a time. The world does not usually speak to the grown-up so directly. Nonetheless, if you observe a plant patiently through the seasons, contemplate its appearance, let it come to life in you again and again, and also study its many details – right down to the chemical composition – then the notes of its song can reveal themselves one after another. Eventually, you will begin to discern a full melody.

It was a great service of Charles Darwin to show that the world and the life in it is not fixed, but in a process of 'evolution' (literally 'unrolling'). Living creatures therefore evolve and come about through an individual development arising out of a common past. Besides his varied and inspiring observations of nature, Darwin also drew on a long line of intellectual predecessors and, on the very first page of his ground-breaking work *On the Origin of Species*, he mentioned Goethe as one of the proponents of the same idea. However, this idea actually predates the era of natural science and arose out of ancient philosophy, religion and ultimately, mystery wisdom.

In the 13th century, the Islamic mystic Jalal ad-Din Muhammad Rumi spoke of how we have ourselves passed through the realms of nature in a long process of evolution, and that a long way still lies before us until we return to the spheres from which the world once arose:

I died as a mineral and became a plant,
I died as plant and rose to animal,
I died as animal and I was Man. Why should I fear?

When was I less by dying?
Yet once more I shall die as Man, to soar
With angels blest;
but even from angelhood I must pass on:
to become what I don´t understand –
HIS holy breath.[2]

Darwin perceived the 'preservation of favoured races in the struggle for life' in the 'survival of the fittest' and 'natural selection'. In contrast, Rumi understood that sacrifice and death lead to a gradual ascent. A similar philosophical idea can be found in Christian thinkers. Insights into the evolution of the earth are described in a wonderful way in the writings of Rudolf Steiner[3], the founder of anthroposophy and anthroposophical medicine. He unites natural and spiritual science and offers a way of achieving our own direct perceptions of the inner aspects of the world around us.

The human being has already passed through all the realms of nature that are 'below him' and in this sense are related to him. Thus it makes sense that there is always something in nature that can help us when something is 'lacking'. In this book, Chapter 1 shows how this applies quite literally, right to the details of biochemistry and the hormonal system, and describes how certain plants actually produce substances which correspond to hormones in our body. If we lack these, they can be replaced by a specific plant. In other situations, the same plant in potentised form can stimulate the regulation of a pathological endocrine condition. But plants are also able to stimulate healing processes at other levels, which cannot be so directly understood in a material way.

This is naturally not to say that all medicines should be made only from plants. In this book, which is really a book about plants, you will find a chapter with a description of gold as a remedy (see Chapter 38) as an example of how minerals (or in this case, a metal) are linked to us and can become medicines. In addition, the description of the bee demonstrates an animal with therapeutic properties (albeit one which is particularly well connected to plants). In fact, medicines can be obtained from all the realms of nature. Nonetheless, plants are the mainstay for treating ourselves in daily life, which is why they form the principal focus of this book. Even nowadays – according to the World Health Organisation – more then 60 % of all illnesses worldwide are primarily treated by plant medicine.

To avoid any misunderstanding right from the start: if all substances have their origin in the 'primordial word', then this applies equally to penicillin (originally a natural substance, which was produced from a fungus) and also the surgeon's knife. I value plant remedies for treatment whenever they can reasonably be used, because they generally encourage our own powers of healing. This certainly does not mean that other remedies should be avoided when needed.

It is obvious that plants can help us. Just as importantly, we have a duty to them which goes beyond protecting them in nature or growing them in the garden. This duty may be explained by a reference in one of the wonderful stories of the eastern Jewish Hasidim, brought to us by Martin Buber. Many of the plants described in this book are so mild that we can drink them as tea without any harm. Some, however – for example, monkshood *(Aconitum napellus)*, greater celandine *(Chelidonium majus)* and Christmas rose *(Helleborus niger)* – are poisonous and should never be consumed as food. They have to be specially prepared and used with precise knowledge of the correct dose in order to have a beneficial effect. Yet as a rule, the poisonous plants produce the most powerful remedies.

Medicinal plants like these appear in the stories told by Martin Buber. Once upon a time, the daughter of Rabbi Baruch of Mesbiz was seriously ill and had to take a tincture made from a medicinal plant. Her father asked himself why people who were ill were given poisons to make them better, and in the end provided the answer himself. Rabbi Baruch said to himself: 'The sparks which fell from creation into the *qliphoth* (impure husks) and changed into stones, plants and animals, they all rise up to their source through the sanctification of the pious who work on them in holiness, who make use of them in holiness, who consume them in holiness. But how can the sparks which fell into the bitter poisons and poisonous plants be redeemed? So that they do not remain cast out, God has intended them for those who are ill, for each who is the bearer of the sparks which belong to the roots of their soul. So the sick person is himself a doctor who heals the poisons.'[4] Perhaps studying the inner being of plants also contributes to collecting the 'sparks' concealed in them, so that in this sense they only find their goal when human beings make use of them and transmute them.

In this book, the description of the plant itself is followed by an explanation of its therapeutic use. Where appropriate, a description is given of how to collect and prepare the plant yourself. An outline is also provided of its status in phytotherapy, homeopathy and anthroposophical medicine (the focus of my medical practice), but without any claim to completeness. Instructions on self-treatment are given where this is appropriate, while in cases of more serious illnesses these notes on aspects of the plant's efficacy (potentially in combination with other plants and substances) are simply for the reader's information. One or another of these may also be of interest to the expert.

As a rule, an expert should be consulted in cases of more serious or ongoing health problems. It is normally helpful to have a general practitioner or local pharmacist who knows you well and – if they have studied this area – can judge which plant remedies (if any) are suitable for a specific illness.

I hope that this book will provide useful information, but in particular I hope it will stimulate the reader's own experience of the varied and wonderful world of plants which surrounds us. If in this process you discover a 'magic word' and hear the 'singing' of the plants with your inner ear, then that would give me particular pleasure.

Marcus Sommer

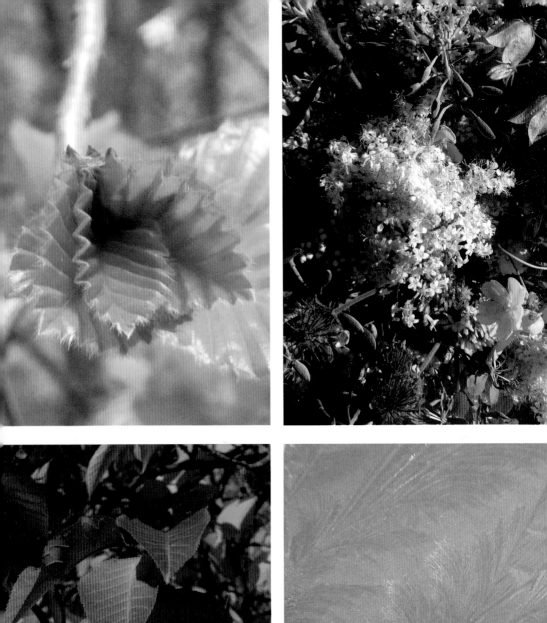

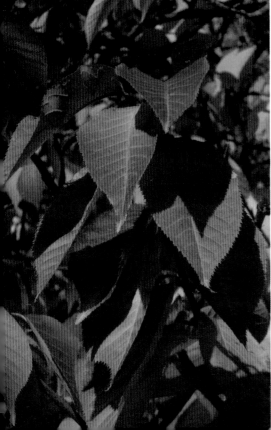

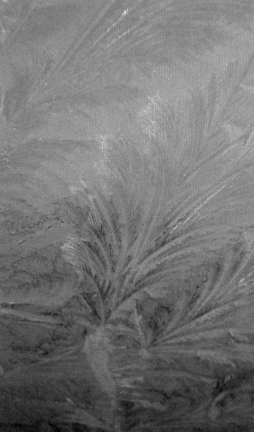

CHAPTER 1

Our Inner Herbal Garden

Even nowadays every intensive care unit uses drugs that originated from plants, a fact that few people are aware of. The painkiller morphine is still obtained from poppy juice, most antibiotics are produced from fungi (organisms at least similar to plants) and many cyctostatics used to treat cancer were discovered in plants such as the yew tree – a relative of the periwinkle, the American mayapple and many others.

Why should plants in particular be of such help to us? Their effects were often known to native healers and medicine women, but in most cases they only became part of 'scientific medicine' by chance.

A hundred and fifty years ago, there were still blank areas on the map, especially in Africa. Brave and ambitious men like David Livingstone set out to fill in these gaps in knowledge. Livingstone followed the River Zambezi and, while searching for its source, discovered the Victoria Falls. He had to be accompanied by a doctor on these expeditions to treat any tropical diseases and injuries from accidents or the weapons of the natives who felt threatened by the intruders. The doctor on Livingstone's expedition was called John Kirk (unfortunately, it is not known whether he was an equally adventurous ancestor of the captain of the same name who commanded the space ship *Enterprise* hundreds of years later!). The following short story is recorded in the expedition diary. Dr Kirk had a cold with a slight fever and a rapid pulse. As a conscientious Scotsman of regular habits, he never failed to brush his teeth every morning, even in the jungle. An odd taste on his toothbrush did not bother him as he regularly took bitter-tasting quinine to prevent malaria, and sometimes stirred it in a glass of water with his toothbrush. He noticed

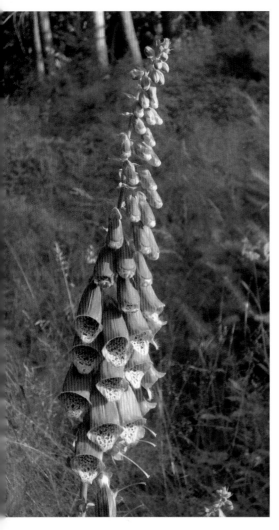

Foxglove (Digitalis purpurea),
which was methodically introduced into
medicine by William Withering, contains
substances related to strophanthin which
are produced in our own bodies.

that the palpitations caused by his fever had disappeared after his morning ablutions and he felt calm and decidedly well. He began to ponder the cause of this.

And then his objectivity and thoroughness (qualities that distinguish every good scientist) became apparent. He noticed that he had carelessly stored a sample of a highly potent arrow poison, which the natives used to hunt animals (and also unpleasant humans), in the same bag as his toothbrush.[1] The poison causes the heart to contract and eventually come to a standstill. However, in a smaller dose (such as the residue of poison accidentally stuck to the toothbrush), the substance increases the strength of the heart and lowers a too-fast pulse. Kirk and Livingstone suspected that the poison could be useful as a medicine – and this proved to be spectacularly correct. They found that the main constituent of the poison was crushed seeds from a vine with the botanical name of *Strophanthus*. Later, the actual toxin, strophanthin, was isolated from these seeds, a substance which has much in common with the active ingredients in our native foxglove *(Digitalis)*.

For many decades these cardiac glycosides were such a crucial drug for the treatment of the heart that the famous German pathologist Professor Naunyn, one of the most noted doctors of his day, said that he would not wish to practise medicine without them. It was only a few years ago that they went out of fashion, partly because a study had shown that, even though patients with cardiac insufficiency felt better when given digitalis glycoside, on average they died sooner.

In anthroposophical medicine, *Strophanthus* continues to be used in a potentised form. Rudolf Steiner, the founder of this form of medicine, pointed out over 80 years ago that a remedy made from the seeds of this vine can counterbalance the 'negative effects of civilisation'.[2] In a potentised form the substance has indeed proved very effective in treating stressful conditions such as exam anxiety, stage fright and similar, but I have often wondered how this is connected to the familiar effect on the heart.

In recent years it has been discovered that strophanthin not only exists in the form of a phytotoxin, but is also produced in our own bodies. This occurs primarily in the adrenal gland. This gland also produces the well-known stress hormone, adrenalin, as well as cortisone, a substance which is likewise involved in adapting to stress.[3] Strophanthin is also produced in the brain and even in the heart itself and is now regarded as a hormone – a substance present in the blood through which various organs communicate with and influence one another. It is now known that strophanthin production increases in situations such as a sudden demand on physical performance (in sport, for instance) and then appears in the bloodstream in the high concentrations which medication aims for. The heart's capacity is increased by the body's own strophanthin, the hormone enabling higher performance.

However, constant overproduction of strophanthin has detrimental effects similar to those of constant stress. For example, it causes the heart muscle to thicken. It is suspected that continuous overproduction of strophanthin is involved in the development of some types of high blood pressure. In such cases, a potentised form of strophanthin could have a regulating effect.

It has since been discovered that large quantities of medicinal cardiac glycoside are harmful if the body is already making excessive amounts of strophanthin due to chronic stress or illness. However, if the amount of strophanthin produced by the body is too low, then supplying an external source of the phytotoxin can be useful. This is yet another topic which brings us to Rudolf Steiner, who once said

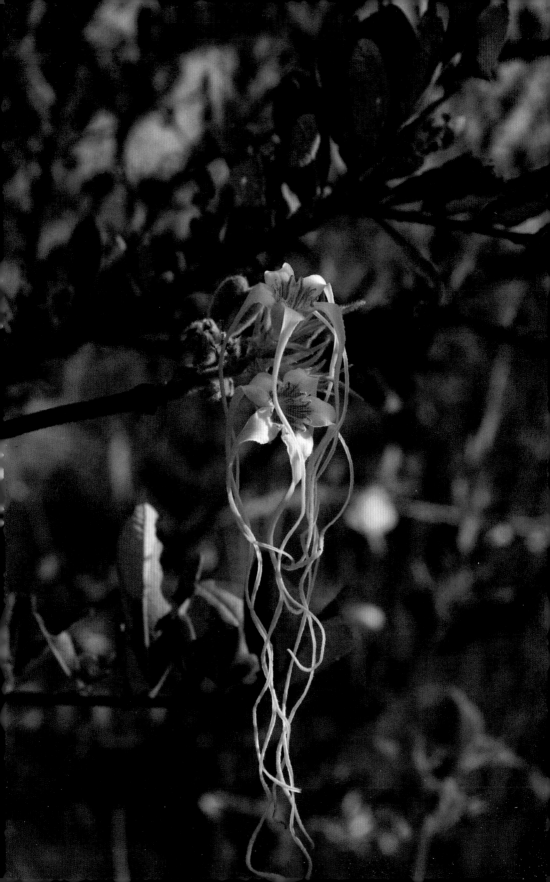

something that must have sounded very poetic and perhaps rather strange even then: 'if a plant is lacking from a person's "inner garden", then he must be given it as a medicine'.

Nowadays we know from the most up-to-date research that we ourselves produce a substance that was for decades known only as a phytotoxin. It has been discovered that we also produce the toxins found in foxglove, and that substances are made, similar to those in the poppy, which act like morphine and help with our ability to bear pain. Conversely we have inner 'organs of perception', known as receptors, which react specifically to these substances. Anthroposophical scientific knowledge has shown that there is a deep connection between nature and the human being, that they have a common origin and develop together. The naturalist Lorenz Oken, who lived at the time of Goethe, described the human being as a 'concentration of nature' and nature as a 'human being spread out and revealed in his parts'. Current scientific research confirms this view and teaches us respect for knowledge based on a more comprehensive perception of reality, even though it may at first appear rather absurd and even strange.

Strophanthus

The Strophanthus species of use to medicine *(S. kombé, S. gratus)* grows in Africa. The product used in Europe is mainly imported from Malawi. Imports to Europe have been repeatedly blocked by political tensions and conditions amounting to civil war in the areas where the vine originates. Another problem is the hot and humid climate, which causes the seeds to spoil easily. Concentrated strophanthus preparations in particular are often difficult to obtain. Fortunately, the situation in Mali has now eased and it has been possible to set up projects geared towards sustainable production which safeguard nature and ensure fair treatment for the producers. Drying plants operated by solar power should prevent the contamination of plant material by fungal toxins, leading to hopes that the availability of strophanthus preparations will stabilise.

Flower of Strophanthus kombé.

Concentrated strophanthin preparations

Strophanthin is absorbed into the blood via the mucous membranes of the mouth or the intestine only to a minor degree. Therefore, for conditions of acute *heart strain* it was mainly administered by injection in the past. These types of ampoule preparations are almost unobtainable nowadays. Concentrated strophanthin preparations are often only available on prescription. Some pharmacies have specialised in preparing such remedies. There are some reports of positive results with concentrated strophanthin preparations in the prevention of heart attacks and treatment of angina pectoris, and they are said to be useful for helping to cope with stress. But there is still considerable debate as to the suitability of this therapeutic approach.

Strophanthus oil

The heart-stimulating alkaloid strophanthin dissolves well in water but poorly in oil. This is why the oil obtained from the strophanthus seeds contains only small amounts of it. Nevertheless, it is used to manufacture Oleum Strophanthi forte capsules (Weleda). The important thing about these capsules is not just the action of the strophanthin (which is of course present) but the fact that this oil comes from the seed of a medicinal plant. Rudolf Steiner pointed out that seeds can have a special effect on the heart. Fats and oils also represent the highest level of heat concentration which a plant can produce and, conversely, we can release particularly large amounts of heat from these substances. The heart is also the centre of warmth in our bodies, producing a great deal of warmth at every moment of our lives and passing this on to our blood. This is another way in which strophanthus oil has a special effect on the heart. The Oleum Strophanthi forte capsules are used for cardiac insufficiency and for the complementary treatment of angina-pectoris pain and functional cardiovascular conditions.

The capsules are available on prescription only, so a doctor must be consulted before using them. A common dose is one capsule 2–4 times daily.

I have repeatedly observed, especially in the case of older patients with less severe forms of *cardiac insufficiency* which can manifest in slight shortness of breath during exertion or in heart-related sleep disturbances, that Oleum Strophanthi forte capsules have led to an improvement in their condition. It is also often necessary to effectively treat high blood pressure in the patient.

Potentised strophanthus preparations

In my experience, potentised strophanthus preparations are often more useful than the concentrated ones. Weleda supplies Strophanthus kombé, ethanol. Digestio D3 as prescription-only ampoules, and Wala produces rhythmised preparations in D3 (prescription only), D4, D6 and D10 as ampoules and D3 and D6 as globules under the name Strophanthus kombé e semine. The remedy is often used in this form for treating an *irregular heartbeat* when the pulse rate is too slow and also for mild symptoms of a *cardiac insufficiency (weak heart)*. Aurum/ Strophanthus (Wala) can also be given for the same indications. This preparation combines Strophanthus D5 with potentised gold, Aurum D9. (Weleda also produce a very similar remedy.) For older patients with clear symptoms of *cardiac insufficiency* I have repeatedly found a considerable improvement in the overall condition by giving this compound along with Cardiodoron 1% ampoules (Weleda). It goes without saying that serious heart conditions should not be treated without the advice of a doctor.

Whilst administering strophanthin as a substance can be seen as a kind of replacement for an insufficient strophanthin production by the body, potentised strophanthus is often effective in cases where there is a chronic over-production of endogenous strophanthin. This can take the form of overly strong physical reactions to prolonged emotional stress, which can result in an *increase in blood pressure*, for example. This effect is involved in the indications and preparations described below.

For *stage fright* and *exam nerves* taking Strophanthus e semine D6 (up to 5 globules hourly) has proved successful. Presumably in this case both the effect on the adrenal glands (which produce several stress hormones) and the calming down of the circulation play a role. In the case of stage fright there may be a certain parallel to the orthodox medicinal use of beta blockers which lower the pulse rate and produce a general calming effect. I find Aurum/Valeriana comp. (again, up to 5 globules hourly) even more effective for exam nerves than pure strophanthus potencies. This remedy also contains potentised gold (which helps the patient to become more centered) potentised valerian, potentised hawthorn (*Crataegus*), which also acts on the cardiovascular system, and cactus. The advantage of this remedy compared to conventional alternatives (such as sedatives and beta blockers) is that it does not interfere with emotional and mental alertness and capability. Aurum/Valeriana comp. has also proved useful for air travel as it eases the unpleasant bodily symptoms of *jetlag*. It is also especially beneficial in *operations* as it results in significantly improved post-operative stability and tolerance of anaesthetic. The usual dosage for this is 10 globules 3 times daily, from three days before the operation to up to four days after it.

I had a memorable experience of the efficacy of a potentised strophanthus preparation on my own body. The contraction of the heart muscle is normally controlled by stimulating waves which start from the right atrium of the heart at regular intervals and systematically spread out over the whole heart. I had unexpectedly developed a premature heartbeat which started from the ventricle, so that my heartbeat 'stumbled'. I experienced this irregularity as extremely annoying and unpleasant, particularly as it was accompanied by an abnormal sensation in the stomach and chest and a feeling of weakness. Up to this point I had always reassured every patient in whom I had diagnosed this irregularity that it is almost always harmless. But now I understood that when you suffer from this condition, all you want is to return to your normal, calm heartbeat as soon as possible.

I tried a number of things, but nothing I did for myself had any effect. I finally went to a colleague for advice (unfortunately doctors have a tendency to want to treat themselves). Georg Soldner, my friend and colleague in the next room, suggested: 'Well, you have taken an interest in Strophanthus for so long – perhaps *that* will do you good.' He prescribed Strophanthus comp. Wala for me. This remedy

---

is similar in composition to Aurum/Stibium/Hyoscyamus, which is often used for an irregular heartbeat (and which I had already tried without success). It contains potentised gold and antimony, plus henbane. In place of the last named, Strophanthus comp. ampoules are made using Strophanthus D4 (D2 in the globules). I injected this remedy under the skin and a few minutes later my heart was beating regularly again. As no treatment had worked for over ten days, this effect seemed like a miracle to me. My heartbeat remained regular (apart from a few minutes in a severely stressful situation) without any further need for medication. Besides revealing the powerful healing properties of Strophanthus, this experience also showed me that you often need someone else to suggest a cure when your efforts at self-treatment are not sufficient. In retrospect, I suspect that stressful situations that I did not want to acknowledge were also responsible for my temporary heart complaint. A cardiologist whom I subsequently consulted on the matter used the remedy for other patients with similar symptoms and reported with delight that it also frequently helped his patients to a remarkable degree.

CHAPTER 2

Bulbs

Even when it is still cold outside, they are already stirring under the earth, and, in a few slightly warmer spots, flowers are bursting forth. We are talking about bulbs. When the first flowers appear very early in the new year, most of these come from bulbs: snowdrops and crocuses as well as daffodils and tulips. Bulbs contain warmth, which sometimes even enables the plants to thaw the snow around the shoot a little.

Our culinary bulbs – onions – only flower in summer, but we can experience the warmth in them as well. In their fresh, uncooked state they burn on our tongues, and when we chop them up they make us cry, reminding us of the effect of a smoking fire. Both the hot taste and the stinging eyes are due to substances containing sulfur, which vaporise easily and can therefore irritate the mucus membranes.

In nature, sulfur is found where the heat from the depths of the earth reaches the surface: in volcanoes or sulfur-rich geothermal waters. For example, magnificent glowing yellow sulfur crystals were formed in the crater of Vesuvius. If you put a flame to them they melt and start to burn. The gas produced – sulfur dioxide – has a pungent smell and burns our mucous membranes. It is not surprising that people pictured hell heated by burning brimstone. The old English word 'brimstone' means 'burning stone', and the fact that a mineral – a 'stone' – burns is really incredible and shows what internal heat it contains.

Onions are not the only culinary plants containing sulfur. Mustard does as well, for example. It also tastes hot, its smell can bring tears to the eyes and when it comes into contact with the skin, it causes reddening and a very hot sensation, which is sometimes used for treating illnesses where a warming action is needed. Mustard is traditionally served with meat dishes and makes them easier to digest.

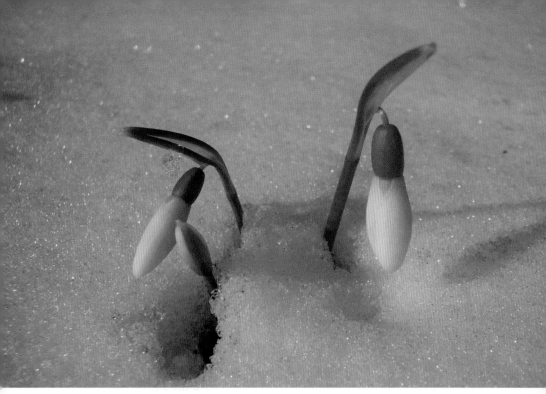

The snow is melted by sprouting snowdrops.

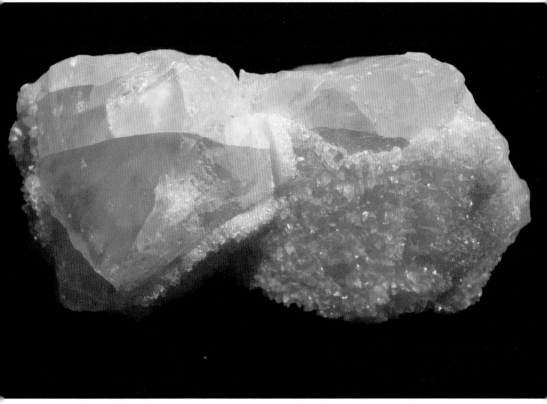

Sulfur crystal from Etna.

In fact, digestion can be viewed as an extended process of cooking and transformation. One purpose of cooking food is to make it more digestible and to start the process which is completed by our digestion. This makes it easier to understand why onions play such a major part in cooking. Hungarian cookery cannot be imagined without them, including the famous goulash recipe, which has spread throughout much of the world. The original recipe for goulash uses the same quantity of onions as meat and in many parts of the world meat is likewise prepared with a lot of onions. Unlike the modern trend to fry a tender steak quickly, in earlier times preparing meat was a lengthy process – it still is in many countries today. Tough kinds of meat such as mutton only become soft and palatable after being marinated. One method consists of mixing the cut up meat with chopped onions and leaving it to stand for at least half a day. The 'sulfur forces' in the onion are then able to perform a kind of cooking process without heat, making the otherwise tough meat soft and appealing. Onions can even improve the taste of vegetarian food and it is not without reason that braised onions often accompany dishes which are otherwise difficult to digest. However, it is no secret that onions themselves are hard to digest for some people and betray their sulfur content by the aroma of the digestive gases. However, they are also more digestible when heat-treated by cooking and in particular by frying. Another method is to add hot spices, such as those used in Indian cuisine, which produces delicious and digestible dishes.

The warming power of the onion is also used therapeutically. A hard *cough* with phlegm which simply refuses to loosen up and needs to be 'melted', as it were, was treated effectively by our grandmothers using onion juice or onion syrup (see page 30). I often hear that these old home remedies are still being used to this day. Naturally, treating oneself in this way does not replace examination by a doctor if a cough persists over a longer period than would normally be expected, or if chest pains, high temperature or other worrying symptoms are also present.

In ancient medicine – as is still the case in Chinese medicine today – whole groups of illnesses were regarded as 'cold illnesses'. *Arteriosclerosis* is one such disease. It occurs when fats, which should be dissolved in the bloodstream, are deposited on the walls of the blood vessels, even forming crystals at times (in a similar way to water freezing). It is often reported that a diet rich in onions (and its close relative, garlic) can help prevent these deposits. Additionally, onion can produce healing effects when applied directly to the skin. Many mothers know the 'onion bag' as an effective first aid measure for *earache.* The vapour from the onion produces a warming effect and promotes the circulation in the ear, thus counteracting inflammation (see page 30). Of course, this treatment is no substitute for medical attention. In addition, the unavoidable 'side effect' of the smell of onion is not to everyone's taste. Another application of onion to the skin is perhaps better known: for a *bee* or *wasp sting,* placing a cut and slightly crushed onion on the affected area of skin can quickly ease the symptoms (see below). A well-known principle of homeopathy is that patients are given potentised preparations of substances which, in a healthy person, create the same symptoms from which the sick person is suffering. Under its scientific name, *Allium cepa,* the onion plays an important role in homeopathy for *colds* when they are accompanied by watery eyes.

So we see that the forces of warmth, which the bulb family reveal even in nature, have many uses. It is no surprise that the onion has long been a highly prized medicinal and culinary plant. It has even been found as a burial object in the royal tombs of Egypt and ancient writings specify how many onions the slaves who built the pyramids or the Roman soldiers should receive as payment. This plant can also be more valuable to us than we imagine.

Onion (*Allium cepa*)

Nutrition, phytotherapy and external application

While the onion can bring the benefits of warmth, it can also act as an anti-inflammatory. In particular, in the case of *bee stings,* it can be observed that after carefully removing the sting from the skin using a pair of tweezers, the swelling and pain quickly subside if a newly cut and lightly crushed onion is placed on the affected area. It can be beneficial to use a new onion after 10–15 minutes. The effect is equally good for *wasp stings.*

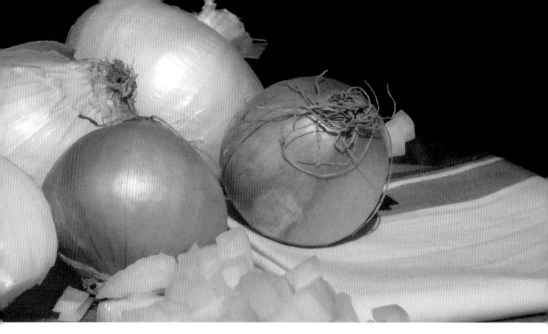

All the items needed for an onion bag are easy to obtain.

The onion also has an anti-inflammatory and pain-relieving effect for *inflammation of the middle ear* when applied as an *onion compress*. This condition should always be treated under medical supervision. When the problem first occurs and as a complement to the doctor's treatment, it is beneficial to chop an onion finely, wrap the pieces of onion in a handkerchief and press this firmly so that the juice runs out before applying the damp pack to the ear. The compress can be heated by placing the onion bag in a sieve over boiling water. The bag is then held or tied against the affected ear until the symptoms start to improve.[1]

There are various recipes for making *cough mixture* from onions. The simplest method is to chop one or two onions, stir in two tablespoons of honey and leave the mixture to stand overnight. The honey 'draws out' the onion juice. Strain it through a sieve and take one teaspoon several times a day. The juice obtained in this way must be freshly prepared at frequent intervals as it only keeps for one or two days.

A more labour-intensive method is to boil 500g (1 lb) of chopped onions with 500 ml (2 cups) of water and 225 g (8 oz) of sugar until a thin syrup is produced. This can be kept in the fridge for at least a week. Take one teaspoon of the syrup several times a day (up to once an hour for more severe coughs).

It is possible that a diet with plenty of onions can slightly reduce cholesterol and blood pressure, and it may inhibit blood clotting. However, the scientific findings on this are contradictory and research is not yet complete. Supposedly, though, onion can contribute in a limited way to preventing *arteriosclerotic vascular diseases* and their consequences such as *heart attack, arterial occlusive disease* and *stroke*. Scientific findings have appeared just recently which verify that hydrogen sulfide produced in the body from sulfur-rich foods such as onions and garlic expands the blood vessels.[2] This expansion leads to a reduction in blood pressure and prevents vascular sclerosis. Such results provide scientific proof for the effects which herbal medicine has attributed to onion and garlic from time immemorial. What is new, however, is that these foods are also supposed to have a protective effect on nerve cells and promote *memory*. Another outcome of the effect of blood-vessel expansion is that *erectile function* is enhanced. The 'sulfur effect' of the onion family is also said to counteract the *ageing process* in numerous ways.[3]

In cell cultures, onion extracts inhibit the growth of intestinal cancer cells. An inhibitory effect on cancer cells has also been shown in animal tests. However, there is still no clear proof of efficacy in this connection for human beings.

Potentised onion

In homeopathy, onion is used under the name of *Cepa*. The corresponding preparation made by the anthroposophical pharmaceutical company Wala has the complicated but botanically correct name of Allium cepa e bulbo ('e bulbo' meaning that the medicine is obtained from the bulb and not from other parts of the plant).

I almost always use the globules in potencies of D3 or D6. For colds with a *runny nose* (also for *hay fever*) that make the area around the nose painful, this remedy can be very helpful if 5 globules are taken hourly and allowed to dissolve slowly in the mouth or under the tongue. In most cases any accompanying *irritation of the eyes* also improves.

Onion in compound remedies of anthroposophical medicine

Due to its warming effect on the one hand, and anti-inflammatory and decongestant effect on the other, onion is contained in several medicines for internal and external treatment of *injuries, superficial inflammation* and *muscle* and *joint pains.*

In Symphytum comp. globules and ampoules (Wala), combined with potentised comfrey *(Symphytum)*, arnica and tin *(Stannum)*, onion relieves the pain of *broken bones* (fractures) and assists the healing process. This remedy can also be used for *tendonitis, bruises* and *sprains,* at a dose of one ampoule 3 times a week or 5–10 globules 3 times daily.

In drop form there is Symphytum comp. N (Weleda) which also contains arnica and onion but in combination with rue *(Ruta)*, marigold *(Calendula)* and witch hazel *(Hamamelis).* In the early phase after an injury (in the first one to two weeks) I usually prescribe the Weleda remedy (15 drops 3 times daily) because the plants it contains are more effective at reducing swelling and enhancing healing of the wound. I follow this with the remedy from Wala, which has a greater solidifying and stabilising effect. The latter has proved successful for the treatment of vertebral pain caused by micro fractures in *osteoporosis.*

A basic remedy for the treatment of *osteoarthritis* and the aches and pains caused by it is Cartilago comp. (Wala) which is available as ampoules, globules, suppositories and ointment. They all contain onion, birch, tin (*Stannum* being the metal for the cartilage) and an organ preparation of cartilage to promote regeneration. The role of the onion is to enable 'sulfur forces' to become active. Many arthritis patients find that sulfur baths ease their aches and pains. Interestingly, cartilage is one of our body's most sulfur-rich tissues. Its weight is composed of almost 50% chondroitin sulfate, a sulfur compound which can absorb up to 40,000 times its weight in water. Food supplements containing chondroitin sulphate are often recommended for the treatment of osteoarthritis. Another (and in my opinion often more effective) 'sulfur therapy' is provided by Cartilago comp. For long-term treatment a dose of 5 globules 3 times daily is recommended, accompanied by application of the ointment in the evening. For more severe pain, injections of the same preparation can be given for a short period.

Onion, arnica, comfrey and tin form the basic ingredients of Articulatio talocruralis comp. (Wala) which can help the ankle joint, with lower potencies of ankle joint cartilage promoting regeneration and higher potencies combating inflammation. It also contains an organ preparation of periosteum and the sciatic nerve. This remedy is often amazingly effective for *osteoarthritis of the ankle* and I have seen how it has enabled patients who have already been advised to have an operation to fuse the joint and become largely symptom-free without having to undergo surgery.

The anti-swelling, anti-inflammatory and stimulating effects of onion are also the reason for its use in the production of Mercurialis Salbe (ointment) (Wala), along with marigold (*Calendula*) and dog's mercury (Mercurialis). This ointment is beneficial for various forms of suppurating processes of the skin.

Finally, onion, along with a whole range of other potentised substances, is contained in Narben Gel (scar treatment gel) from Wala which counters any tendency for the scar to spread and makes the area more elastic if the gel is rubbed into the affected skin twice daily. An extract of onion as the active agent is also contained in a herbal ointment Contractubex, which is often recommended by plastic surgeons to treat scars.

CHAPTER 3

Yarrow

Every spring brings opportunities for coming into contact with yarrow. Beautiful coloured Easter eggs can be made by sticking intricate yarrow leaves firmly to the surface of the egg using thread (or an old nylon stocking). The egg is then dyed by boiling it together with onion skins (for a yellow ochre colour), brazilwood, cochineal or turmeric. When the leaves are removed, the leaf shape – which looks very much like a fern – appears as a light negative image against the darker dyed shell.

If we look at the shape of the leaf on the egg, or at the leaf itself, we are amazed by its regularity and delicacy. The creative force displayed in this leaf can be found in almost every meadow. Unlike a 'standard leaf' (for example, from plantain or a beech tree) the yarrow's leaf is divided once and each leaf is subsequently divided a second time. There is often even a third generation of smaller leaves with a lanceolate 'tooth' at the end of each. An expert silversmith could not shape his work more beautifully and symmetrically than this plant shapes its perfectly divided leaves. Other plants whose leaves are drawn out into fine rays (such as dill or chamomile) appear almost untidy in comparison. There may be a link to the yarrow's perfection in the German name *Schafgarbe* which comes from the Anglo-Saxon *Gearva*, meaning 'finished, perfect, beautiful' and is applied to a plant 'which makes an absolutely beautiful and stately impression'.[1]

The plant's flowers are also attractive, even if they are not a spectacular single flower like the rose or the lily. Looking more carefully at the inflorescence which is composed of white or sometimes pink-tinged florets, you notice that what appear to be single flowers are themselves made up of florets in line with the principle of the daisy family. As with the leaves, we find a progressive subdividing pattern

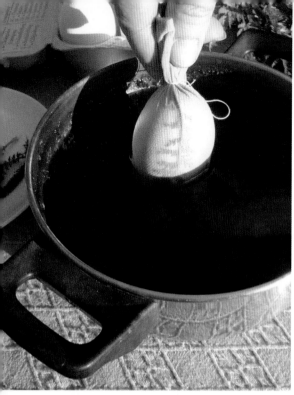
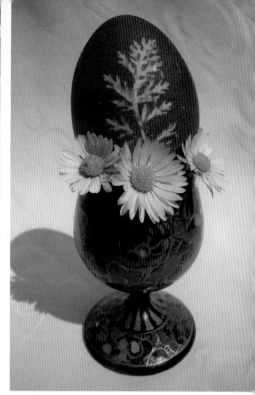

After soaking in the dye bath secured by a nylon stocking, the leaves become an Easter motif.

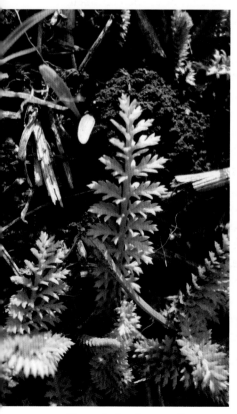
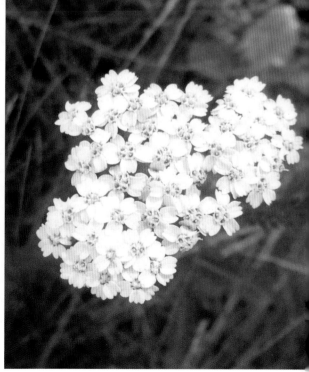

Yarrow leaf and yarrow flower.

into which the individual elements fit, producing a beautiful overall form.

The German name for yarrow, *Schafgarbe*, also contains the word *Schaf* ('sheep'), and sheep are indeed fond of it. But how can this plant be of use to humans? In turning it into a medicine, we strive to use the formative forces revealed in its wonderful shape to stimulate the patient's own formative forces. Where there is a *wound*, the body's order has been thrown into disarray and needs to be restored. In Greek mythology, the centaur Chiron, who is the source of all medicinal knowledge, recommended that the hero Achilles treat his wound with yarrow (scientific name *Achillea millefolium*, which roughly translates as 'Achilles' thousand-leaved plant').

The first thing a wound needs is to have the bleeding stopped, and this is indeed one of yarrow's therapeutic effects (one of the English names for the plant is actually 'nosebleed'). While the blood in our veins is amorphous, liquid and lacking in form, when it escapes from its natural pathways it has to coagulate. This requires the development of fine webs of fibrin. Perhaps the plant can help to stimulate this development process. In any case, it has always had a good reputation for the treatment of *bleeding*, and I have observed that injecting ampoules of potentised preparations of yarrow can alleviate serious *bleeding tendencies*, for example in pathological processes of the mucosal membranes.

Where else can this medicinal plant be used? Its Lower Austrian name of 'tummy-ache plant' is a clear indication of this. It can be helpful as a tea for *cramping stomach pains* (also in relation to *menstruation*), for *diarrhoea* and *upset stomach*. The yarrow's particular relationship to the intestine can almost be seen by looking at it, and ancient medicine attached great importance to these kind of visible signs of similar characteristics which were known as signatures. The *signum* (i.e. sign) of the intestine which is similar to yarrow is its structure. At the most basic level this shows itself as indentations with a surface of fine villi – which are themselves covered with delicate finger-like protuberances. The intestine only functions properly when the structure is regular, right down to the smallest parts. A simple bout of diarrhoea or, more seriously, chronic inflammatory bowel disease (which can even lead to bleeding) brings this intricate work of art into disarray. Yarrow is very beneficial for most of these disorders, even if it cannot alleviate or actually cure every one of them.

If this makes you think that ferns with similar structures can also have a beneficial effect on the gut, you would be right. There are indeed fern preparations that are successfully used for the treatment of intestinal diseases. However, be warned! There are also poisonous ferns, so expert advice is definitely required. Naturally, this kind of similarity (such as the fine divisions of the leaf form on the one hand and the division of the structure of the intestine on the other) can only be an outer – and at times misleading – sign of a relationship between the external world of nature and the inner world or the organs. A modern knowledge of nature can view such visible signatures as a starting point for a possible treatment. In any case, it is important to investigate whether similar formative forces are really at work in both areas, or whether there is only an outer resemblance.

Yarrow is also a very effective and frequently used remedy when applied externally. It plays an important part in anthroposophical medicine. A strong yarrow infusion is used in warm liver compresses for the treatment of many *liver disorders*, which may also manifest in problems throughout the body. Although these are caused by a disturbance to the more subtle functioning of the liver, they do not necessarily lead to measurable changes in laboratory tests. They include *skin problems* but also *sleep disturbances,* accompanied by waking up around 3 a.m. – that is, at a time when basic changes in liver metabolism discovered by physiological research are taking place. Even *depressive mental disorders* with *lack of motivation* can be connected to a disturbance of the liver in certain cases. An anthroposophical doctor may recommend a liver compress with yarrow infusion for all of these different indications of liver dysfunctions. However, he will first try to obtain the most exact picture possible of the whole person in order to make a helpful recommendation for the proper readjustment of the body. I actually know patients whose persistent sleep disturbances only disappear when a liver compress of this kind is applied.

There is another use for yarrow, which does not require expert medical advice. The delicious fresh leaves of yarrow can be added to salads in the spring. These leaves have a bitter and aromatic taste and stimulate the digestive function. For many people they are part of a spring detox, like other bitter-tasting young leaves (for example dandelion, nettle, silverweed, etc.). Bitter herbs appear in connection with fasting, passion and Easter (and also on the plates of Jewish families at Passover). In many districts of Germany, yarrow belongs to Maundy Thursday soup – perhaps not just because of the taste but also because it helps to create inner order.

Yarrow (*Achillea millefolium*)

Phytotherapy – tea and external application

This plant is particularly suitable for collecting yourself. It grows in most wild meadows and there are scarcely any poisonous plants with which it could be confused. However, care should be taken not to collect the plant in places where it has been exposed to pesticides or a lot of exhaust fumes. The most suitable harvest time is in early summer after the flowers come out. Yarrow is easy to process. Just tie the stems together and hang it upside down to dry. It can then be chopped up or broken into pieces by hand before use.

To make yarrow tea, pour one cup of boiling water on to 1 or 2 teaspoons of the dried herb. Leave covered for 10 minutes and then strain. The tea works as an antispasmodic for abdominal pains due to an *upset stomach* or *flatulence,* but can also be helpful for *menstrual cramps.*

Yarrow can also be added to any herb tea for its bitter taste and stimulating effect on the digestive glands or as a cure along with bitter herbs. To the latter can be added some common centaury or cotton thistle, but stinging nettle and dandelion are also suitable additions. If the tea is required for combating a *tendency to cramps* (for example for an *irritable bowel*), then the yarrow can be mixed with silverweed and peppermint. If you want to enhance the anti-inflammatory effect on the mucous membranes, then chamomile flowers, which have a series of uses in common, can be added.

A thorough study has recently verified that the yarrow's relaxing effect can also affect the blood vessels and it can therefore lower high blood pressure. In an experiment, yarrow was as effective as a *calcium antagonist,* a drug of first choice in general medicine for the treatment of *high blood pressure*.[2] This finding needs to be backed up by more extensive observation of patients, but there is already some evidence that yarrow can produce a slight lowering of blood pressure in human beings. If you want to try this out for slightly raised blood pressure or in addition to other measures, then mix the yarrow with birch leaves or horsetail. These increase the excretion of water and salt, thus helping to reduce blood pressure in a different way (see also Chapters 7 and 14). It can also be combined with hawthorn leaves and flowers which also have a balancing effect on blood pressure. As with every other type of blood pressure treatment, measurements need to be made to be certain that an adequate effect is being achieved. A protective effect on the liver against certain liver toxins (paracetamol and carbon tetrachloride) has been verified experimentally for the internal use of yarrow.

If a yarrow infusion is used for a *liver compress*, it should be made stronger (two heaped tablespoons in 500 ml (2 cups) of boiling water). Soak a cloth which can cover the right upper abdomen one hand's breadth above and below the right costal arch when folded and wring out well. Then lay it on the specified region as hot as is comfortable for the patient. Lay a dry cloth over it and cover both with a woollen cloth. A half-filled hot water bottle may also be placed on top. The compress should be kept in place for 20–30 minutes and the patient should remain lying for at least 10 minutes after it has been removed. It has been shown that a hot moist liver compress like this increases the liver function.[3] This can encourage the removal of toxins from the body, which is why regular liver compresses of yarrow are used, for example for *cancers*, often as part of a holistic treatment programme. Incidentally, in experiments using cell cultures, it has been possible to demonstrate that yarrow itself can inhibit some kinds of tumour cells. For other chronic diseases and *exhaustion symptoms*, yarrow liver compresses can be beneficial as they promote the function of the liver, which is the main organ of metabolism and synthesis. Finally, these kinds of compresses are used for *liver diseases* themselves, such as chronic *hepatitis C*.

A stronger infusion with 50–100g (2–4 oz) of dried yarrow per litre (quart) of boiling water is used as an additive to sitz baths for *cramping symptoms in the lower abdomen* and for *haemorrhoids* and *eczema* around the anus. This type of bath can also be used for a *bladder infection*. A sitz bath should normally last 10–15 minutes.

Potentised yarrow

Yarrow is available as a potentised remedy from Wala under the name of Achillea ex herba in D6. I have frequently injected these ampoules subcutaneously for treating a tendency to *mucous membrane* and *tumour haemorrhages* and had the impression that they were most effective. As part of this treatment I sometimes also used Stibium metallicum D6 (Weleda) whose mineral compounds (particularly the mineral antimonite) display a similarity to the yarrow leaf in their finely divided radiating form. The fine fibrin threads produced during blood clotting which finally lead to the arrest of bleeding also have a structure which is related to the metal and the plant. Of course in cases of serious bleeding, the attending doctor must be consulted and a decision made as to whether other measures are possible and necessary.

Achillea (D1) and antimonite (D8) are contained in Achillea comp. drops (Weleda) with horse chestnut (Aesculus D3), witch hazel (Hamamelis D3) and gentian (Gentiana D3). This remedy has proved very successful for painful conditions around the anus such as *haemorrhoids, eczema* and *fissures in the mucous membranes*, if 10–15 drops are taken 3 times daily. However, problems with the anal region should generally be examined by a doctor (which can be done by a proctologist and often by the general practitioner) so that serious intestinal diseases can be excluded.

Sitz baths with yarrow have already been recommended above for *bladder infections*. The plant is contained in a potentised form (as D2) in Cantharis Blasen globules and injection (Wala) along with potentised horsetail (*Equisetum*), an organic bladder preparation, and in Cantharis D5, which is also one of the most frequently used homeopathic remedies for bladder infections. In this case, it is the anti-inflammatory and antispasmodic powers of yarrow which are effective.

Yarrow's particular relationship to the bladder may be clarified by taking a look at a realm which at first seems to be far removed. In his *Agriculture Course*, Rudolf Steiner explained that productive agriculture requires the correct interaction of plants and animals. We know this from the fertilising effect of dung, which has a quite different power than fertiliser made from plant material alone. In biodynamic agriculture (the basis of which was set down in the above-mentioned course) special fertiliser preparations are added in the composting process in very small, almost homeopathically active quantities. These are mostly produced by preparing particular plants with particular animal organs. In the case of yarrow, said to be of particular help in organising the sulfur forces (often linked to inflammation in the human body), the plant is processed along with red deer bladder. This may seem astonishing at first, and only becomes easier to understand when you get to know red deer better. Here it must suffice to say that this choice is also affected by the relationship of this plant to the bladder. I prescribe Cantharis bladder globules for acute conditions with burning pain when passing water and an increased urge to urinate, and give 5 globules every 2 hours. The remedy has also proved effective for the prevention of *bladder infections* by taking 5–10 globules daily. It should be noted that a bacterial bladder infection can progress to the kidneys and then become dangerous. Warning symptoms are back pain around the kidneys, high temperature and a general feeling of being unwell. A doctor must be consulted immediately in this case. This also applies if the condition being treated does not improve quickly or if an obstruction to the flow of urine is suspected (for example, by an enlarged prostate, bladder stones or something similar), because in such cases the condition can quickly spread to the kidneys. In many simple cases, Cantharis bladder globules make a good treatment option if therapy is started early. Cantharis bladder globules have often been able to contribute to a permanent cure even in patients who were constantly prescribed antibiotics to prevent recurring bladder infections.

The relaxing and warming effects of Schafgarbe (yarrow) 5% in olive oil (Dr Heberer Naturheilmittel) as an oil dispersion bath can prove beneficial for a tendency to recurring bladder infections and for cramping pains in the female urogenital area.

Mention was made on page 37 that there are remedies made from ferns for the treatment of *disorders of the bowel action*. These are, for example, Digestodoron (Weleda) or Aquilinum comp. (Wala).

CHAPTER 4

Dandelion

In northern Europe in April the sun can shine quite warmly. When the radiant dandelion flowers appear, it is as though the earth itself had produced a host of little suns. Every child knows the dandelion. Is there anyone who has not played with them at some time and woven chains or little crowns? The only annoying thing is that the hollow stems secrete so much thick white milk, which sticks to everything, making brown stains. There have actually been attempts to obtain a kind of rubber from this milk, as the plant produces such an excess of it.[1]

The short-lived nature of the flowering spectacle need not be a cause for too much regret, as it is replaced by another delight when the dandelion clocks (the seed heads) appear. An architectural perfection, they stand with their silvery globes at the top of each flower stalk. Numerous little rays connect the pointed seeds with their tiny parachutes, giving the plant a mobility and potential to disperse otherwise reserved for animals.

The owners of a carefully tended lawn are not quite so delighted when the seeds end up on their patch, because the dandelion can colonise with no effort at all. If gardeners want to be rid of it, they have to dig it out by the roots. Even when the dandelion root is only as thick as your finger, it is strong and offers tough resistance. If the root breaks, it also exudes plentiful white milk.

The contrast between the dark tap root, which is firmly anchored in the earth, and the extremely delicate white parachutes with their crystal-like structure is certainly impressive. Between the two lies the dandelion's leaf rosette. Its leaves arise exactly at the level of the earth's surface. Everyone recognises these leaves, although no two are alike. Try it out for yourself; pick a hundred, a thousand or ten thousand

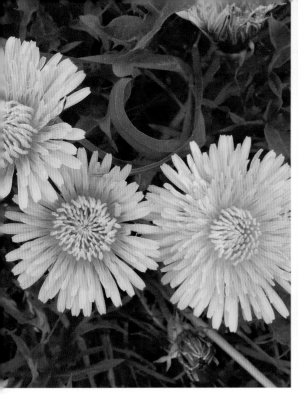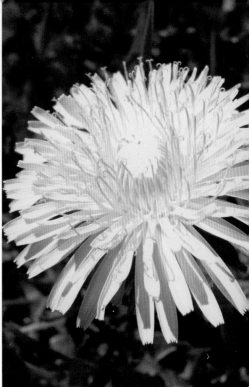

Dandelion flowers can look like little 'suns' in the meadow.

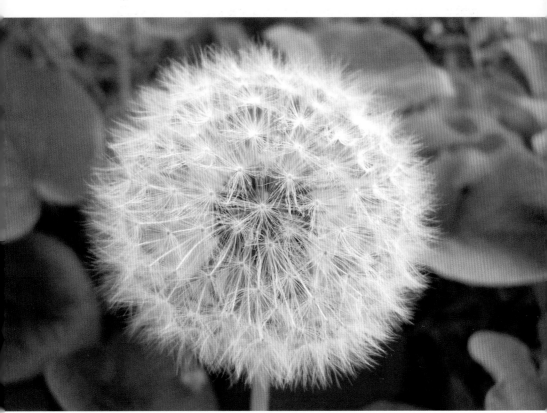

The dandelion seed may remind us of the moon.

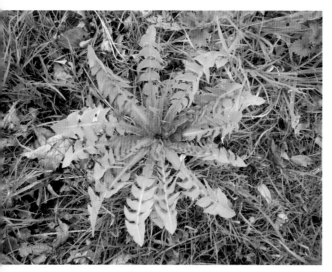

Dandelion leaf rosette.

leaves. No two will be exactly the same. How different this is with the leaves of a beech tree, a birch tree or a rose! The word 'dandelion' comes from the Middle French *dent de lion,* that is, 'lion's tooth'. However, a lion with teeth like this would be a pathetic creature – it would find it very difficult to chew. The teeth of a real lion are a model of order and beauty, but dandelions have a rather unkempt appearance and sometimes it is hard to know whether they are made that way naturally or are a result of injury or being eaten by snails. While on the one hand the dandelion clock appears so orderly, on the other the dandelion leaf is so disorderly. But even if it has been eaten or pulled up, we have no doubt that it can survive. Its vitality is unfailing – the dandelion pushing up through asphalt is proof of the energy it contains.

In recent decades it has been discovered that the dandelion has an irrepressible determination to be individual and that it 'nonchalantly' breaks crucial laws in biology. Reading about it in different books can leave one feeling increasingly confused. In one place it says that the common dandelion *(Taraxacum officinale)* has 25 sub-species. In another place it has 50 sub-species, yet another source records up to 600 – and finally you find the opinion that these are in fact all the same species. The secret lies in the fact that the dandelion reproduces in more than one way. We know from potatoes or the runners produced by strawberry plants that plants do not only reproduce via seeds. However, the dandelion can produce seeds asexually (as well as 'sexually' of course). In the so-called sexual reproduction of most species of plants, and in the actual sexual reproduction of animals and human beings, two chromosomes (one from each parent), which together form a pair, first divide and then recombine. However, in the dandelion, this distinct pair may be missing. Two, three or four chromosomes (as may also happen in other plants) can belong together. The dandelion 'juggles' these different chromosome numbers (in a process called apomixis) quite remarkably, so that new mutations with new characteristics are constantly being produced. This explodes the current concept of 'species', which has previously been applied to all living nature. To overstate this somewhat, each individual plant produces its own species, so that we now refer to a common dandelion aggregate. Although dandelions reproduce asexually (and are thus not dependent on being visited by bees) they nevertheless exude plentiful nectar and therefore form an important source of food for bees at a time when there is not much else for them to eat.

We can see how the dandelion balances out a polarity: energy, vitality and attachment to the earth on the one hand, and openness, delicacy and a crystalline form (in which something almost like sensitivity can be detected) on the other. This is also reflected in a statement by Rudolf Steiner, founder of biodynamic agriculture, who said that the dandelion brings the forces of potassium and silicon into harmonious balance and is therefore of inestimable value for the landscape, and as a fertiliser.[2] He even said that the dandelion is 'the greatest boon' for the area where it grows. Potassium is an agent of vigour and the dandelion contains almost 5%: more potassium than almost any other plant. In contrast, silicon combined with oxygen produces quartz crystals, the most transparent mineral structure on earth. These six-sided crystals also have perfect architecture. Silicon is particularly abundant in the sense organs and it seems to have a special significance in those places where our sensitivity to the surroundings arises. (Sense perception requires a certain 'transparency' so that the effects of the environment can penetrate into us to a certain degree.)

In our bodies, the liver is 'the centre of potassium'. This is where substances are synthesised and a wide range of metabolic processes occur. The liver is also a place where the substances and effects from the outer world which have been absorbed from the gut are subtly perceived and 'tasted' in a certain sense. One can well imagine why the dandelion can be a remedy for the liver in numerous ways. The dandelion has always had a reputation for being a cure for the liver and gall bladder and it is often eaten as a delicate, slightly bitter

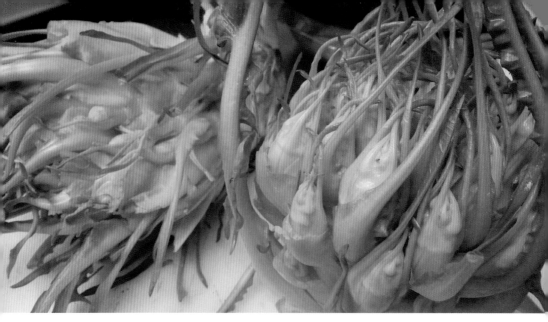

In French cuisine, tasty dandelion shoots are occasionally used in salads or as a fried vegetable.

appetite-stimulating green for a spring detox. A second organ closely connected to potassium is the kidney, which regulates the potassium levels in the blood. Experiments have shown that the diuretic effect of dandelion can equal the strongest drugs are available for this purpose. (This explains the plant's crude French name *pissenlit,* as well as the old Middle English name, 'piss-the-bed'.) Another organising aspect can be experienced on the skin, due to high amounts of silicon. I have repeatedly found that a dandelion gel can improve wide, thick *scars* quite impressively and bring their colour back to normal. A group of doctors (who were also the source of the idea for a gel preparation) around Professor Klas Diederich even discovered effects that proved astonishingly beneficial in individual cancer patients.[3]

So there are many reasons why we can be filled with delight when the dandelion opens its sunny yellow flowers once more.

Dandelion (*Taraxacum officinale*)

Delicate dandelion leaves collected in March and April are an excellent digestive addition to salads for a spring detox. The herb can be collected until May in places where it is not exposed to exhaust fumes and then dried, to be used later as tea.

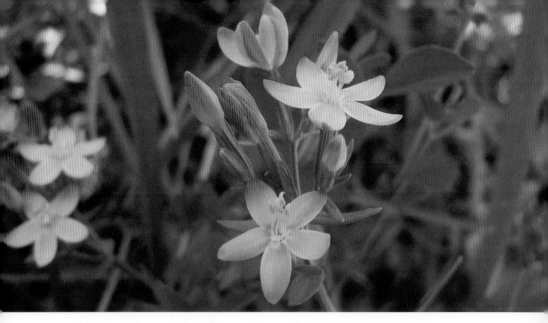

Common centaury, which is often used along with dandelion in bitter digestion-stimulating teas.

Another modern way of incorporating dandelion into a spring detox or including it in the menu throughout the year is the option of using it to prepare green smoothies. Further details are given in Chapter 28 on the stinging nettle.

Dandelion tea

Two teaspoons of chopped dandelion leaves in a cup of boiling water left to infuse for 10 minutes give a strong, bitter-tasting tea which stimulates bile production and therefore assists digestion. The tea also has a diuretic effect, which is why it is good as a preventative for a tendency towards *kidney* and *bladder stones*. However, dandelion is usually used in mixed teas. It is mixed with other herbs both as a digestive (toning and strengthening bitter tea) and also as a diuretic in cases of mild *bladder infections* and for *preventing bladder stones*.

For a bitter tea, a mixture of dandelion leaves, common centaury, blessed thistle, yarrow and wormwood can be used. For a bladder tea, mix dandelion, nettle and horsetail.

External uses for dandelion

For the *scar treatment* mentioned above, apply dandelion gel to the scar once or twice daily after the wound has healed. As this gel is not yet available ready-made, you can have it made up by the pharmacist. One tried and tested formulation contains:

- ⇢ Mother tincture of dandelion (e.g. from Ceres or Weleda) 20.0 g
- ⇢ Glycerol (this moisturises the skin and keeps it supple)   6.0 g
- ⇢ Hydroxypropyl cellulose (as the gel-forming component)   5.0 g
- ⇢ Aqua (water)   ad 100.0 g

The gel should be stored in a tube so it keeps longer.

As mentioned above, Professor Klas Diederich recommended dandelion for the treatment of tumours of the abdominal cavity.[4] At the Rechts der Isar Hospital in Munich good results have been achieved with the additional use of dandelion (besides the normal treatment, primarily surgery) for advanced *ovarian cancer*.[5] Potentised dandelion preparation (see below) was injected and gel applied externally.

Potentised dandelion

The ampoule preparations Taraxacum e planta tota (Wala) D3, D6 and D8 are manufactured from the whole flowering plant of the dandelion. Taraxacum e planta tota D3, D4, D6, D8 and D30 are available as globules from Wala and mother tincture (with 50% alcohol content) from Weleda. These remedies are used for *stimulating liver function* and *bile production* and for *promoting kidney function*. Homeopathy has developed an important guiding symptom known as geographic tongue (where smooth pink shiny areas appear on an otherwise white coated tongue like a map), which indicates the efficacy of Taraxacum for the patient. In practice, however, beneficial effects from Taraxacum can be achieved even in the absence of this specific symptom. Taraxacum supports the liver and kidneys, the main organs for removing toxins. Thus it has a general detoxifying effect, which can be of help for *chronic eczema* and also for easing the effects of *environmental toxins and drugs*. Patients who are drained by *chemotherapy* in particular – for example using Temozolomide (Temodal or Temcad) or Capecitabine (Xeloda) – and also those receiving *anti-epileptic treatment* which places a burden on the liver will have their general vitality significantly improved by the administration of Taraxacum (5 globules D3 2–3 times a day), with Taraxacum Stanno cultum (Weleda) as a possible alternative (see page 56). The compound remedies with detoxifying effects mentioned below also contain Taraxacum.

Good results have recently been achieved with the administration of Taraxacum for *ovarian cancer* recommended by Professor Diederich (see page 48). A daily injection of the D3 into the subcutaneous fatty tissue of the abdomen in addition to the normal therapeutic measures has been successful. Single observations of positive effects have also been made for *gall bladder* and *bile duct carcinomas*.

The great anthroposophical doctor, Dr Heinz-Hartmut Vogel, separated dandelion roots into those harvested in spring and those harvested in autumn, and introduced this into therapeutic practice. He suspected that the spring root Taraxacum e radice (vernale) was suited for treatment of a tendency towards *raised blood sugar* while the autumn root Taraxacum e radice (autumnale) was appropriate for a tendency to *low blood sugar*. The harvest times are at polar opposite points in the course of the year. The autumn root has accumulated a maximum of carbohydrate, whereas the carbohydrate reserves have been used up when the plant starts growth in the early spring. Therapeutic preparations from both types of root are supplied by Wala as D3 and D6 in the form of ampoules only. I have been able to establish that the different tendencies to *blood sugar instability* were stabilised in individual cases when these ampoules were taken orally in the evening.

The last-mentioned remedy makes use of dandelion collected at specific times. I should also like to mention one remedy which makes use of a particular part of the plant: *Lac taraxaci*, the dandelion milk which escapes when the plant is pulled up or cut. As this milk is almost always processed into a medicine in combination with a lichen, its healing powers will be described in the next section (page 52).

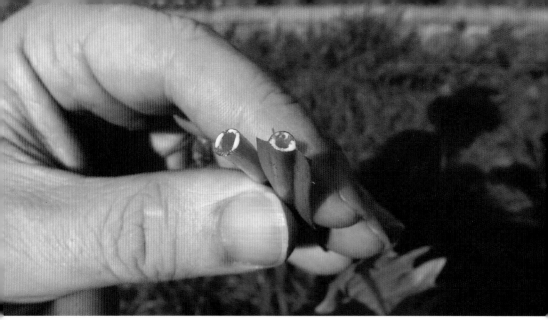

The latex secreted when dandelion stems are pulled up is one of the ingredients in the remedy Lac taraxaci/Parmelia.

Taraxacum in composite remedies in anthroposophical medicine

I recommended a bitter tea mixture containing dandelion for *digestive disorders* earlier in this section. Bitter substances as a whole can support the catabolic and regulating forces of the soul and spirit in the metabolic realm. Thus, for example, *skin rashes* or *headaches* caused by metabolic disturbances can get better. Instead of a tea, a mixture of alcoholic extracts of bitter herbs, such as Amara Tropfen (Weleda), can be used. This mixture contains common centaury, yellow gentian, wormwood, yarrow, chicory, juniper, sage and masterwort in addition to dandelion. The usual dose is 10–15 drops before meals. Where there is a tendency to *feeling overly full*, the remedy can also be taken half an hour to one hour after meals.

The action of Gentiana Magen globules (stomach remedy, Wala) is also based on bitter substances and contains a mother tincture made from wormwood and yellow gentian plus a low potency (D4) of Nux vomica in addition to the dandelion mother tincture. Contrary to its name, the remedy not only affects the stomach but, like Amara Tropfen, invigorates the whole digestive system and can therefore have a beneficial effect on conditions which are caused or aggravated by a deficient digestion. Besides *stimulating the digestion*, this can also have a beneficial effect on *gastroesophageal reflux disease* accompanied by *heartburn* and on *dyspepsia* caused by stress and *toxin burdens* from substances such as alcohol and certain drugs.

An equally generalised *stimulation of the digestive and detoxification functions* is achieved using Chelidonium comp. Tropfen (Weleda) (The comments for the use of *Chelidonium* in Chapter 11 apply to this remedy). In addition to dandelion, this includes stinging nettle, milk thistle, greater celandine and several species of ferns and willows which have a beneficial effect on the processes of movement and excretion. This remedy, of which 10–20 drops should be taken 3 times daily, has also proved successful as a complementary therapy for *tumours*. The same applies to Aquilinum comp. globules (Wala), which also contain ferns, dandelion and greater celandine with the addition of golden rod *(Solidago)* which promotes kidney function and the excretion of toxins via the kidneys. I usually prescribe 5–7 globules 3–7 times a day after the *use of antibiotics,* during *chemotherapy* and for treatment of *skin diseases* related to intestinal disorders.

An effective remedy for rosacea is made from a beard lichen of the genus Parmelia *along with dandelion milk.*

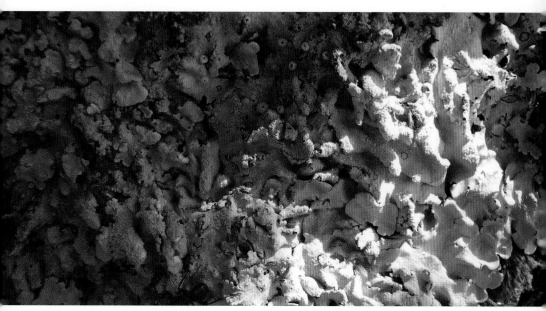

By *promoting liver* and *kidney function*, the composition of Agropyron globules and injection (Wala) has cured many diseases where this option was not at first considered. This remedy is often helpful for *colds* and *infections of the paranasal sinuses (sinusitis)*, in particular the maxillary sinuses. Prolonged exhaustion and poor liver function are often implicated in the latter. This medicine includes couch-grass (Agropyron) which gives the remedy its name, an extremely persistent weed well-known to every gardener and characterised by great powers of resistance. It can give an exhausted patient new energy. Couch-grass also has a positive effect on fluid processes and helps to loosen dry, viscous mucus in the nose and sinuses. By improving liver function, dandelion also promotes the fluid processes, as do the potassium carbonate obtained from beech wood ash and potentised cinnabar contained in this remedy. At the start of treatment I usually inject the remedy into the neck, but treatment can be continued using the globules (5–10 hourly).

I have already mentioned the dandelion latex, *Lac taraxaci*. An understanding of its healing effect and how this combines with another ingredient in the formulation requires a long and rather complicated discussion. However, this is definitely worthwhile, as it brings to light basic principles and processes which play a role in maintaining health in a variety of ways. When these principles and processes do not interact in the right way, we fall ill.

The latex of the dandelion contains substances akin to gums and resins dispersed as tiny droplets in water. These are rather special because resins actually repel water. Everyone who has had resin from a tree on their fingers and tried to wash it off will know this; and it is equally difficult to remove spots of rubber or gum, because using soap does not make them dissolve in water. In its latex, the dandelion manages to combine substances that initially want nothing to do with each other, based on their chemical properties. Producing the latex actually introduces a type of death process into a primary synthetic plant process. The tiny droplets of resin and gum only enter the sap when the cells where they were produced disintegrate. The milk is formed from their contents and the 'normal' sap.

When he was asked about this kind of 'milk', Rudolf Steiner explained that it could promote a rhythmical balance between the 'breaking-down' processes in the body (which create conscious sensations), and the 'building-up' processes (which are active only in the unconscious realm). It was already indicated that the liver is active more in one or the other way at different times. In the first half of the night, certain substances are created in the liver and at the same time the production of bile, which is excreted into the gut and promotes the breaking-down functions in digestion, ceases almost entirely. Blood sugar decreases during the first half of the night because the liver transforms sugar into storage compounds. These are broken down again in the early hours of the morning, releasing the sugar, which makes conscious thought processes possible. However, these forces of consciousness require a breaking down of physical substance. In nature, we usually find the process of building-up and breaking-down divided between the plant and animal kingdoms. Plants synthesise substances (with the help of sunlight) – beginning with sugar, which is then condensed into more solid plant matter. Animals (and human beings), conversely, break these substances down in their digestion and finally transform the sugar back into water and carbon dioxide – which are then available to the plants for synthesis once more. The energy, which comes from the sun and which was incorporated into the original synthesised substances, is then released and is available for human beings and animals for their conscious activity. Processes therefore occur on a large scale in nature which resemble those which occur in our bodies, and in both cases they need to be arranged and related to each other in a rhythmical way in order to remain stable. When we sleep, our conscious mental processes withdraw completely and we are more like plants. Even our growth and the processes involved in the renewal of our organs take place mainly at night. During the day we are engaged as ensouled beings: thinking, feeling and consciously working to form our environment. The processes of physical breaking-down cause us to lose some weight, become 'drier' and more 'formed'.

These opposite processes can be observed right down to a microscopic level. We showed above how these processes are separated over *time* in the liver. In the skin, these processes are separated in *space*. The lower layers of the epidermis contain the cells which enable the skin to renew itself throughout our lives (the famous stem cells). Fine blood vessels extend to just below these cells, taking the nutrients to the epidermis, which has no blood supply of its own. However, this is where abundant nerve fibres and their very sensitive terminals are located. On the one hand, they are responsible for the perceptions of the world we have through our skin; on the other hand, they can make us feel unpleasantly itchy if we have a skin ailment. The further we progress outwards in the epidermis, the more the cells are 'forsaken by life', becoming drier and harder. The stem cells are still more or less spherical but, as they travel outwards, the cells first appear 'prickly' (spinous cell layer) and have already lost their ability to divide – a crucial aspect of their vitality. Even further out, the cells die off completely but still adhere together tightly and protect us by effectively sealing us off from the environment (horny layer). However, even this horny layer finally disintegrates by breaking down into little scales, which are constantly being sloughed off from the surface of our body. In someone who is healthy, the processes mentioned here, ranging from the new cells forming to the point where they die off and are shed, are organised in a very rhythmical manner. This is not so much a daily rhythm as a monthly one (although a daily rhythm is also present in the skin). It takes 28 days from the time an epidermal cell is produced until the moment when it is shed as a tiny scale. This rhythm is disrupted in many skin diseases and the skin either has an exaggerated 'vitality' or the hardening, deadening forces or those creating sensations (e.g. itchiness) are too strong.

Rudolf Steiner once suggested to doctors treating a patient with 'a long-standing irritating outbreak of spots' that they make a medicine from dandelion juice and tree lichen. This sounds very strange and, as far as I am aware, there is no example of a prescription like this in traditional herbal medicine. The observations presented above suggest that dandelion juice can be useful, particularly if a dysfunction of the liver is connected to the skin condition (which is in fact frequently the case). However, it is simply a stroke of genius to add lichen to this. Lichen is not simply a plant. If you study lichens carefully, then you discover that that they contain an alga, for one thing. We might expect to find algae in water, where they are responsible for much of ocean life, for example, producing an incredibly large amount of living substance. The second component of lichen is a fungus. Fungi are not able to synthesise substances in the presence of light as plants do. They live by breaking down matter and so can survive without light but need material created by other living organisms. Fungi are therefore found everywhere where plant material is rotting (e.g. in every compost heap). The alga and fungus are combined in the lichen and permeate each other completely. The alga produces sugar, amongst other things, and makes this available for the fungus. The latter is able to store water, for example, and so allows the alga to climb to a realm above the water which would otherwise remain closed to it. A healthy lichen exists in a balance between the synthesis of matter by the alga and its degradation by the fungus. At a simple level, nature therefore provides a model of what is achieved in us (e.g. in the skin or liver) as a balance between the 'building-up' activity of the life-forces and the 'breaking-down' activity of the soul-forces. The symbiosis (literally 'living together') of the alga and fungus in the lichen can be destabilised if the lichen is constantly very wet – the alga can then get the upper hand. In contrast, if the lichen is constantly drying out, the alga dies off and only the more drought-resistant fungus survives. We might therefore anticipate that the lichen can influence disturbances in the fluid balance of the skin.

These detailed observations allow us to have some understanding of the unique substance made from dandelion latex (*Lac taraxaci*) and tree lichen (*Parmelia*). The dandelion component is itself produced by a process of cell breakdown in a higher plant, whereas the lichen is more than a plant and represents the successful association of opposite life processes. Both these components stimulate our ability to promote the regulation of the life-forces and formative-forces in their rhythmical balance. Dandelion juice may do this mainly at the level of the formation of substance. The lichen does it by coordinating and balancing the activities of the life-forces and the forces of sensation and shaping. In any case, the remedy proved of lasting benefit to the patient mentioned above to whom Rudolf Steiner's advice applied.

The corresponding preparation is available nowadays as *Lac taraxaci* D10/Parmelia D10 as drops and ampoules from Weleda. A group of dermatologists has looked into which skin disorders it is particularly helpful for. Someone who made particular use of this kind of knowledge was the anthroposophical dermatologist Lüder Jachens.[6] For example, it is thanks to him that we know that this remedy is very often of benefit for *rosacea,* a skin disease of the face where redness and small spots develop in the centre of the face around the nose, middle of the brow and below the eyes, sometimes even resulting in disfiguring redness and coarsening of the skin on the nose. The existence of this remedy is a blessing for patients suffering from this skin disease, as it is otherwise difficult to treat. It is also sometimes helpful (along with other remedies) for acne, inflammation of the hair follicles and various types of eczema, and it can sometimes also bring about an improvement in psoriasis. The main characteristic of these skin diseases is that the anabolic forces associated with the blood are too strong and not enough form is being introduced by the drying and structuring forces. Quite frequently, it is also necessary to prescribe the patient an ongoing treatment for the liver. The dosage for Lac taraxaci D10/Parmelia D10 is usually 10 drops 3 times daily, or injection of one ampoule under the skin 3 times a week for serious cases. As skin diseases usually require detailed knowledge of the disease processes in the body as a whole, and because additional instructions on skin care and lifestyle may be needed, a full medical examination is usually a prerequisite.

Dandelion grown on soil enriched with metals

Taraxacum Stanno cultum is an example of the time-consuming process of manufacturing preparations from plants grown on soil enriched with metals. This process, in which a medicinal plant is intentionally combined with a metal, not when the pharmaceutical product is manufactured, but rather in the garden, is unique to anthroposophical pharmacy. After various processes for making salts of the metal have been carried out in the laboratory, the potentised metal preparation is added to the soil (this process will be described in detail in Chapter 28). In this case, the metal being processed is tin (*Stannum*). Tin is the metal used in anthroposophical medicine and pharmacy because of its relationship to the liver and also because of its generally therapeutic effect on fluid processes. Dandelion is grown on this soil and the plants are then made into compost. The compost is used to grow dandelion again and the plants are once more composted. Only the third generation of dandelion, grown on the second batch of compost, is processed into a medicine.

Taraxacum Stanno cultum Rh D3 (Weleda) has an even better

effect than pure potentised dandelion for patients being treated with anti-epileptics (particularly valproate) in order to combat their side-effects (especially drowsiness and poor concentration and changes in liver function values), something that the paediatrician Georg Soldner was mainly responsible for pointing out. The dose prescribed is usually 10 drops 2–3 times daily.

The remedy has also been successful for chronic illnesses aggravated by poor liver function. This applies particularly to the *rosacea* mentioned above which causes small red patches and pimples on the skin of the face (particularly the nose), but also for *psoriasis* and *rheumatic conditions,* if there are also disturbances in the fluid processes such as a dry mouth, a sensation of thirst and wrinkled skin which point to liver disorders. This remedy is also recommended for a *liver disorder,* indicated by stools that are too light in colour.

CHAPTER 5

Peppermint

Everyone has seen peppermint tea bags. But, when out for a walk on a really hot day, have you ever come to a place where your feet sank into the marshy ground and it smelt mouldy and musty – and suddenly you were wide awake, because you were hit by a bright and refreshing aromatic smell? Perhaps you then glanced down at the ground and noticed that the pleasant clean scent came from the plants with the grey-green leaves that you had just trodden on. Maybe you thought to yourself: 'I know this smell from somewhere or other,' rubbed the leaves between your fingers, smelled them once more and suddenly realised: 'It smells of peppermint!'[1]

If you had put a leaf in your mouth and chewed it, it might have tasted a bit bitter, but your mouth – dry from walking – would have filled with a wonderful cool freshness. You might have wondered how such freshness could be produced in such a swampy, musty place. You can find examples like this time and again if you pay attention: the one-sidedness of the plant's environment appears to provoke something like a response in the plants which grow there, which balances out this 'one-sidedness'. Peppermint and the essential oil it produces actually have a mild disinfectant effect (in other words, an effect which counters the mould formation), so the plant is sometimes used for superficial infections that are threatening to spread. Washing the skin with cold peppermint tea can also help to clear up spots.

Peppermint grows mainly in places where water accumulates in the soil, and in earlier times this was also seen as a sign of its hidden power: its potential use for human beings. When you have a *head cold*, the blood becomes congested in the mucous membranes of the nose, they swell up and this can lead to further problems. Because the nasal sinuses and the

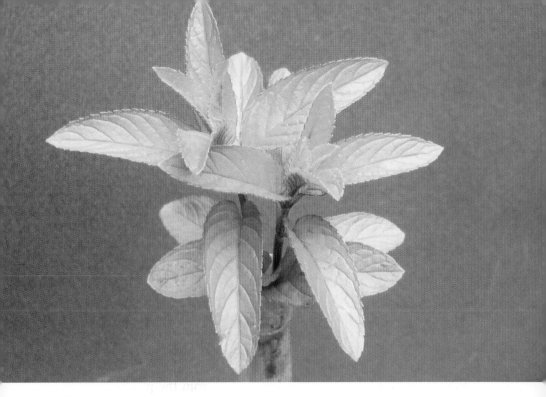

Peppermint.

ear are no longer properly connected with a free exchange of air, they are at risk of infection. Reducing the congested nasal mucosa can be achieved merely by inhaling essential oil of peppermint or by rubbing an ointment containing peppermint oil below the nose. However, care must be taken with small children as there is a risk that, if their sense of smell is stimulated too strongly, this can produce a reflex respiratory arrest. The cause of this (fortunately very rare) effect is not any toxicity of the peppermint but the intensity of the smell itself.

The peppermint as such is non-poisonous. Even with minimal botanical knowledge, you can carry out the experiment described above and chew a leaf without danger (of course, it is not generally recommended to chew any leaf indiscriminately). If you have ever found some of the small pale mauve flowers on the plant, you will have noticed that these have a tube with two symmetrical lips on the lower part. These are the reason for the Latin name of this plant family, *Labiatae*, (from *labium* – 'lip'). You can study the characteristics of these flowers particularly well on deadnettles *(lamium)*, because they are relatively large and abundant.

Remarkably, the family has no poisonous plants as such. The

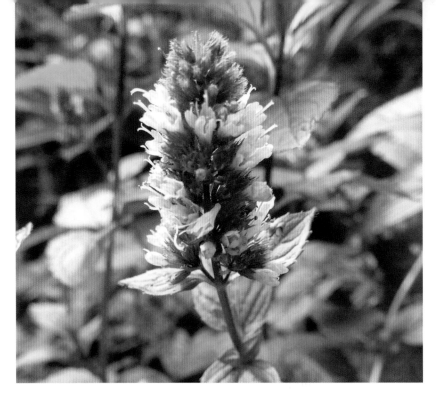

Flowering peppermint.

majority of its members are distinguished by aromatic scents which contribute both to their use as herbs and to their efficacy in promoting healing. Some of the best known examples are basil, thyme, rosemary, oregano or sage.

When you taste a mint leaf, however, another quality distinguishes it from other members of the family; after chewing a fresh leaf, your tongue and gums feel quite cold and a little numb. Try this out and will find that even if you eat something like pepper after chewing a leaf, you can hardly even taste it – it will not produce the same burning sensation as normal. It is not really possible to distinguish subtle flavours of food just after drinking peppermint tea or brushing your teeth with toothpaste containing peppermint oil. This is probably why many homeopaths are suspicious of this plant. It is easy to understand that the subtle effects of remedies and therefore the efficacy of homeopathic medicines is impaired if the mouth has been numbed by peppermint oil before taking the remedy. But this anaesthetic effect can also be put to good use. Some family doctors prescribe an ointment or powder with peppermint oil or its main constituent, menthol, from the pharmacist for itchy skin conditions.

Perhaps the well proven rubbing of peppermint preparations into the temples for some types of headache, especially tension headaches, may also be linked to the above-mentioned numbing effect.

However, what is best known and most widespread is the use of peppermint tea (apart from its use as a beverage, particularly in Arab countries for its cooling effect) for slight *stomach upsets*. Perhaps, as with many other slightly bitter-tasting herbs, this may be partly due to a digestive effect which aids the flow of digestive juices. However, it may well be that the slightly anaesthetic effect alleviates unpleasant irritations of the stomach.

This may be connected to the way peppermint oil can benefit an area for which there are scarcely any proven remedies (but which should only be applied by a doctor or at least an experienced therapist). Some people suffer from recurring and variable abdominal pains for which no 'organic cause' can be found, even after careful medical examinations. The latter include ultrasound scans of the upper abdomen (to look for gall or kidney stones), gastroscopy and enteroscopy (to look for ulcers, inflammation or tumours) and laboratory tests. The patient is thus usually diagnosed as having irritable bowel syndrome. It is assumed that incorrect movement sequences and spasms in the intestinal wall are involved. It may be that these inappropriate movements are partly triggered by an oversensitivity of the intestinal wall to stimuli from the content of the intestine. At least some patients obtain relief from peppermint preparations – however, as stated, this initially requires careful exclusion of more dangerous causes and supervision by a doctor. Peppermint can then play an important role, along with regular meals, a reduction in stress, chewing well, increased movement and perhaps special movement therapies such as curative eurythmy.

Peppermint (*Mentha piperita*)

Medicinal peppermint was produced by crossing several types of wild mint and contains particularly high levels of the fresh-smelling active substance menthol. It not only has anti-inflammatory and anti-bacterial properties, but also stimulates the cold receptors in our skin, which is the reason for the cooling sensation and numbing effect of peppermint

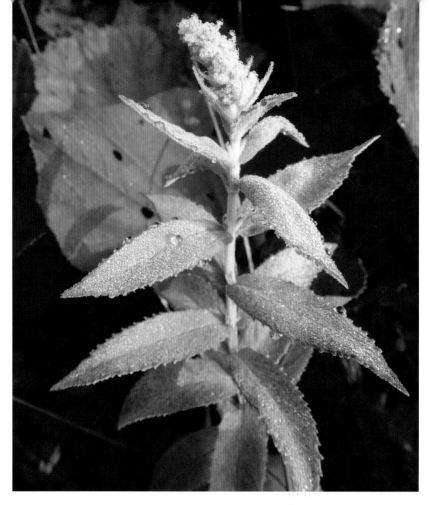

While peppermint has been bred from several natural ancestors, there are a series of naturally occurring species of mint – such as Mentha longifolia *here – which are used in tea and for seasoning due to their flavour.*

preparations. True peppermint does not grow in the wild but is a cultivated plant. It can also be grown in the garden, where it should be given a site which is not too dry. It can be picked fresh for making tea or harvested in June or July before it comes into flower. Tie several stems together and hang them up to dry. It is best to harvest the plants in the morning as some of the essential oil evaporates in the heat of the sun.

The peppermint might be one of the very few plants to which a special museum is dedicated and – amazingly – there are two for peppermint: one in Eichenau, Germany, the other in Lyons, NY, USA. Decades ago both towns cultivated peppermint in the surrounding wetlands.

Peppermint tea

Pour one cup of boiling water over about two teaspoons of dried leaves and cover, so that the essential oils do not evaporate. Let stand for 10 minutes.

Drink a cup several times a day for *upset stomach, slight biliary disorders or diarrhoeal diseases*. For acute conditions with a tendency to vomit, a sip can be taken every few minutes.

When peppermint tea is used purely for enjoyment it should be exchanged for a different tea after a few weeks. Drinking it for too long can itself lead to abdominal problems in some sensitive people.

The cooled tea can be used for washing the face to treat minor skin blemishes. Skin irritations can also be soothed by compresses.

In the case of the abdominal pains mentioned above, it can be useful to mix peppermint with chamomile flowers and yarrow leaves.

Peppermint oil

Distilling peppermint with steam produces peppermint oil, which has the same properties as the whole plant but with additional effects due to the high concentration. It has been shown that *tension headaches* can be relieved by rubbing a few drops into the painful region of the head. Studies have shown that peppermint oil is just as effective for this as chemical analgesics. Apparently, even the ancient Romans knew of its efficacy in treating headaches, as it was common practice to wind peppermint round the head at feasts in order to prevent a hangover. High quality peppermint oil can be obtained under various trade names in pharmacies and often in drug stores.

Tension headache is the commonest type of headache and is experienced as pressure, often like a ring clamped around the head. If a headache appears suddenly, is particularly bad or is accompanied by unusual symptoms (for example, disturbed consciousness or vomiting where there is no known tendency to migraine), then it is essential to seek medical advice.

Using Oliven-Pfefferminz-Öl demeter (Dr R. Heberer Naturheilmittel) has also proved effective. This oil is intended for use with an oil dispersion bath device. This was designed by Werner Junge, following the ideas of Rudolf Steiner. It is a kind of small turbine made of glass with a receptacle for oil (usually a mixture of olive oil and the medicinal plant substance). The water flowing in carries the oil to the turbine, where the oil and water are thoroughly mixed by the action of the turbine (see page 135).[2] This oil is then as finely dispersed as the fat droplets in milk. If you lie in water with an oil dispersion of this kind, much of the medicinal plant substance becomes active through the skin, and relaxing warmth processes are stimulated. For migraines and headaches, dispersing a smaller amount of the peppermint-olive oil mentioned above in a gentle flow and letting it run over the head has proved successful.

Whilst this application has a therapeutic effect, there is also a Demeter peppermint lemon oil which tends to be used for its stimulating and gently toning effect on the skin and connective tissue and is found to be especially beneficial in hot weather.

For *colds* with a *blocked nose*, rubbing some peppermint oil under the nose can ease the breathing. It should not be used for small children and infants as it can cause reflex breathing disturbances (see page 59). In *irritable bowel syndrome* (IBS, *colon irritabile*) feelings of discomfort such as pressure and spasm occur in the abdomen. Irregular bowel movements such as diarrhoea or a tendency to constipation are also frequent. In most cases these symptoms are harmless, but they can also be a sign of more serious abdominal disease such as chronic inflammation (for example *ulcerative colitis* or *Crohn's disease*) or even a tumour. In any case, medical advice should always be sought for these symptoms.

IBS appears to be due to an oversensitivity of the nerves in the intestine. Peppermint can be of benefit here. Sometimes even peppermint tea is sufficient, and at times the condition can be improved by taking 2 drops of peppermint oil on a sugar lump or in some water. A combination of peppermint and caraway oil, which is released in the small intestine, has shown to be very effective in studies even with patients with severe symptoms of functional dyspepsia.[3] One basic remedy for IBS is adequate (gentle) movement such as walking. Curative eurythmy can also be very helpful. Adequate peace and quiet at mealtimes and thorough chewing are also necessary for a long-term cure.

CHAPTER 6

Daisy

Wherever you find people, you almost always find daisies, and as children we loved this little plant, wove chains out of it, used it to decorate a birthday table, or picked the flowers with the yellow hearts and the white rays sometimes tinged with pink. There is something cheerful about this plant which is called *tusendfryd* – 'a thousand joys' – in Norwegian, but simply 'daisy' in English. Its scientific name is *Bellis perennis,* which means something like 'perennial beauty'.

In fact, it flowers almost the whole year round and the little flowers winking up at the sky can even be found under the snow, or they open shortly after it melts. This reveals this little plant's special power – it can assert its own rhythm in the face of the sun and its seasons. It overcomes cold by its own powers of warmth. (In this it resembles mistletoe, which is also able to flower in the depths of winter.)

Another aspect of its strength is revealed by the fact that the plant is often to be found in places where people walk, animals graze or the lawnmower is in use. Such places offer it enough light, but not much protection. On the other hand, it appears to recover quickly from its injuries. Some places without any grass are covered in a dense carpet of daisies. If you look carefully, you often see a strong original plant in the centre with daughter plants spreading out from this in rays or rosettes. From these, new generations of plants can radiate in turn, so a 'spreading rhythm' is visible.[1] If we look at the flowers very carefully (ideally with a magnifying glass) we can see that the inner yellow part of the flower has hundreds of tiny florets side by side which are crowded together in a strict order when in bud, like the hexagonal honeycomb in a beehive. However, on opening, they reveal tiny flowers with five surprisingly sweet-smelling petals. Let us

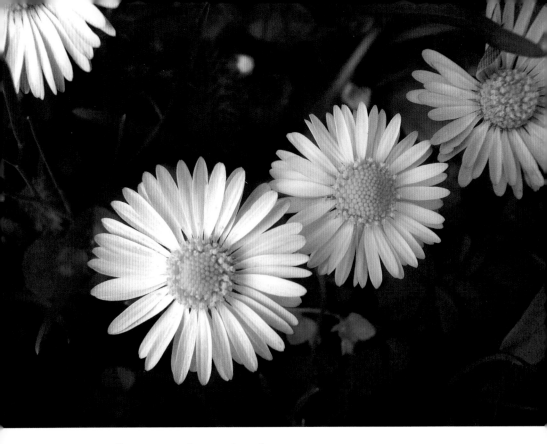

Daisies flower in many lawns and meadows.

continue our careful observations and look in more detail at the green leaves lying on the ground. In many plants the leaves on the ground are simple and undivided, but are increasingly divided and complex the further up the stem towards the flower you go. The leaves of the daisy all look practically identical. They are always rather reminiscent of the rounded succulent seed leaves, which are the first to open when the seedling emerges from what at first looks like a dead seed. This seedling can be so strong that it breaks up asphalt and forces open cracks in rock. The similarity of daisy leaves to cotyledons is also a sign of the powerful primal nature of this plant.

If, after this initial study of the plant, we try to find a region in the human body where similar movements are at work and where the plant might be of benefit, then we might think of organs with a continuous power of regeneration and a certain primal quality. The result of testing homeopathic medicines and long years of experience show that both the skin and the uterus can benefit from the daisy's healing effects. At first glance, the two organs could not seem more different: hidden deep within the body or turned totally outward; designed for supporting and nourishing future life or setting a boundary and forming a sheath. However, they do have something in common: both regenerate within 28 days, in the same rhythm which takes place in the heavens from one full moon to the next. This rhythm is obvious in the case of the uterus, even though it can fluctuate somewhat around this average in individual women. The mucous membrane of the uterus is regenerated within a month (this word again contains the moon) and is then sloughed off during menstruation. A comparable process takes place in the skin, but less obviously. It takes exactly 28 days from the formation of a new cell at the base of the epidermis to the time it is shed as a small dead scale. This rhythm is disrupted in some skin diseases. The disruption is most obvious in the case of an *injury* from outside. The regenerative processes then have to speed up in order to heal the damage. The homeopathic preparation *Bellis,* made from the daisy, can be of help in this.

There are some similarities between the daisy and the well-known plant for treating wounds, arnica (see Chapter 23), which also produces a rayed composite flower. In Britain, where arnica, a typical inhabitant of high mountains, is absent, the daisy has even acquired the title of 'our own arnica'. However, *Bellis* is equally renowned for follow-up treatment of damage to the womb after childbirth or operations, leading to it being given the other title of 'womb arnica' in homeopathy. Extract of daisy, which is characterised by a feeling of purity, can also help to clear up *blemished skin*.

Traditionally, the small white shining flower was recommended for lightening freckles and *liver spots*. Whenever patients suffering from blemishes ask me about this, I always recommend pressing the fresh juice from the plants and dropping it on to the places to be lightened in the evening, or applying some of the crushed plant. (Of course, whenever new dark spots appear, which could conceal a melanoma, a doctor must be asked to examine these). Previously, I was forced to say that there was no proof of efficacy. However, there have since been frequent reports of success and, moreover, it could not do any harm. Now there is scientific evidence that daisy extract can in fact suppress the development of dark skin pigmentation very effectively and the enzyme in the skin cells that it inhibits has even been identified.[2]

Thus the plant of our children's games has risen to scientific eminence. The joy that it radiates and the help that it gives us remain unchanged.

Daisy (*Bellis perennis*)

Use of the fresh plant

As mentioned above, the leaves and flowers of the plant can be pressed between the fingers and laid on freckles, which will become lighter with regular application. Investigations have shown that *liver spots* should also lighten if extracts of daisy are applied regularly.

Daisy flowers are edible and are therefore suitable for decorating salads, quark with herbs, etc.

Medicinal plant extract

You can make *daisy essence* yourself by placing 20 g (1 oz) of finely chopped daisies (leaves and flowers) in a jar with a good seal in double the quantity (40 g, or 2 oz) of 20% ethanol for at least two weeks. To extract the constituents more thoroughly, place the plant material in a mortar and crush well in alcohol. Shake the jar with the plant and alcohol mixture well every day. Finally, squeeze out the liquid. A makeshift way to do this is by emptying the contents of the jar into a coffee filter bag and squeezing it well between a plate and a wide jar with a flat bottom. The essence can be dropped on to skin blemishes twice daily.

Acne Water from Wala and Clarifying Toner by Dr Hauschka contains daisy essence alongside other medicinal plant extracts (for example, marigold and kidney vetch).

Potentised Bellis

In homeopathy, Bellis (often in D6) is used for *open wounds* (in contrast to arnica which tends to be used for closed injuries with bruising). While this does not replace a proper external treatment of the injury, Bellis perennis D6 (5 globules 3 times daily) can also be given internally, and this usually leads to a noticeable improvement in healing and a reduction in pain.

The preparation Symphytum comp. (Weleda) contains *Bellis* in addition to comfrey *(Symphytum)* and arnica. It is suitable in the initial phase after *breaking a bone* to ease the pain and stimulate healing. I generally prescribe 10 drops 3 times daily for the first fortnight. Later, I tend to give the Wala preparation of the same name which contains potentised tin instead of *Bellis*, the former to stimulate the growth of new bone (see also page 32, Onion).

CHAPTER 7

Birch

People have strong feelings about birch. It is easy to understand why anyone with a pollen allergy who finds it hard to breathe when early birch pollen is released might dislike this tree. Others get annoyed by the tiny gliders released by the trees in July when the seeds are ripe, which cover the streets and find their way into the house through every little crack. However, I am an unreserved admirer of birch trees. As a child, I lay for many an hour in the shimmering shadows of three birches which were planted soon after my birth and gazed up at the sky through their constantly moving leaves. Later on, 'paper' could be created from the white bark, on which my two brothers and I attempted to paint with difficulty. Somehow, we three felt closely related to the three birches. We even tried to use their impressive growth as an incentive for our own.

There was really no more convincing sign of spring every year than the wonderful pale green of sprouting birch trees with their initially crumpled, resinous, sticky and bittersweet-tasting leaves. The delight felt by others about the 'special green of May' was shown in our town by the paths to the Lutheran and Catholic churches being decorated with leafy birch branches at Whitsun and Corpus Christi. In my memory, these decorations were always bathed in sunshine, making them glow – although there must have been wet days back then as well.

The birch's life cycle shows a curious similarity to that of human beings. Like us, it has a long youthful period with the initial emphasis on growth and development. Only when it is around 15 to 20 (very

Birches in spring.

70

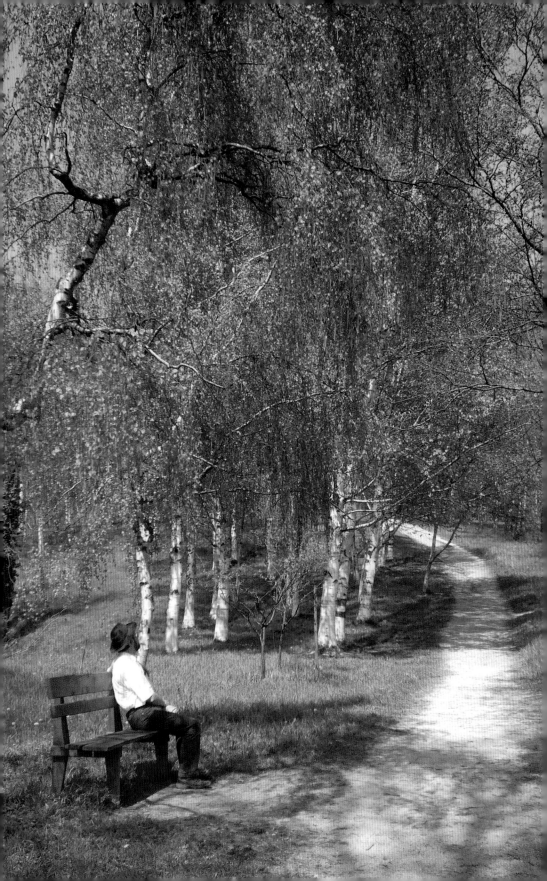

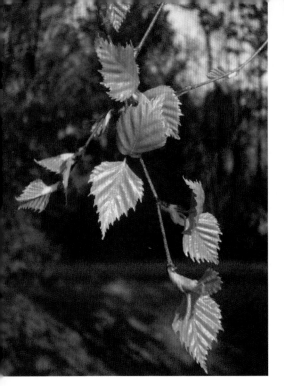

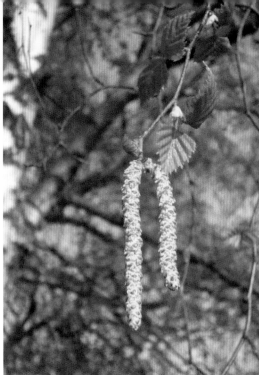

Birch leaves.

Birch flowers.

rarely as early as 10) years old does the birch start to flower and become sexually mature. Compared to other trees, it does not get old; its maximum age of 120 years comes close to the greatest age a human being can reach. However, at a hundred it is already frail and aged. But each autumn when the birch prepares for the 'little death' of winter, it demonstrates just how successful a withdrawal from life can be. The trees appear like golden waterfalls in the October light.

There is scarcely any other tree that dominates such vast regions. It only grows in the northern hemisphere, but here it covers huge areas of Scandinavia, Poland and Russia, all the way to Japan. In these regions, the birch can survive winter temperatures down to -70°C (-95°F). In the harsher areas of the far north and in the mountains, our silver birch is often replaced by the knee-high dwarf birch whose leaves turn a shining red after the first frost and set the *Fjell*, the Norwegian high mountains, ablaze before the snows fall.

In the Altai region of Central Siberia, where Russia, China and Mongolia meet, I came to know the birch as a useful resource for the people living there. The district was very poor and people could not afford to have many imported products from other regions. In spring, the local people bored holes into the bark of the birch, or simply cut off branches and put the cut ends into bottles. Huge amounts of sap ran out of the cut trees for two weeks – up to 10 litres (2 gallons) per day! The sweet sap, which it was claimed had medicinal powers, was fermented and provided the basis for 'wine' and 'champagne' which were enjoyed in the village. In Finland, birch sap is used in a similar way, but also as a hair tonic and to stimulate water excretion.

It is easy to believe that birch trees, which often grow on damp soil and carry large amounts of water from the soil into the air, are rulers of the water cycle. It has been proved at the biochemical level that birch leaf tea actually increases a hormone in the blood (atrial natriuretic peptide, or ANP), which stimulates the excretion of salt and water in human beings. Birch leaf extracts inhibit its breakdown (by neutral metallopeptidase), which leads to increased water elimination. Birch leaf tea is therefore good for a 'flushing treatment' for mild *inflammatory symptoms in the urinary tract and kidneys* and as a preventative measure when there is a tendency to form *kidney stones*.

The mechanism described for increasing water excretion can also produce a slight *lowering of the blood pressure*. There is a second way in which birch does this. It inhibits the angiotensin-converting enzyme (ACE)[1] and therefore has the same effect as the most frequently prescribed drugs for reducing blood pressure, ACE inhibitors. In orthodox medicine both effects are often combined in one tablet (Ramipril plus, for example). The birch provides a natural example of this kind of process. So it is easy to see why it has always been claimed that birch counteracts *sclerosis* – that is, hardening (of the arteries). Rudolf Steiner recommended birch particularly often when there was a need to counteract extreme sclerotic processes in the body (in relation to the blood vessels, the joints in cases of *arthritis* and for *cataract* in the lens of the eye or *otosclerosis* in the ear).

Whilst most trees become fixed and inflexible, birch remains supple, even when very old. Perhaps this is why it has always been claimed that birch sap and preparations of birch leaves can counteract *rheumatic complaints* and *arthritic tendencies* and are important as part of a spring detox.

Another effect of birch is easy to experience. In birch woods you

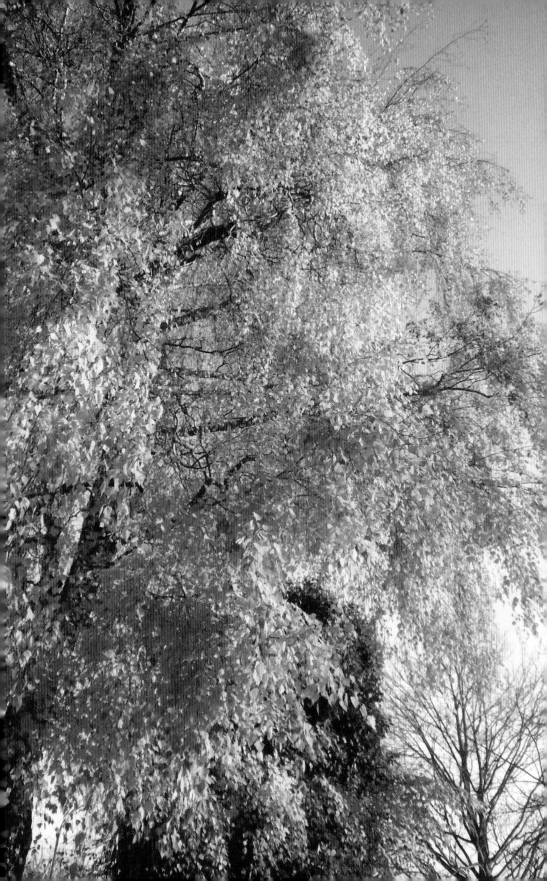

sometimes see fallen tree trunks lying around, but if you give these a kick they just collapse, because they are really nothing more than a hollow tube of bark. Birch wood rots quickly while the shiny white bark lasts 'forever' and is almost never attacked and decomposed by fungi and bacteria. This is why, in Russia and Finland, birch bark is used for making storage containers for foodstuffs. Food keeps longer in these than in other types of containers, because the preserving effect is 'transferred' to them. I do not know whether shoes made of birch bark help to reduce the tendency to athlete's foot, but I could imagine this to be the case. The white substance in the bark, the *betulin* (from the Latin *Betula,* meaning 'birch') has an anti-bacterial and anti-fungal action, which is why it is also good for the prevention and treatment of *inflammatory skin diseases*. It is particularly helpful in those parts of the body where there is skin-to-skin contact (like the groin, or underneath nappies) or elsewhere where there are warm, moist conditions which favour microbial growth. Luckily it appears that betulin – unlike birch pollen – does not to trigger any allergic reactions.

The white bark can also be seen as a type of sun protection for the tree. Interestingly, betulin and the related betulinic acid can have a beneficial effect on photodamage to the skin. It has even been shown in cell cultures that they induced malignant skin cells to dissolve while the healthy skin cells remained unaffected. Maybe even those people who get annoyed by the birch can come to see why it can also be admired and loved.

Birch (*Betula pendula*)

Birch leaves can be harvested in May or June, either from your own trees if you have them, or with the permission of the owner. They dry relatively quickly if spread out loosely in a warm airy place. The leaves are particularly efficacious if some of the sticky resinous substance surrounding them when they first open is still attached.

A birch in autumn can look like a golden waterfall.

Birch leaf tea

Pour a cup of boiling water over one tablespoon of the leaves and leave to stand for at least 10 minutes.

This tea increases the excretion of water, and can be used as a 'flushing treatment' for a tendency to *urinary tract infections* and also for a tendency to *kidney stones*. It can also be used for a (slight) tendency to *fluid retention (oedema)*. The mild effect in reducing blood pressure has already been mentioned (see page 73).

Because birch also stimulates the excretion of waste, including uric acid, it is often used for the naturopathic treatment of *gout* and *rheumatic diseases*. However, birch leaf tea can also be used as an accompanying measure for the treatment of almost all sclerotic – that is, hardening – diseases, or as a spring detox to help counteract the increased hardening tendencies in the second half of life.

Birch extract

Birch extract is available in ready-to-use formulations for mild *irritation of the urinary tract* and *prevention of bladder stones* in the form of effervescent tablets such as Uroflan effervescent tablets or Urorenal effervescent tablets. In addition, birch extract is contained in various herbal combination remedies.

Tonics and elixirs

Birch elixir (Weleda) is made by boiling birch leaves with sugar and is often recommended for a spring detox. Dilute 1–2 teaspoons in water and add a little lemon juice to taste. This preparation can be taken daily in spring for 2–4 weeks, for instance to accompany a gentle fast. Because many toxins stored in the fatty tissue are released during a fast and more uric acid is produced, it makes sense to stimulate the excretory processes.

Wala Kidney tonic (Nierentonikum) can be used in a similar way, but this also contains juniper berries which enhance the excretory effect. I also prescribe this remedy if I wish to bring down slightly *raised blood pressure*. During the manufacture of the kidney tonic the plants undergo rhythmical light and dark periods, are stirred and left to stand, and are finally subjected to a heat process.

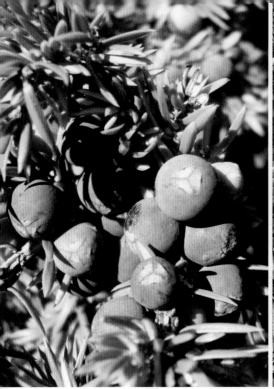

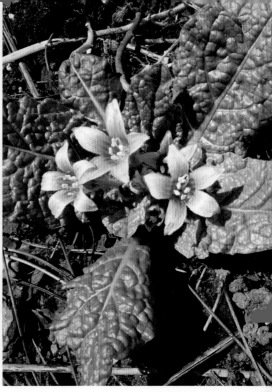

Birch leaves are often combined with juniper berries due to their diuretic and 'cleansing' effect.

Mandrake (Mandragora officinarum) *is often combined with birch for treating joint conditions.*

If you want to help counteract excessive *sclerotic processes* such as *arteriosclerosis* or a tendency to *raised blood pressure,* then Scleron tablets (Weleda) should be taken for 4 weeks (1 tablet at night) followed by Kidney Tonic (Wala) for 4 weeks.

The manufacture of both the Weleda birch elixir and the Wala kidney tonic includes a boiling process. Rudolf Steiner pointed out that birch preparations like these work particularly strongly on the metabolism. If you wish to focus the effect of birch in the head (for example, for treating *otos clerosis,* a disease which affects the auditory ossicle) then a cold extract of birch leaves is required. I have no experience with this type of preparation method, but perhaps potentised birch preparations would be appropriate for these symptoms. This may apply particularly to substances produced by the Wala rhythmic process, or as a Rh preparation because these use rhythmical cooling processes as an important stage in manufacturing the remedy.

Potentised birch

Birch leaves are processed on their own to produce Betula e foliis D4 ampoules (Wala) and Betula folium Rh D3 (Weleda) plus Betula D3 ampoules (Abnoba). Like birch leaf tea, these remedies are used for *rheumatic diseases* and to *stimulate excretion*.

More commonly, birch is used in compounds with other medicinal substances. It is almost always aimed at promoting excretion and therefore counteracting tendencies to concretion, the build up of inorganic material in tissues.

In this form, it is commonly used for *muscle* and *joint problems*. One preparation of this kind is Betula/Arnica comp. (ampoules and globules; Wala) which includes both the birch leaves and bark along with arnica, ant extract and sulfur. This remedy has proved particularly successful for muscular problems around the shoulder joint *(periarthropathy, periarthritis humeroscapularis)* where it is especially effective if injected by the doctor or alternative practitioner and combined with physiotherapy or curative eurythmy.

Arnica/Formica comp. ampoules (Weleda) combining birch bark, formica (ants) and arnica have a similar composition to the Betula/ Arnica comp. (Wala).

In Betula/Mandragora comp. (Wala), birch is combined with mandrake *(Mandragora)*, potentised galena and meadow sweet. This remedy often has a good pain relieving effect in a variety of more acute *rheumatic conditions*.

I often prescribe Cartilago comp. globules or ampoules (Wala) for *arthroses* in order to reduce pain and prevent further deterioration. In this remedy, birch is combined with gold, tin, ant and an organ preparation which directs the action to the joint cartilage. In acute cases the remedy can be injected close to the joint (possibly along with mistletoe, which can have a regenerating effect on the joint but must be administered only by experienced practitioners because of possible side effects). The globules are suitable for long-term use, the recommended dose being 5–10, three times daily.

Cartilago/Mandragora comp. (Wala) is an option for *acute inflammatory joint conditions* where potentised silver and antimonite combat excessive destructive inflammatory processes. *Mandragora* (which was depicted on objects buried with the Egyptian pharaoh

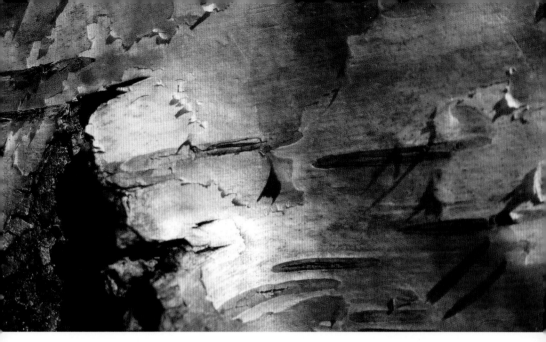

Birch bark

Tutankhamen who suffered from a hip joint complaint) can also alleviate the pain.

Mandragora comp. (Weleda), which can be used in a similar way, is a combination of birch, mandragora, arnica, ant, horsetail (which, like birch, promotes excretion) and an organ preparation for the meniscus of the knee joint. As a general rule, *joint inflammation* should not be treated for too long without specialist advice. The more severe the condition, the sooner an expert should be consulted.

Compounds including birch bark are often used for treating *vascular sclerosis* and its after-effects. On the tree, birch bark is characteristic of hardening processes on the one hand, but on the other displays a particularly strong relationship to the light.

Wala Secale/Bleiglanz comp., available as ampoules and globules, is composed specifically for this type of application. Besides birch and potentised galena, this contains potentised tobacco (which in its pure form is one of the major causes of sclerotic vascular disease) and ergot *(Secale cornutum)*. Like tobacco, ergot in its raw state leads to constricted arteries, but in its potentised form it expands the blood vessels. Lastly, the remedy contains an organ preparation that directs the action to the arterial blood vessels. In this remedy, birch primarily promotes excretion but also has a mildly relaxing effect. This remedy is used in cases of a tendency to *vascular spasms* but also for *peripheral artery occlusive disease,* which is primarily caused by tobacco abuse. Good results have been repeatedly observed, even in serious cases where amputation is being considered. Obviously, serious conditions like this require (specialist) medical attention.

Secale/Retina comp. (Wala) has a similar composition, but the organ preparation directs the action to the retina of the eye. It is mainly used for *circulatory problems inside the eye.*

Birch for external use

In recent years birch preparations have become increasingly popular for treating external conditions. Over the last few decades new health benefits of the substance contained in the birch's white bark, *betulin,* have repeatedly been discovered. Betulin has an inhibitory effect on bacteria, fungi and viruses, and helps to promote the healing of wounds. It can kill tumour cells in the skin without damaging healthy cells and the 'sun protection' constituent of birch can benefit photodamaged skin and combat light-induced roughening and hardening *(actinic keratosis).* The anthroposophical pharmacist Dr Armin Scheffler rendered this substance a great service by being the first to extract it from birch bark on a commercial scale. He also discovered that powder obtained this way was easy to make into ointments and creams, as it acts both as an emulsifier and preservative in such preparations. It has no toxic effects and does not trigger allergies. Various ointment preparations have been produced, which are sold by Birken GmbH under the name of Imlan.[2]

This ointment is particularly efficacious in moist regions such as the nappy area or where skin rubs against skin (for example, due to a very large bosom or a pendulous belly-fat apron), where *skin injuries (intertrigo)* occur, which may be accompanied by *fungal infections.* Imlan has also been successful in treating *poorly healing wounds* and – as already mentioned – *chronic photodamage.*

Birch leaves also play an important role in external treatment. Oil dispersion baths with Betula e foliis W 5%, Oleum (Wala) are helpful as a complementary therapy for *rheumatic joint conditions* and *skin complaints.* For rheumatic *pain in the muscles and joints* and for pain caused by sport and overexertion, embrocations can be made using Birken Rheumaöl mit Arnica (birch based rheumatism oil with arnica; Wala) if required. Besides birch, it contains stinging nettle, extract of burdock root, ant and arnica. For patients who are allergic to arnica (which occurs rarely) there is a version without this plant Birken Rheumaöl ohne Arnica (birch based rheumatism oil without arnica).

An oil introduced into medical practice very recently is Birkenrinde 10% in Olivenöl (Dr Heberer Naturheilmittel) which has given good results for flaky skin conditions (particularly for psoriasis). However, it is also used for a tendency to dandruff, for which it is applied in small amounts directly to the scalp by means of an oil dispersion bath device, for example in the shower. This oil has a very strong smell, which not everyone likes.

Arnica comp./Apis ointment by Weleda is recommended for inflammatory conditions in *joints with arthritic changes* (activated arthroses). It contains a decoction of birch leaves, arnica, mandragora, a small amount of the painkilling monkshood and an extract from bees.

With a similar name but a very different composition, Arnica comp./Cuprum (Weleda) is an oil containing warming copper, arnica flowers, birch leaves, marigold flowers and essential oils of rosemary and lavender. This remedy has a very warming effect and can help in cases of *muscle tension*.

It is clear that birch is a good partner in many medicinal compounds (despite the large range included, not all of them been described here). In all these, birch often has the task of stimulating excretory processes and therefore ensuring that 'deposits', which have sometimes been set in motion by the other ingredients in the compound, are removed from our bodies before they lead to new problems in other places.

CHAPTER 8

Cowslip

After a hard winter, every spring flower we come across brings delight: the white snowdrop, the delicate wood anemone, the radiant dandelion. But one flower in particular appears to be surrounded by an unusual cheerfulness and childlike purity. The cowslip reminds many people of their own childhood.

There are two species of cowslip: the sulfur-yellow oxlip, which is found in damp places, frequently in woodland and scrub from where it often shines forth even in April, and the true cowslip. The latter's flower is darker, orangey-yellow in colour. On each of its five petals, close to the flower tube that unites them, there is a shining orange-coloured nectar guide which shows the bumble bees and butterflies the way to the fragrant nectar. The cowslip has a much stronger scent than the oxlip. The nectar guides look as though the yellow in the rest of the flower has been concentrated into them, contracted – and the yellow looks like the diluted 'expanded' orange. If you take time to look at a flower, you may be able to sense something like a rhythmical pulsation between these qualities of contraction and expansion.

The true cowslip flowers slightly later than the oxlip and prefers drier, warmer sites such as sunny slopes. Its Latin name *Primula veris,* which roughly means 'first little one of the spring,' is not quite appropriate, as several other flowers (including other relatives of the cowslip) appear long before the cowslip opens its flowers. Its flowering period peaks in May, and the last flowers can still be found in June. The yellow of the true cowslip is very beautiful. So it is not surprising that in places in Central Europe where cowslips are abundant, their flowers are used for dying Easter eggs.

The leaves are also unique. The flowers number up to thirty, all

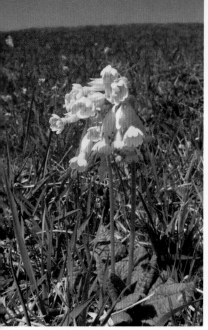

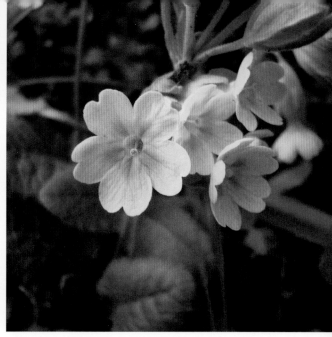

Cowslips in unimproved grassland.

Dark nectar guides on the petals are characteristic of the medicinal cowslip.

arising from a point at the top of the leafless stem about 20 cm (8 in) above the ground and either turning to one side or (more rarely) forming a true spherical head. The leaves also arise from a point, not raised above the ground but directly on the surface of the soil where they form a rosette. Whilst the leaves of most other plants are smooth, those of all Primula species are divided into small domed areas. From above, they look a little like a carpet of foam made of closely-packed bubbles. The main active agents in the medicinal plant are in fact foaming agents, known as saponins (from Latin *sapo* – 'soap'). The other group of medicinal ingredients are the flavonoids, which simply means yellow substances. The flavonoids have a slight anti-inflammatory effect while the saponins are strongly mucolytic. The plant's root (or rhizome, to be botanically correct) contains particularly large amounts of these substances. This pale yellow rhizome spreads out just beneath the surface of the soil. When dried, it produces a smell that is slightly reminiscent of chewing gum. This is caused by the anti-inflammatory methyl salicylate, which is indeed used for flavouring chewing gum.

In traditional herbal medicine, cowslip tea (from the flowers, leaves or root) is used to break up thick *phlegm in the bronchial tubes*. Cowslip is often mixed with other plants because – at least in the

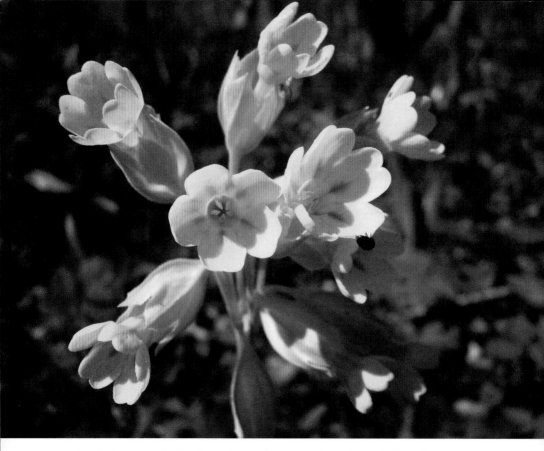

The inflorescence of Primula veris *may form a complete sphere, which can have a radiating quality like a little sun.*

case of tea made from the root – gastric irritation can occur at higher doses. Common remedies for *inflammation of the sinuses* and *bronchitis* (Sinupret forte, Bronchipret, etc.) contain extracts of cowslip, which help to liquefy viscous mucus in the nose.

In anthroposophical medicine, cowslip is also used for completely different diseases. For instance, a very elaborate process is used for producing a medicine from cowslip by growing it in soil fertilised with gold. Gold might appear to be a very expensive fertiliser, but in fact the expense is due less to the cost of the metal (which is only used in traces) than to the laborious processing. The gold is added to the soil in a very fine dispersion (using gold salts whose orangey-yellow colour resembles the nectar guides in the cowslip flower). The cowslips grown on this soil are composted. The cowslips grown on this are themselves made into compost and only the third generation of plants grown on the 'gold cowslip compost' are used to prepare the medicine.

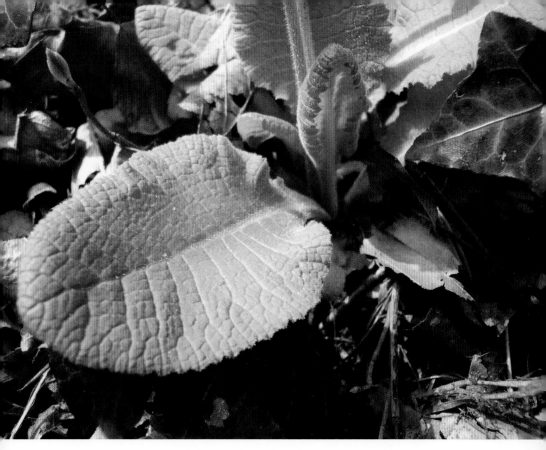

The sections of the cowslip leaf appear slightly domed.

This is mainly used for treating *cardiac diseases*, for which potentised gold is also an option in homeopathy and anthroposophical medicine. It is as though potentising the medicine – which is otherwise done in a pharmacy laboratory – is performed by the plant itself.

Cowslip can be turned into a heart medicine even without gold fertiliser. In anthroposophical medicine, along with preparations made from thistles, for example, cowslip is transformed into a basic remedy for treating the heart (Cardiodoron). I have seen this treatment lead to impressive recoveries in cases of serious *heart disease*. This is really amazing, as cowslip on its own is not known as a heart remedy and thistles normally produce liver remedies. But perhaps this is just where the secret lies: a large proportion of the blood which flows into the right chambers of the heart comes from the liver and is then sent on by the heart to the lungs. The blood that flows into the left chambers of the heart comes from the lungs and then flows to the rest of the body. The cowslip first has an effect on the lungs (for example, as an expectorant, and even the plant's leaf form resembles the alveoli). The thistle works on the liver. Perhaps this type of remedy helps to relieve the heart when it is under strain from the organs to which it is connected. At any rate, the cowslip is held to have a 'heart relieving' effect in a different way. Hildegard von Bingen claimed that it has a cheering effect on the soul; so it could be beneficial for *mild depression*.

Apart from illness and medicine, we can sense the 'cheering effect' on our heart when we come across the cowslip, smell its scent and delight in its colour. Perhaps this is why it is a symbol of the Virgin Mary, creating a piece of 'heaven on earth,' which is also why the plant is called

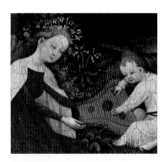

Himmelsschlüssel ('key to the heavens') in German. It is depicted by an unknown painter of the late Middle Ages growing in the Garden of Paradise between the feet of Mary and the playing child.

The cowslip is shown in a central position in the Frankfurt Paradiesgärtlein *(about 1410, Städel Museum, Frankfurt am Main).*

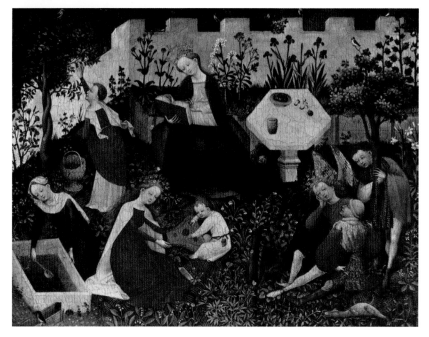

Cowslip/Oxlip (*Primula veris/Primula elatior*)

The oxlip *(Primula elatior)* is more abundant on the continent of Europe and Siberia than the cowslip *(Primula veris)*. In Britain the cowslip is native to all but northwest Scotland, while the oxslip is rare outside East Anglia. The cowslip has deep yellow flowers and orange nectar guides, and the oxlip has paler narrower calyces and no extra spots in the flower.

General herbalism rarely distinguishes between these two species and both are used mainly as a cough remedy for *loosening phlegm.* Collecting the flowers is generally not worthwhile as very large amounts have to be picked in order to obtain a reasonable quantity. However, if you use them only in mixtures (which is recommended in any case) and can therefore make do with smaller amounts, a handful of the flowers will make a pretty spring bouquet and a pleasant tea. Of course, this assumes that there are a sufficient number of plants growing (in your own garden, for example), so that collecting them does not do any damage. After drying them quickly, the flowers must be stored in jars with a good seal so that as little as possible of the scent is lost. However, I would tend to advise against collecting the roots (which is done in autumn) because drying roots properly is more difficult than drying the tender quick-drying flowers. Moreover, collecting the roots kills the plant so that the attractive species is depleted at this location.

Cowslip tea

Cowslip tea has an expectorant effect but is not suitable for a dry cough. The tea is therefore particularly good in the second phase of a *cold* with a productive cough and also useful for *chronic bronchitis.* The cowslip flowers are usually combined with other mucolytic medicinal plants.

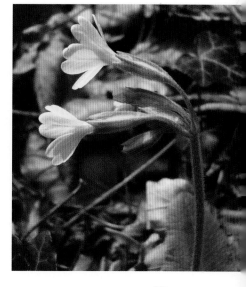

The oxlip (Primula elatior) *is also used for teas. It has a paler colour and its calyces are narrower than the more deeply coloured medicinal cowslip* (P. officinalis) *which is used for anthroposophical medicines.*

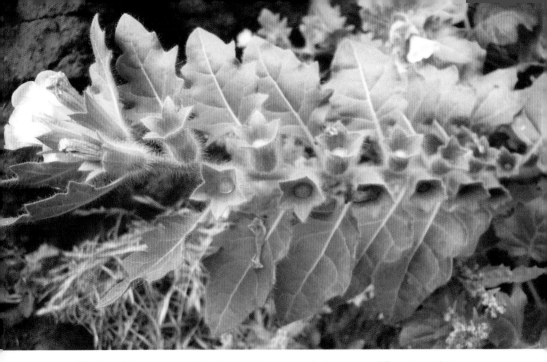

Henbane (Hyoscyamus niger), *with its very regularly structured form, is used in combination with cowslip and cotton thistle for regulating heart function and circulation, along with ribwort plantain to regulate muscle function.*

Suitable species are mullein flowers, ribwort plantain or thyme, for example. If you want to achieve a particularly powerful effect, then cowslip root can be used, but this can sometimes cause slight problems in people with sensitive stomachs. Add 2 level teaspoons of the mixed herbs to one cup of boiling water and leave to stand for 10 minutes, then drain. Drink a cup of this tea several times a day. A little honey can be added to taste.

Herbal medicines

A whole range of proprietary medicines intended for loosening mucus in *bronchitis* or *inflammation of the sinuses (sinusitis)* contain cowslip extracts. Examples of these are Sinupret (forte) (with, for example, gentian root, verbena and elder flowers), Bronchipret (which contains thyme leaves), and a number of others.

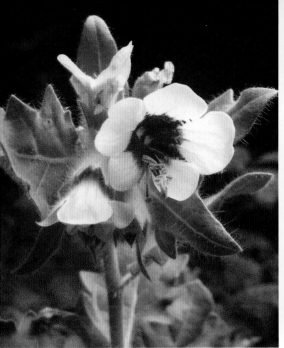

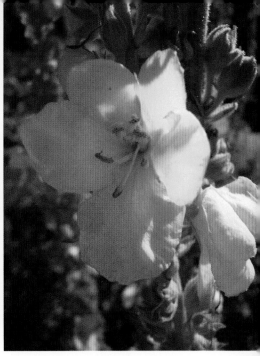

Flower of henbane (Hyoscyamus niger).

Mullein (Verbascum) *is a good addition to an expectorant tea for a cold with a productive cough.*

The cowslip in anthroposophical medicine

Earlier in this chapter, we described how the small yellow cowslip with its rounded leaves and the large purple-flowering cotton thistle with its pointed leaves are processed into cardiovascular medicines. Throughout life, the heart exists in a rhythm between expansion and contraction, and it thereby gives the blood an impulse and impetus for movement. The blood, in turn, first flows towards the inside of the body and is then exposed in the lungs to air from the outside world. Disturbances in this rhythmical balance can manifest as *arrhythmic episodes*, which are experienced as the heart beating irregularly. They can also manifest as a failure to adapt the blood pressure to different needs (such as *blacking out* or *feeling faint*), or a slight tendency to *raised blood pressure.* Cardiodoron (Onopordon comp., Weleda) is then often an excellent remedy which may, however, have to be taken for a time before its effect develops fully. This remedy is really a model for the kind of anthroposophical medicine in which plants or individual substances with opposing tendencies are combined in a pharmaceutical process with the aim of stimulating a rhythmical balance in the body.

89

Cardiodoron can therefore be helpful for a tendency both to *low* and *high blood pressure* and likewise for a *too slow* or *too fast pulse*. In addition to the contrasting plants mentioned, this remedy contains a small amount of Hyoscyamus (henbane), a plant which appears particularly rhythmically structured, and which has a poisonous effect in larger quantities (for example, by accelerating the heartbeat). In the small amount added here, it has a stimulating and balancing effect on the processes of the patient's 'rhythmical system'. Cardiodoron (Onopordon comp.) drops and Rh tablets are prescription-only medicines in many countries, as are the 1% and 5% ampoules.

In the doctor's hands these ampoules are sometimes amazingly efficacious, even for more serious heart conditions. My colleague Hubertus Magerstädt gave me the idea of injecting these ampoules along with my other heart treatments. It has often allowed me to avoid an otherwise necessary hospital admission, especially in the case of some elderly patients. This increased my admiration for the lovable cowslip and, equally, for Rudolf Steiner, who was the first to recommend processing this plant (which no one before him had used for heart and circulatory problems) into such an efficacious medicine.

Primula comp. (Wala), which is suitable for roughly the same fields of application, is made from the same plants but in a lower concentration, and may not require a prescription. The plants mentioned above for Cardiodoron are used along with some others which act on the heart (sea squill and lily-of-the-valley) for the remedy Primula/Convallaria comp. (Wala). It is recommended for the *onset of cardiac insufficiency* but has also been successful for *circulatory problems due to infectious diseases.* I would recommend consulting an (anthroposophical) doctor for all these conditions, which is why I shall not give any further information on self-medication here.

Plantago-Primula cum Hyoscyamo ampoules (Weleda), prescription only in many countries, also contain cowslip and henbane with the addition of ribwort plantain (Plantago lanceolata, see Chapter 13) instead of cotton thistle. Plantain is about the same size as the cowslip but in many ways appears its polar opposite. It has already been mentioned that the cowslip leaf is rounded and has a network of domed segments, which make it appear crinkled. In contrast, the ribwort plantain's leaf is marked by parallel veins and appears to be stretched. There are also polar aspects when it comes to the constituents of the two plants. While Cardiodoron and related products influence the rhythmical processes in the cardiovascular system, Plantago-Primula cum Hyoscyamo regulates muscular tension. This remedy can therefore be an extremely valuable aid for patients who suffer from *spasm (spasticity)* of the musculature in neurological diseases such as *multiple sclerosis, stroke* or *infantile cerebral damage.*

> Following a stroke, one female patient had suffered hemiplegia for 15 years. Her arm and hand were bent in a spasm, too stiff to use and getting in the way, and the paralysed leg was the same in its cramped extended position. Years of physiotherapy had made almost no difference to this condition. After injecting this remedy, a marked relaxation set in so that it was possible to begin curative eurythmy. The patient's family also noticed a psychological effect and the woman's husband, who was normally rather sceptical, commented, 'I have never seen you as relaxed as this!'

This remedy is often very efficacious for *muscle spasm in acute back conditions* (also for *slipped disc*), something that was pointed out to me originally by my colleagues Freimuth and Andreas Hessenbruch and Irene Stiltz[1].

Further information about this remedy is given in Chapter 13.

CHAPTER 9

Pasque Flower

Our gardens have long been home to a multicultural society as peaceful as it is colourful. Scarcely a single one of the bright splashes of colour in which we so delight in spring is of native origin. However, the arrival of some of these plants was accompanied by conflict. The fascination with tulips, for example, was quite extreme in earlier times. It is now hard to imagine that sometimes people sold house and home just to own a single bulb of a particularly coveted variety (until the bubble burst in 1637). Then again, even today, stock exchange values and real ones also differ enormously at times.

However, some spectacular spring-flowering plants originate from our own soil. Amongst the most heart-warming is the pasque flower or *Pulsatilla* (whose name comes from the Latin *pulsare* – 'ringing', referring to its similarity to a bell). Although it may almost disappear in the garden amongst the other magnificent flowers, our hearts are lifted when we come across it in spring on a dry sunny spot out in the country.

There are scarcely any larger or more colourful flowers in the wild in Spring. Sometimes the flower reaches a diameter of 5 cm (2 in). Anyone who carefully lifts the deep purple bell to glance inside the flower cup will be amazed by the radiant yellow colour on the elongated, densely-packed stamens in the centre of what may at first seem rather a melancholy plant. It is not just the colour that expresses a complete polarity: the enveloping petals and the taut stretched stamens are also opposites. If the stem has not yet emerged far from the soil but the flower is already open, it is almost like looking into an eye, which looks innocently back at you. It is amazing how early in the year this occurs. All around, winter has left clear traces: the grass is brown

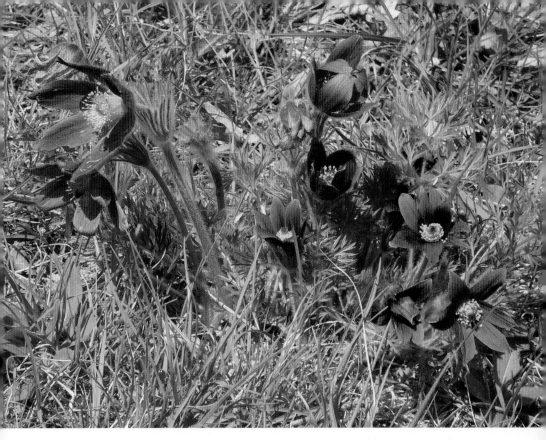

Pulsatilla is often found in groups in the wild.

and flattened and scarcely anything is stirring in the plant world when
Pulsatilla has already opened. Sometimes it even opens its flower 'eye'
in February.

The rather thick buds are already formed in late summer and wait a
long time until the first warming rays of the sun kiss them awake – just
like the prince and sleeping beauty in the fairy tale. Snow White lies in
the coffin of glass (that is, of liquefied and hardened silica). The buds
and flowers of *Pulsatilla* also have a siliceous aspect. They are covered
with a coat of fine white hair, although I do not know if there is a higher
level of silicon in these hairs, as there is in our hair. This is the case in
many plants; many hairs are not only for protection but are also a sign
of sensitivity (just think of a cat's whiskers). In *Pulsatilla* it is not just
the flowers but also the incredibly finely structured leaves which are
surrounded by a fringe of lustrous hair. The flowers are protected by
them, and one secret of their early flowering is that it is often more
than 10°C (18°F) warmer inside them than in the surroundings. The

93

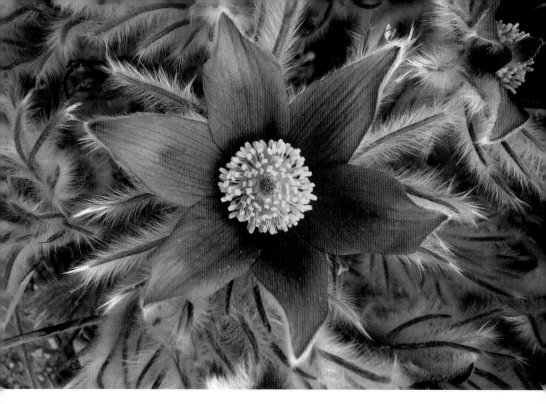

The Pulsatilla flower is surrounded by the downy hairs of the sepals.

coat of hair insulates them like a covering of down and the feathery sepals (which are also covered in hair) add to this, until the warmth of the sun is finally captured by the dark flower. Apparently, metabolic processes in the flower also release additional heat, so that *Pulsatilla* is able to open at a time when the air around it is so cold that other plants are still hidden in the ground. But even a few clouds or the cool of the evening cause the flower to close again and turn downwards.

A few weeks after the purple and yellow beauties have flowered, a site with *Pulsatilla* looks quite changed: dishevelled hairy heads now stand in the wind. The seed heads – called 'wild man' in some places – seem to have been formed by an inversion of the bell-shape. By inverting the analogy as well, we could well call them 'gentle maiden.' When the seeds (which are several centimetres long) are ripe, they are caught by the wind and can travel a good distance on it. But this is not all: the seeds have appendages which stretch and curl during the course of the day, enabling the seed to 'crawl' a little, even with no wind. The stretching and curling are driven by dew during the night and drying during the day. In addition, the seed can bore its way

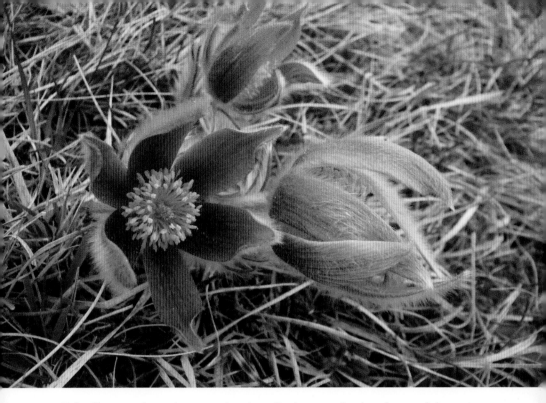

Pulsatilla seems almost shy on opening, immediately prepared to bow down and close again.

into the soil with up to nine rotations like a corkscrew. It seems that movement is important to *Pulsatilla*.

Pulsatilla was probably used as a medicinal plant even in ancient times. Hippocrates, the forefather of modern-day doctors, used it to regulate the menstruation of his female patients. This plant was and still is a renowned help, especially when menstruation does not get going properly in a young woman. In homeopathy, *Pulsatilla* is still an important remedy for *menstrual problems* and *gynaecological disorders*. But it is also related to the male reproductive tract. Time and again *inflammation around the testicles and epididymis* has responded rapidly to the administration of homeopathic Pulsatilla. This may be connected to the emphasis on the flower in this plant (which is, after all, the plant's reproductive organ).

On the other hand, ancient herbal wisdom knew of the effect of pasque flower on the eyes. It is said to have repeatedly brought great improvements to serious *sight defects*.

Pulsatilla is not used in herbal medicine nowadays, but in homeopathy it is one of the most important remedies. It is used

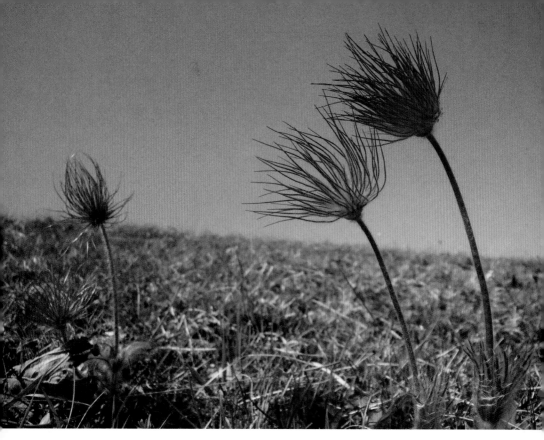

The Pulsatilla seed head is called a 'wild man' in some places.

with great success for certain cases of *inflammation of the eyelid and conjunctivitis*. In view of the unusual relationship to movement demonstrated by the seeds, it is no surprise that Pulsatilla can have a beneficial effect on *joint disorders*. I previously would never have believed that serious *rheumatic diseases* could be permanently cured by it. However, my paediatric colleague, Georg Soldner, has used it with success on several occasions. When a child who has suffered pain and swollen joints for years can run around happily again, then I am seized by great gratitude and amazement for such a powerful healing plant. However, this should not awaken false hopes, because it does not happen every day, even to my talented colleague, and Pulsatilla does not always help, although in suitable cases it may.

But what constitutes a suitable case? A number of things are linked to this, but very often what homeopaths call the 'Pulsatilla constitution'. They have discovered that preparations of the plant particularly help gentle compliant people who are likeable on good days but also quickly become tearful when in pain, even touchy and irritable (like an ill child) and whose sense of well-being definitely requires movement and cool fresh air. These patients often have variable moods and can be cheerfully enthusiastic at one moment and then despondent and despairing. The physical symptoms are also often not stable but change polarity and fluctuate from place to place. Are these descriptions not somewhat reminiscent of the 'atmosphere' surrounding the plant?

It never ceases to amaze me how careful study of a plant allows something of the healing power or – as the doctors in ancient times would have said – its 'virtue' to be discovered.

Pasque flower (*Pulsatilla vulgaris* & *Pulsatilla pratensis*)

Phytotherapy

The pasque flower is no longer used in phytotherapy. This is linked to the fact that the fresh plant is poisonous due to protoanemonin, a substance previously called Pulsatilla camphor, which gives the plant a hot burning effect irritating the skin and mucus membranes. Although this substance disappears quickly when the dried plant is stored, its effects were never completely predictable.

For this reason it is not suitable for self-collection and, in addition, the plant is an endangered species and is protected in many countries. However, many garden centres supply it as a herbaceous plant for the garden, where it will grow perennially on a sunny nutrient-poor site and delight us with its beautiful flowers in the spring.

Homeopathy

In homeopathy, unlike phytotherapy, Pulsatilla is a very important remedy. In fact, it is one of the most important homeopathic medicinal plants. Homeopaths say that it is a polycrest – in other words, a remedy that helps a large number of conditions. In homeopathy, Pulsatilla is used in a range of potencies from very low (down to D3) to very high. The former tend to be used for localised symptoms (for example *gynaecological complaints),* the latter for treating *psychological disturbances,* amongst other things. However, it must be borne in mind that, at lower potencies where the substance still has an effect, similar problems to those arising with the dried plant can occur if it is stored for longer periods, i.e. it gradually loses its efficacy. This appears not to be the case for higher potencies (at least above D12).

Medicines which are used according to constitution are generally prescribed by a homeopath and are less suitable for self-medication as they require an assessment of the total picture of the patient. The constitutional aspects of Pulsatilla have already been described above. Pulsatilla is prescribed particularly often for women but it appears that, in recent decades, many men also display more of what were traditionally thought of as 'feminine' traits and *Pulsatilla* can help them too. Characteristic traits are 'gentleness', 'softness' and 'mildness'. The renowned homeopath Georgos Vithoulkas once described this constitution as follows: 'A soft, polite being with sensitive feelings. Optimistic, but easily disheartened, can never be aggressive or cruel. Does not wish to impose.'[1] This is a telling characteristic which appears to match the impression given by the plant itself. The tendency to changeability in these traits is also expressed here (optimistic – yet easily discouraged). The type of condition that responds to *Pulsatilla* often improves with gentle movement (ideally outdoors). People with this kind of constitution often have a longing for cool fresh air, although they also have a tendency to be chilled easily.

In general a great *sensitivity to pain* and *tearfulness* are also typical. This can apply equally to a child with *inflammation of the middle ear* and a woman with labour pains in childbirth. Many gynaecologists and midwives recommend taking low potencies of Pulsatilla (for example, D6) in the weeks before the birth to make the *birth* easier. However, this should not be done as self-treatment but following individual expert advice, particularly as very low potencies can also have a stimulating effect on labour. If the patient wishes to influence the time of birth (whether using a 'labour drip' or very low potencies of Pulsatilla) then there must be a very good reason in order to justify

Once they are dry, the seeds of Pulsatilla can be carried away by the wind, thanks to small fine hairs.

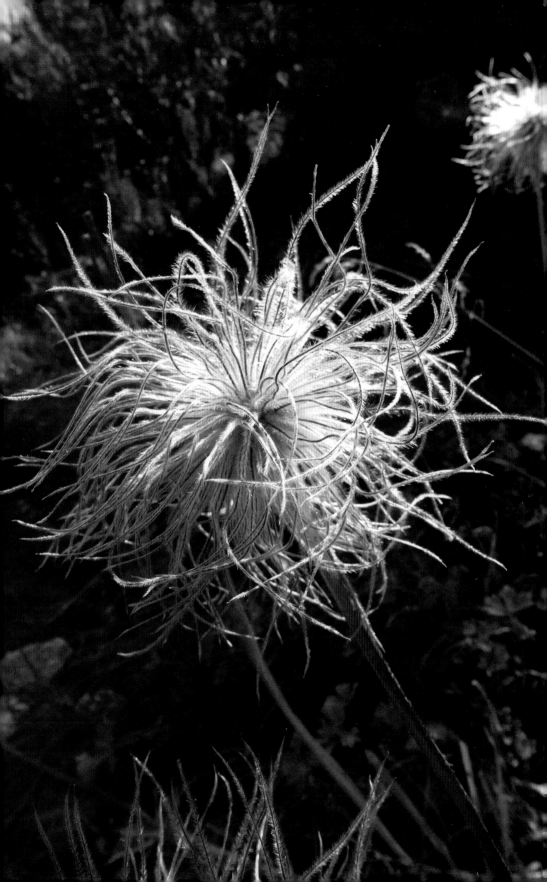

this. The birth is normally initiated by the child, who influences the mother's hormonal processes, which in turn trigger the contractions. The first impulse therefore comes from the child, so that it is born when the right time has come. It is typical for a 'Pulsatilla constitution' that menstruation does not get going in puberty. Likewise typical are a rather light bleeding or a *tendency to discharge.*

Rheumatic complaints which often move about are also typical. Further characteristics are *intolerance to (fried) fat* and the tendency to venous stasis symptoms (for example *varicose veins*).

Local symptoms which can be cured by Pulsatilla are slight (i.e. not irritating or burning) *mucous discharges* (for example *conjunctivitis* or *vaginal discharge*).

Anthroposophical medicine

Weleda manufactures its Pulsatilla medicines (Pulsatilla vulgaris D1, D2, D3, D4, D6 drops) from the whole flowering plant as is customary in homeopathy, while Wala uses only the flower (Pulsatilla e floribus D4, D6, D30 globules, D4 ampoules), which guides the effect more in the direction of the metabolic and genital organs. These single low potency remedies are often used to *stimulate ovary function* (and thus *menstruation)* or *contractions,* but also for *mucosal catarrh.* High potencies are given for *psychological disturbances* (for example for *depressive moods).*

The renowned anthroposophical doctor Friedwart Husemann developed an original idea for a remedy. He used a low potency (D4, D6) of *Pulsatilla* when he wished to strengthen patients who had too little of their own warmth and were susceptible to infections, because the plant can develop with great vigour at a time when it is still inhospitably cold. In addition to this application he was also very successful in treating *inflammation of the male genital region* (testicles, epididymis, prostate), a result which has also frequently occurred in my practice. Once again, these are illnesses which are not suited to self-treatment (for example, because treatment which is not effective enough can lead to fertility problems, so very careful supervision is necessary).

The same restriction applies to Bryonia comp. (Wala) which is used in the form of ampoules or globules for inflammation, especially of the female genital tract. In this remedy, potentised *Pulsatilla* flowers are prepared with potencies of bee *(Apis)*, bryony *(Bryonia)* and deadly nightshade *(Belladonna)*; in other words, remedies which all produce an anti-inflammatory effect.

In this context I should also mention Melissa/Phosphorus comp. (Weleda), which contains *Pulsatilla* along with a number of other plants (for example, Agnus castus, lemon balm, and marjoram) because its production entails the application of another important principle of many anthroposophical medicines. Besides medicinal plants and mineral or metal ingredients, these often contain potentised organ preparations. These organ preparations can have an enlivening effect on the relevant human organs if they have become chronically weakened. These medicines cannot be replaced by others in this respect. Usually cattle are used as donor animals. They are kept on Demeter farms under strictly controlled conditions and then processed in a separate slaughterhouse. Numerous procedures and checks ensure the manufacture of completely safe and hygienic preparations. In the case of Melissa/Phosphorus comp. it is the corpus luteum from the ovary which is used. This organ produces gestagens which are active during pregnancy and in the second half of the menstrual cycle. Insufficient production of these gestagens – for example, in the years before menopause finally sets in – can lead to a *shortening of the menstrual cycle* and *mid-cycle bleeding*. This remedy can often be very efficacious in such cases. Again, it goes without saying that this remedy normally has to be prescribed by a (specialist) doctor who first has to determine the cause of the abnormal bleeding.

The stimulating effect of *Pulsatilla* on the venous system and therefore its effect in treating *venous stasis* is the basis for the pasque flower's use in a range of other composite anthroposophical medicines. For instance, Pulsatilla e floribus is found in several Disci preparations by Wala. (*Disci intervertebrales* is the scientific name for the intervertebral discs and also denotes the relevant organ preparation which is contained in each of these composite medicines.) They are used for the treatment of *spinal disorders* (see also Chapter 14). The spinal canal contains a dense network of veins. If the blood in these veins becomes congested, this can contribute to dull, pressing pains in the back – particularly the lower back – which can typically be eased by gentle movement (compare the characteristics of *Pulsatilla*). This is the cause of some of the back pain associated with the menopause. It can be treated using Disci comp. cum Pulsatilla (Wala) which is available as globules, ampoules and ointment. There is a similar composition under the name of Disci/Pulsatilla comp. cum Stanno (Wala), also available as suppositories.

The effect of *Pulsatilla* on the venous system is also very important for its use in Hirudo comp. (globules and ampoules, Wala). In this remedy, pasque flower is prepared with other medicines which have a proven effect on the venous system, especially on the veins in haemorrhoids: horse chestnut *(Aesculus hippocastanum)*, witch hazel *(Hamamelis)* and peony *(Paeonia officinalis)*. This is accompanied by a preparation from the leech *(Hirudo)*, whose saliva – which it secretes into the wound when it bites – contains enzymes which dissolve the blood clots and have an anti-inflammatory effect.

A special feature of many anthroposophical remedies is the use of potentised metals. The metal used in Hirudo comp. is mercury *(Mercurius vivus)* in a highly potentised and therefore non-poisonous form. This mercury has a special relationship to all fluid processes – in this form, it can bring fluid processes back into movement when blocked. This composition is used, for example, for treating superficial *inflamed veins (thrombophlebitis), varicose veins* and *haemorrhoidal problems*. In these cases, it is important to exclude potentially dangerous diseases with similar symptomatology (for example diseases of the deep leg veins or the intestinal mucosa) before treatment. The usual treatment is by subcutaneous injection once per day or 10 globules 2–3 times daily. As this overview shows, *Pulsatilla*, the purple-flowered relative of the yellow meadow buttercups, has an astonishingly broad therapeutic sphere of activity. This delicate plant reveals itself as a powerful healing agent.

CHAPTER 10

Wild Strawberry

Most people can recall a few plants that they particularly liked as children. My guess is that these may often be the cowslip, the daisy and the wild strawberry. When I ask adults about these three plants, a dreamy look often comes over their faces. I suspect that this is because the thought of these little plants warms their hearts, just as it warms mine. These plants belong to completely different families and have little in common with one another except that they are so small that they do not grow any higher than a small child's knee. I cannot really say why these plants seem so likeable, but they seem to have a kind of friendly aura.

If you ever find shiny red strawberries in an undergrowth of green wood sorrel, dog's mercury and bilberry, this moment of happiness can stay with you for the rest of your life. This moment is a special joy for a child, because the berries are just the right size for a child's mouth. Compared to cultivated strawberries, wild strawberries seem to be like something from a doll's house, where everything is two sizes smaller than in real life. But their smell and taste are much more powerful than many of their large-fruited cousins. Last but not least, the wild strawberry is simply a beautiful plant. The threefold, slightly shiny leaves with their delicate veins are not only immediately recognisable, they are also attractive. This applies in like measure to the flowers. Their gently-domed, yellow centres and five pure white petals make them easy to identify as members of the rose family. But we are not fully satisfied until we find one of their berries. The colours of the red berry and the green leaf complement each other perfectly and thus intensify each other.

Unlike other edible fruits, whose seeds lie in the centre of the fruit

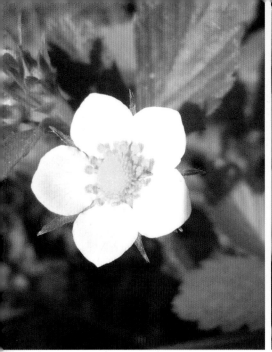
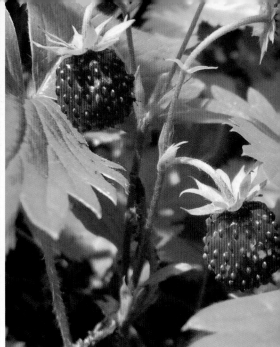

Strawberry flower and fruits.

surrounded by juicy flesh, the seeds of the strawberry are on the surface of the fruit and feel rough on the tongue. The appealing flesh of the fruit is formed by the receptacle. The small brown 'seeds' are actually the fruits (or 'nutlets' to a botanist). What we think of as the fruit is really a 'false fruit', or more specifically, an 'aggregate accessory fruit'. But as children we were not interested in these botanical subtleties. The only difficult decision was whether to eat the berries straight away as we picked them, or to save them up and then enjoy them all at once.

One would not at first suspect that the wild strawberry also has healing properties. In fact, even in otherwise comprehensive volumes on medicinal plants, the plant is not usually included. An exception is found in the work of Sebastian Kneipp (1821–97), the priest and skilled naturopathic healer famous for his cold water therapy, who also worked with medicinal plants. It seems he had a very intuitive knowledge of plants. He recommended tea made from wild strawberry leaves for sickly children. This tea was also recommended at times for *diarrhoea* because the leaves contain tannins. Rudolf Steiner also recommended wild strawberry leaves for those prone to diarrhoea.

In fact, the wild strawberry is used regularly in anthroposophical medicine even today. In a lecture, Steiner referred to it as a 'glorious plant' which 'works in a manner which is quite simple yet tremendously

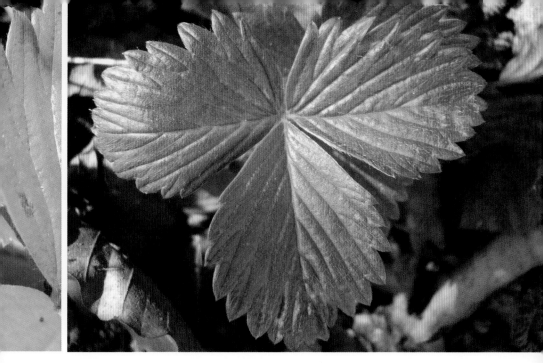

Strawberry leaf.

instructive'. He recommended the wild strawberry even for *anaemia*. There are many remedies for anaemia, but he noted that the strawberry works especially strongly in the periphery of the body.[1] Could this be related to the unusual placement of the strawberry's seeds on the periphery of the 'fruit'? In any case, I have found that using a medicine made from strawberry fruits and nettle leaf (which is also beneficial in cases of *anaemia*), can bring a rapid improvement in the symptoms of iron deficiency, especially on the body's periphery. Examples of these symptoms are poor healing of wounds to the skin or (particularly characteristic) small cracks at the corners of the mouth. A strong tendency to having cold hands and feet can also be a sign of anaemia and may be improved using a remedy of this kind. A scientific study has shown that eating strawberries can increase the amount of iron absorbed from food. (However, the lemon beats the wild strawberry when it comes to this effect.)

Rudolf Steiner gave a further recommendation for the strawberry. He suggested making a remedy for the liver from dried strawberry leaves mixed with dried grape leaves. A medicine based on these two leaves has been developed for the adjunctive treatment of cancer. Who would have thought that this simple berry could help in the treatment of such a serious condition?

Now, I don't imagine that the strawberry will ever replace established and reliable cancer treatments. Nevertheless, it is amazing what can be found in scientific studies in this field. Strawberry extracts can prevent the development of cancer cells caused by chemical carcinogens (substances which produce cancer). They can also stop the formation of new blood vessels in tumours which require these in order to have enough nourishment for their increasing size. Quite a number of tumours and leukaemia cells are disintegrated (a process called *apoptosis*) by strawberry extracts.[2] These extracts also appear to exert a certain protective effect on genetic material. Even tumour cell lines which had become resistant to certain cytostatic drugs still appeared to react to strawberry extracts. The strawberry also seems to work powerfully against free radicals which are involved in various medical conditions (not the least of which are tumour formation and liver disease).

The value of experimental observations like these should not be overestimated. Conditions in the human body are different to those in a cell culture. But it can do no harm to eat strawberries more often. Moreover, as we learn more, our respect for the strawberry as a medicinal plant grows.

This also applies to another effect demonstrated recently: extracts from wild strawberry leaves improve the blood supply to the heart muscle. It is claimed that blood flow to the coronary vessels increases by three quarters due to this type of extract. This dilation of constricted blood vessels in the heart is really impressive.[3] This is scientific proof of what we have known since kindergarten days: the wild strawberry opens your heart.

Wild strawberry (*Fragaria vesca*)

You can easily collect and dry wild strawberry leaves yourself for use in a tea. To dry them, lay them out in semi-shade away from dust and turn them from time to time. When they have dried to the point where they crumble between your fingers easily, store them in an airtight container.

Phytotherapy

Tea made from wild strawberry leaves can be used for cases of *summer diarrhoea*. Add 1–2 teaspoons of the crushed dry leaves to a cup of boiling water and leave to infuse for 5 minutes. A cup of this tea can be drunk several times a day. If the diarrhoea is more serious, then the salts which have been lost (particularly potassium and sodium) also need to be replaced by drinking an electrolytic replacement solution (also called oral rehydration solution). If the diarrhoea is so bad that the overall condition is seriously affected, or if it is accompanied by severe stomach pain or other alarming symptoms such as blood in the stool, then obviously a doctor should be called in. The same applies if small children or frail elderly people are afflicted.

Strawberry leaves mixed with raspberry and blackberry leaves make a fine caffeine-free homemade tea. This can be drunk in the evening without disturbing sleep.

Homeopathy

The wild strawberry is used in homeopathy in low potencies under the name of *Fragaria vesca* to treat a tendency to dental plaque and inflammation of the gums. I have no experience of this use and therefore cannot speak about its efficacy.

Anthroposophical medicine

It has already been noted that wild strawberry fruits with nettle leaves can be helpful for many symptoms of *iron deficiency* such as feeling cold, poor hair or nail growth, slow healing of skin wounds or a tendency to cracks at the corners of the mouth. One remedy which combines these two medicinal plants is Anaemodoron (Weleda). I usually prescribe 10 drops taken 3 times a day. For a particularly strong effect and especially if the patient suffers from tiredness – which can also be a sign of iron deficiency – I prescribe a mixture of Anaemodoron with gentian extract (for example Gentiana lutea, decoctum D1, Weleda), usually in equal parts (also see chapter 25).

Wild strawberry leaves and grape leaves form the basis for the liver remedy Hepatodoron (Fragaria/Vitis comp.), which is dealt with in detail in Chapter 30. That chapter also describes Vitis comp. (Weleda) which is used especially for the adjunctive treatment of cancer to help promote liver function and detoxify the body. In addition to strawberry and grape leaves, this preparation contains the metal antimony and a compound of calcium and formic acid.

Both the fruits and leaves of the wild strawberry (in addition to numerous other plants such as rosehip, wood sorrel, spinach, etc.) are contained in Nervennahrung (medicinal honey) made by Wala. This remedy promotes anabolic processes in a number of ways and can help with overcoming *exhaustion*. The normal dose for this remedy, which consists largely of forest honey, is one teaspoon, in warm tea or on its own, once or twice times daily.

The little strawberry 'nutlets' which sit on the outside of the strawberry are also used in a potentised form. Thanks to the initiative of individual doctors who have become particularly involved in this, these strawberry seeds have been developed into a prescription only medicine by the Weleda pharmacy in Germany. It is hoped that this remedy will be particularly helpful in treating *diseases of the liver*. There is no widespread experience of its use to date. Nonetheless, it is clear that the therapeutic use of even a very familiar plant can be further evolved. The wild strawberry still offers new opportunities for making use of its many medicinal properties.

CHAPTER 11

Greater Celandine

Greater celandine is not one of the best known medicinal plants, yet most people will have noticed it. Like the stinging nettle, it is a plant that follows people. Native to Europe and western Asia, it was also introduced widely in North America. It likes to grow beside roads, and on building sites and waste dumps where human activity has opened up the ground and waste has introduced fertilising nitrogen. With its size of up to 75 cm (30 in), the greater celandine raises itself above the normal meadow species. However, it is primarily its glowing yellow flower that draws attention to the plant. The flower is composed of four petals which tower above the pale green of its (slightly blue-tinged on the underside) leaves. The leaf has a very characteristic and unusual shape. It appears distinctly subdivided but, unlike ferns or the yarrow, it does not give the impression that this is due to an indenting and formative force from outside. Instead, the rounded swelling lobes produce the feeling of a force in the plant, which is constantly pushing towards to the periphery.

This impression is strengthened if we tear off a leaf or stem: a shiny orange-coloured milky juice, latex, wells out, almost like blood does when we cut our finger. We have seen this milky sap in the dandelion, whose flower colour is similar to the bright yellow of the greater celandine. But the dandelion's sap is white and thus seems innocent and harmless compared to the sap of the greater celandine. The sap of greater celandine has a burning, bitter and nasty taste and is in fact poisonous – like the sap of the opium poppy, with its analgesic, antispasmodic but also addictive ingredients such as morphine and papaverine.

The greater celandine does indeed belong to the poppy family. In

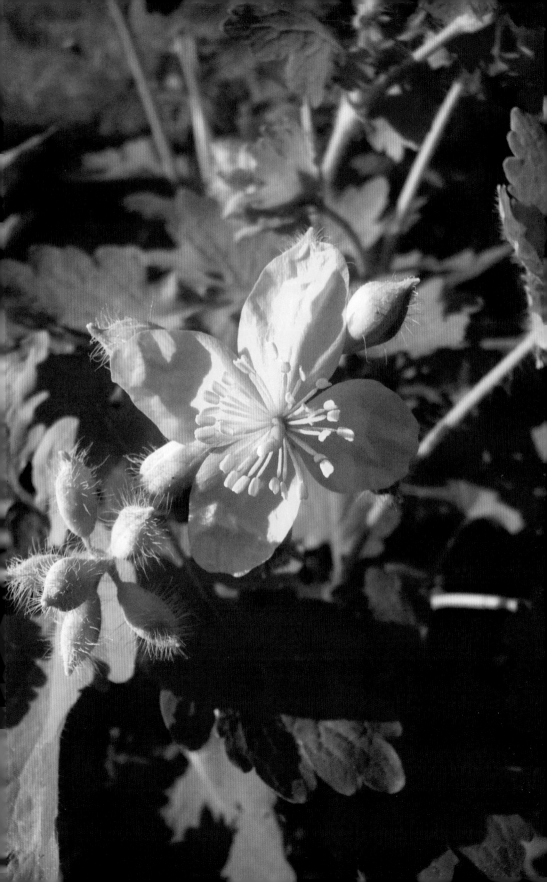

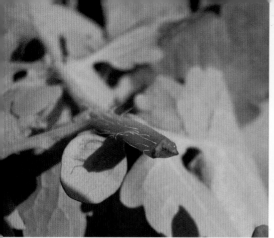

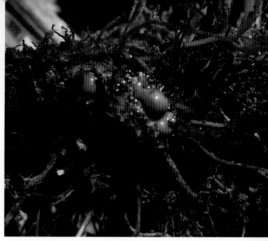

Coloured juice leaks out from the broken-off stem.

A broken root exudes an intensely coloured sap.

addition to the latex, these plants have their strong rough hairiness in common. Like the poppy, greater celandine contains alkaloids, which are nitrogenous, and often very complicated substances. These can also have an effect on our psychological state. Years ago, I found over 20 compounds of this kind in the sap of greater celandine using chromatography – a relatively simple method of analysis for separating substances. At the time, I thought this plant was a proper little pharmaceutical factory. The occurrence of the alkaloid class of active substances in particular may also be related to the fact that the plant loves nitrogen so much.

For a long time, latex was viewed as a breakdown product in plants. However, it is not as simple as that. If you look at it using high magnification under an electron microscope you will see that, on the contrary, it is filled with the cell organelles which are responsible for producing protein: the ribosomes. The plant also needs nitrogen for producing protein. The latex contains large numbers of other organs of synthesis such as mitochondria (which are often called the 'power plants' of the cell). From a biological angle, the latex is actually teeming with life, so that our first impressions of it are confirmed in the laboratory.

Greater celandine has achieved eminence, not only in science but also in art. Albrecht Dürer was famous for portraying nature very precisely. Well-known examples of this are his portrait of a hare, part of a meadow and also an illustration of the greater celandine. There may be a deeper reason for the master having paid so much attention

Greater celandine flowers showing the cross-form of the petals.

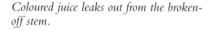

111

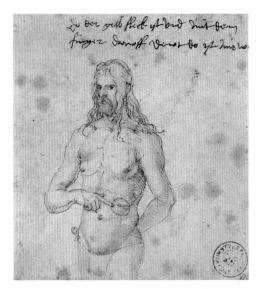

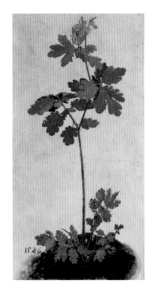

Dürer's self-portrait as a sick man (Kunsthalle Bremen). Written above the drawing it says: 'Do die gelb Fleck ist ... do ist mir weh' (Where the yellow spot is ... that's where it hurts). If Dürer had drawn his mirror image, then this would be the position of his gall bladder.

The famous picture of greater celandine by Albrecht Dürer (Albertina, Vienna).

to the greater celandine. In any case, in medical circles there is a second famous picture by Dürer: this is a self portrait of the painter (dated 1510) in which he is pointing to an oval drawn under his rib cage and coloured yellow. A caption on the picture announces that he has a pain there. It is assumed that Dürer was sending a message to his doctor. But what was wrong with him? The discussion about this has never come to a final conclusion. Some claim that the painter was indicating the place where the spleen is located. It is indeed located on the left side, covered by the lower ribs. But the spleen actually lies more to the side than on the picture and usually it does not hurt, even if there is something wrong with it. So it seems more reasonable that the painter depicted a mirror image of himself, as he painted what he saw in the mirror. The place indicated would then lie on the right side of the body and the gall bladder (which is actually often painful) is located there, filled with a yellow fluid. This fluid, although produced in the liver – the 'centre of our metabolism' – is collected in the gall bladder and expelled suddenly when it is required for digestion (for example after a fatty roast). If the biliary tract becomes obstructed it can even result in jaundice, producing a yellow colouring of the skin and the whites of the eyes.

This is exactly the colour that we have seen, not only in the flower but also in the latex of the greater celandine, and this plant is renowned as a cure for gall bladder diseases. It not only contains analgesic and relaxing alkaloids which can be helpful for bilious colic, but it has also been known to have an anti-inflammatory effect and assist the biliary flow. So experts believe that Dürer was suffering from a disease of the gall bladder and after his 'pictorial consultation' was probably prescribed greater celandine. It is thought that the famous picture of the greater celandine is an expression of his thanks to the helpful plant. It can no longer be proved whether this is really true, but it is certainly possible.

However, greater celandine is not only a gall bladder remedy. Its scientific name is *Chelidonium*. This apparently comes from *chelidon*, the Greek name for the swallow. Some think that the reference to the swallow comes from the fact that the plant starts to flower when the swallows return in spring. The ancient herbalist Dioscorides provided a more poetic explanation: that swallows use the plant to open the eyes of their blind offspring. No ornithologist can confirm this, but there is still an element of truth in it. Chelidonium is a good remedy for the eyes and it is used to make eye drops which for *dry eyes*. In such cases the eye lacks particular fats which help to protect the sensitive cornea from drying out. Interestingly, the most important function of bile consists of enabling the absorption of fats into the body. In addition, greater celandine can cure hardening of the skin (*warts*, for example), and this may have lead to the assumption that it may be able to release the initially closed eyelids of the newly hatched birds.

The use of greater celandine sap in folk medicine to help remove warts has been confirmed inasmuch as it has been shown that the plant inhibits the spread of viruses – and warts are caused by viruses. But Chelidonium also inhibits the production of skin cells, which is excessive in the case of warts. It also inhibits the growth of some other tumours. However, self-treatment is not advised as greater celandine sap sometimes irritates the skin and taking large quantities internally has caused liver damage in particularly sensitive people. But in moderate doses and under professional supervision, Chelidonium is one of nature's most powerful remedies.

Greater celandine (*Chelidonium majus*)

General remark

It has already been mentioned that in rare cases, using concentrated greater celandine preparations, particularly in combination with substances which are harmful to the liver, has resulted in (very rarely serious) liver damage due to inflammation of the liver. At potencies of D4 and higher there are no concerns about this due to the very low content of the Chelidonium alkaloids. However, with concentrated preparations (D3 and below) it is generally recommended to avoid taking medicines containing Chelidonium along with substances known to be potentially harmful to the liver. Concentrated Chelidonium preparations like these should also be avoided if the patient is known to have previously suffered from liver disease. Other contraindications are pregnancy and breast-feeding. There is no adequate information recorded for young children on the use of some preparations, so in this case it is important to check the relevant information on the package insert, or speak with the attending doctor.

If concentrated Chelidonium preparations are taken for more than four weeks, it is recommended that the liver function test results are checked.* Symptoms of the adverse effect of a drug are often not easy to distinguish from those of the original disease being treated, but can be recognised by a change in lab results.

This remark applies in principle to all the remedies described below, and is not repeated for each one.

Phytotherapy

The use of concentrated preparations of greater celandine for gall bladder complaints was very common for a long time but has declined sharply in recent years. Many preparations have disappeared from the market entirely after there were several reports of serious liver disease following their use. This is certainly due to individual oversensitivity (idiosyncrasy), which can lead to toxin-related liver inflammation.

* Alanine transaminase (ALT), aspartate aminotransferase (AST), gamma-glutamyltransferase (GGT), alkaline phosphatase (ALP) and bilirubin.

The consequences are described in more detail in the 'General remark' opposite.

A case of temporary liver damage has been reported even with the use of celandine tea.[1] Because the uptake of the alkaloids from the tea are difficult to calculate, and the use of celandine tea is quite uncommon, I shall not discuss this any further here.

Homeopathy

The use of Chelidonium in homeopathy usually covers potencies of D4 and above, which are not likely to have any toxic effect on the liver. Incidentally, the possibility that long-term use of concentrated Chelidonium can damage the liver is, in the sense of the similarity rule in homeopathy, a decisive reason for accrediting Chelidonium in potentised form with the ability to treat *liver diseases*. The diseases that homeopaths treat with Chelidonium are mainly related directly or indirectly to malfunctions of the liver and *gall bladder* which are expressed, for example, in pain around the inferior angle of the scapula. But pain can also occur in this area from, for example, a *lung infection* in the right lower lobe of the lung, and I have often found that prescribing potentised Chelidonium (in addition to the other necessary measures) was of noticeable benefit.

Anthroposophical medicine

Chelidonium is available as a single remedy not only from homeopathic pharmaceutical manufacturers but also from anthroposophical pharmaceutical companies. While the homeopathic pharmacy principally uses the root of the greater celandine, anthroposophical applications make a greater distinction between the individual parts of the plant. These are harvested at different times when they have their optimum potency. Wala processes rhythmised mother tinctures of the flowering plant (that is, the above-ground parts which are harvested in early summer) into globules in D3 and D6 and ampoules in D4, D8 and D30.[2] In accordance with the knowledge that flowers principally act on the human metabolic system and leaves on the rhythmic system (for example on the lungs), these remedies are mainly used to produce an effect on the metabolic organs (for example the liver) or (in the above-mentioned sense) to treat a *lung infection*. In contrast, the preparation made from the root (which contains particularly high amounts of alkaloids in autumn after the leaves have died back and is a remarkably strong orange colour) acts mainly on the nerve and senses system. Potentised Chelidonium root can, for example, cure *headaches* which are connected to the liver and gall bladder system.

I once had to treat a patient who had suffered from severe migraines for decades. This patient had already undergone many types of treatment and the migraines had become so bad that they had a significant impact on her life. When taking a careful medical history I discovered that, during a migraine attack, the patient's stool was always noticeably light in colour. This was a crucial indication, as bile is the main pigment in our stool. During her migraine attacks the patient obviously had a malfunction in the secretion of bile.

Bile is a very aggressive substance which dissolves the fats in our digestive tract. However, if bile enters the abdominal cavity this leads to a serious and life-threatening inflammation. It is nowadays assumed that, during a migraine, inflammatory processes in the blood vessels of the head (which then irritate pain fibres in the nerves) play an important part in migraine attacks. An anthroposophical view of the theory of disease tells us that in illness, a process which would be normal at one place in the body has moved to another place where it becomes pathological. So for our migraine patient it can be said that the bile process is too active in the head region and too weak in the digestive system.

In order to free the nerve-sense processes, I prescribed Chelidonium e radice (that is, from the root) D30 as an injection (injections are particularly effective for blood vessels, which undergo inflammatory changes in their walls during a migraine). In order to stimulate the action of bile in its natural place, the patient was also given an organ preparation made from potentized bile (Fel Gl D8). From the first administration of this combination the patient remained free from attacks. After a few months, when the treatment was stopped, the headaches started again but were less severe. When the treatment with Chelidonium and Fel was resumed, the condition went away again and never recurred, although no migraine medication has been taken for many years now. Obviously the gall bladder function is now so stable that no additional assistance is required.

Since then I have been able to relieve a whole series of patients from years of migraine symptoms by this method, if the same combination of stool discolouration during the migraine attacks is present.

Turmeric, which is also important in cooking for making food more digestible, is often a partner of Chelidonium in medicines to improve the functioning of the gall bladder.

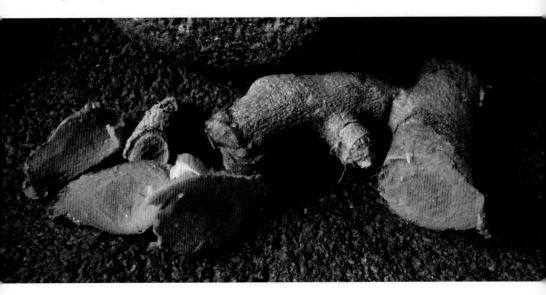

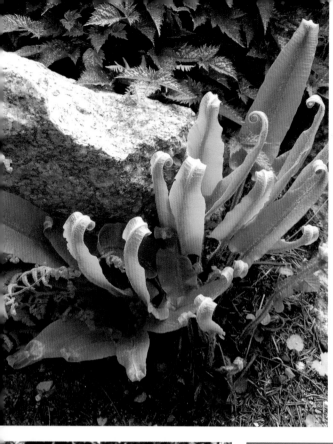
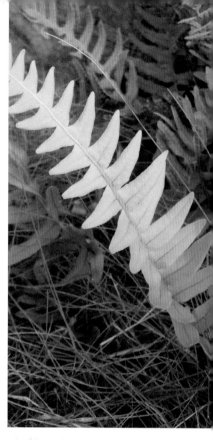
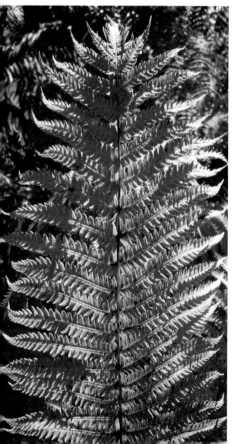
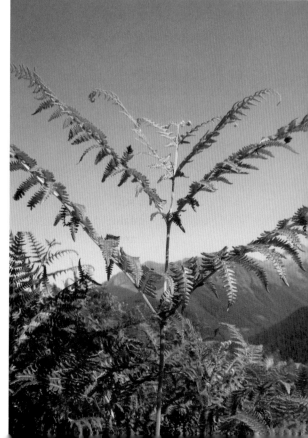

While in this case it seemed right to use the Chelidonium root in order to target 'misplaced bile processes' in the head, there is a remedy containing potentised Chelidonium flowers which acts wholly on the digestive system. This is Aquilinum comp. globules (Wala) which is often helpful for *disturbances to the intestinal function* (for example, after taking antibiotics). Like the digestive preparation Digestodoron by Weleda, this contains a combination of various species of fern (hart's-tongue fern, Dryopteris species and bracken) along with greater celandine flowers (to regulate gall bladder activity), dandelion (which also assists the liver and gall bladder – see also Chapter 4), and golden rod *(Solidago)* which is detoxifying and promotes excretion by the kidneys. All these plants are contained in the D4 potency. This remedy can be used for intestinal problems after antibiotics at a dose of 5 globules 3 times daily. However, it should be noted that serious disorders (for example severe pain or blood in the stool) after antibiotic treatment can be due to an abnormal colonisation of the intestine with the pathogen *Clostridium difficile* and a resulting severe inflammation of the gut which requires special treatment. For this reason, a doctor must always be consulted for any severe stomach pain after antibiotic treatment. Aquilinum comp. has also proved successful for other diseases (for example of the skin) where it is suspected that disturbances to the intestinal function are involved.

Based on what was written above about selecting the correct part of the plant, it initially appears odd that a key gall bladder remedy in anthroposophical medicine, Weleda's Choleodoron (from *chole,* Greek for 'gall') is made from roots. Besides Chelidonium root, it includes turmeric root, which we may have used in the kitchen – it forms one of the main ingredients in curry power. Like greater celandine, this plant has a bright orange root. While not tasting quite as hot as Chelidonium, it is still aromatic and a little bitter. In a certain way there are 'flower qualities' present in the roots of both plants, due to the colour and aroma. Turmeric also promotes digestion and is

Ferns are contained in several medicines along with Chelidonium. Their main role is to help to regulate the functioning of the intestine. The fern used for this is the undivided hart's-tongue fern, Phyllitis scolopendrium *(top left), the singly pinnate common polypody,* Polypodium vulgare *(top right), the bipinnate male fern,* Drypoteris filix-mas *(bottom left), and bracken,* Pteridium aquilinum *(bottom right).*

particularly stimulating to bile production, while also being a strong anti-inflammatory. It is used a great deal in Indian medicine but has also become popular in European medicine, after it was discovered that turmeric apparently has both a preventative effect against cancer and is also beneficial to a certain extent in treating cancers. Concentrated turmeric preparations are still at the stage of advanced experimentation but have shown good effects in treating tumours both in animal experiments and also in human beings. In his book, *Anticancer: A New Way of Life,* the renowned physician and author, David Servan-Schreiber (1961–2011) dealt with the way that turmeric can be used as a spice to prevent cancer.[3]

It is noteworthy that both roots contained in Choleodoron not only act on the gall bladder but also have a certain effect in combating *tumours.*[4] It is remarkable that, long before this side of the aforementioned roots became known, Rudolf Steiner recommended preparing Choleodoron by combining the two root extracts using a pharmaceutical process similar to the one used for obtaining a cancer remedy from the summer and winter sap of mistletoe (see also Chapter 35). There are many aspects to cancer, but one is that living tissue occurs in the tumour which is too hard and too 'physical' (and in fact most cancerous lumps are detected by palpating due to their excessive hardness). The original principal area of application for Choleodoron was for the treatment of *gallstones.* The aim was to dissolve something in the body that had become too hard. In our digestive system, the forces of dissolution are normally dominant and in the head the formative and hardening tendencies predominate (even into its overall form and function). When stones are formed in the gall bladder (in the digestive system), a 'head-like' pathological hardening tendency has to be overcome. Experience and insight have shown that roots actually act on the region of the head. Yet the roots of Chelidonium and turmeric are filled with substances related to digestion. This can explain how, in a concentrated form, these can help in illnesses in which the hardening forces of the nerve-sense system (which normally predominate in the head) are excessive, leading to the formation of stones in the gall bladder, an important digestive centre. This is the inverse of the migraine example described above, where the head appeared to be suffering from pathological 'gall forces' and was brought relief by a high potency (D30) of Chelidonium.

120

But Choleodoron can also be used to treat less severe hardening processes in the form of a *tendency to spasm in the gall bladder and biliary tract (bile-duct dyskinesia)*. Spasms of this kind do not only result in a hardening of the musculature of this hollow organ. Influences with their origin in the 'upper human being' (such as excessive stress or irritation) can have a pathological effect in the 'lower human being' by upsetting the gall bladder. There is an intimate connection between the 'upper' and 'lower' human being. It has been known for millennia that psychological factors can influence the gall bladder and vice versa; ancient Greek medicine saw an excess of bile as being responsible for the choleric temperament, for instance. We also know that *diseases of the gall bladder* can be triggered by acute stress or anger. In such cases, Choleodoron drops can have a relaxing effect and stimulate the flow of bile, thus restoring healthy conditions in the digestive system.

Finally, Choleodoron and similar remedies can be used to treat hardening tendencies in our blood vessels, which can progress to *arteriosclerosis*. Bile acids (able to dissolve gallstones which consist mainly of cholesterol) are actually made by our bodies from cholesterol. If more bile acids are produced as a result of treatment with Choleodoron to stimulate bile production, this lowers the cholesterol level in the blood which, along with other measures (for example, increased exercise and a low-fat diet), can lead to a reduction in the tendency for cholesterol to be deposited in our blood vessels. This effect can also be achieved by the use of artichoke preparations, which likewise stimulate bile production (see Chapter 18). Roughage from wheat bran or Psyllium husks binds bile acids in the gut so that they are removed from the body and have to be produced again, resulting in cholesterol being removed from the blood. The cholesterol-lowering effect of this kind of gall bladder treatment can thus be further increased.

All these disease tendencies should be treated by an experienced doctor, firstly because they often require more than a single remedy and secondly because the long-term administration of Choleodoron (which contains quantitatively significant amounts of Chelidonium) requires the liver values to be monitored for the reasons described above. However, it is obvious that this plant is a basic remedy for various sclerotic diseases.

Wala also produces remedies for treating symptoms of *spasm in the biliary system*, such as Chelidonium/Colocynthis, which is available as ampoules and globules. This contains the whole medicinal plant in a mixture with the Chelidonium root and flowering plant, along with potentised colocynth, a relative of the pumpkin which has close links to symptoms of *spasm in the abdominal region*. This remedy contains low potencies of Chelidonium (D2) and Colocynthis (D3). When used for *acute pain around the gall bladder* this remedy can sometimes give amazingly quick pain relief. Nevertheless, the cause of such pains should be determined by medical examination.

Chelidonium capsules (Wala) also contain all the parts of the greater celandine along with extracts of chicory *(Cichorium)*, Berberis, Colocynthis, relaxing peppermint oil and other medicinal plants. These capsules can be taken to stimulate the digestion if the gall bladder is hypoactive (underactive) and also for conditions due to irregular or cramping movements in the biliary tract.

It has already been mentioned that greater celandine can be helpful for *dry eyes*, and that this is partly due to the fact that eyes with a tendency to dryness are no longer adequately protected by a moisture retaining lipid layer produced by special glands in the eyelid. Chelidonium can help to restore the body's ability to deal with these lipids. Weleda make Chelidonium D4 eye drops for this purpose, supplied in a multiple dose container.

Wala manufactures Chelidonium comp. eye drops which, besides extracts of the flowering plant and roots of Chelidonium (D3), also contain a rose flower extract (D3) rhythmised with Ruta (rue, D3) and larch resin (D5). These ingredients also support the functioning of the internal eye muscles, which can be strained from long periods of 'close work' (at the computer screen or by prolonged reading), contributing to a feeling of tired eyes. These eye drops are supplied in single-use containers with the advantage that preservatives are not required. Both kinds of eye drops are usually dropped into each eye twice daily or when required. Ongoing eye complaints or those accompanied by sight defects should always be investigated by an ophthalmologist.

Treatment for *enlargement of the thyroid gland* (goitre) should also be mentioned as another specific indication in anthroposophical medicine for the use of greater celandine. This application also goes back to

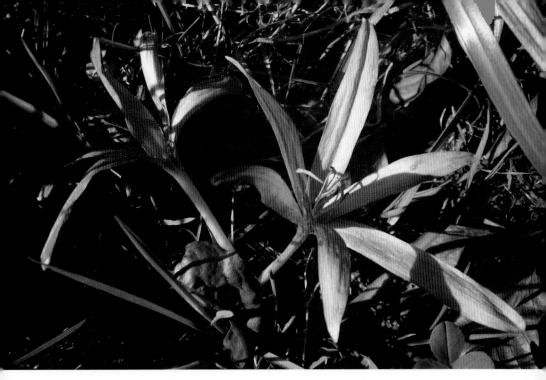

The autumn crocus is used with greater celandine to treat diseases of the thyroid.

Rudolf Steiner, who recommended a combination of greater celandine and autumn crocus *(Colchicum autumnale)* for treating enlargement of the thyroid. This disease is often due to iodine deficiency but it can also be caused by an *overactive thyroid* (for example in Basedow's disease) or, in rare cases, by cancer of the thyroid. A rapid increase in thyroid size always arouses suspicions of a malignant cause. However, every enlarged thyroid should be investigated by medical examination, which usually includes a blood test for thyroid hormones and an ultrasound examination. In the case of a simple enlargement of the thyroid without any additional dysfunction, treatment with Colchicum comp. ointment (Wala) or Thyreodoron ointment (Weleda) may be considered. These ointments, which are applied to the throat area, contain a preparation of greater celandine flowers. I am not aware of any application of the flowers of this plant outside anthroposophical medicine. However, this unusual use of Chelidonium makes sense if you consider that the thyroid hormones regulate the activity of almost our entire metabolic system, and flowers are related to metabolism.

Certain factors have to be taken into account when using these ointments (which are in any case usually only available on prescription and therefore subject to medical supervision) as they contain

Colchicum extract. For example, they should not be taken over longer periods along with certain cholesterol reducing drugs (statins such as Simvastatin, Atorvastatin, Sortis, Zocor and others) as this can lead to symptoms of muscle weakness. Care is also recommended in combination with immunosuppressants such as those used after transplants or for autoimmune diseases. However, my colleagues and I have repeatedly observed that it has indeed been possible to cure goitre using treatment with these ointments.

In relation to Chelidonium I would finally like to comment further on the possibility of modifying the effect of a plant by growing it in soil enriched with a metal. It is first necessary to identify the metal to which the plant has a particular 'inner relationship'. In the case of stinging nettle, many 'gestures' of the plant indicate that it has a relationship to iron. By fertilising the plant with iron, it can be used to create a remedy that is particularly suited to supporting the iron forces which are required for treating anaemia caused by iron deficiency (see Chapter 28). Greater celandine also has a connection to iron. This is indicated by the form of the Cheidonium flower. The plant displays an obvious cross made of four yellow petals. Since ancient times the number four and the cross are seen as a sign of 'Mars forces' and of iron. In our blood we find an iron atom in the middle of the haeme molecule which is functionally the most important part of haemoblobin, carrying oxygen to our body (again, see Chapter 28 on the stinging nettle for more about this). While stinging nettle improves iron metabolism and helps blood production (and so can be used in anaemia), celandine, on the other hand, can be used in cases of haemoglobin disintegration and excretion of bilirubin (the 'waste' produced in that process).

The relationship of greater celandine to bile can also be seen as a connection to iron. Its bitterness and the colour of its sap are similar to bile, and it has already been described as an 'aggressive' substance that serves to 'conquer' the food which has been eaten in the digestive process. However, bile is also connected to the blood, which is only able to be the bearer of oxygen in us because it contains iron (this is why iron can help to improve anaemia). Specifically, it is the red blood pigment, haemoglobin, that contains iron. This is incorporated in a specific way, with one iron atom in the centre of each haemoglobin molecule, so the iron is surrounded by exactly four 'vinyl groups', as

A haemoglobin molecule.

they are called. These hold the iron as though in a net. Again, we have the motif of the number four with iron at the centre of the intersection. When red blood cells containing iron become old or damaged and are broken down, then this produces the yellow bilirubin, which is excreted in the bile and gives it its colour – the same colour which we see in greater celandine.

There is a not uncommon hereditary condition (which cannot actually be called an illness) known as Gilbert's (or Gilbert-Meulengracht) syndrome. This involves an excretory deficiency in the bile pigment bilirubin. It is mostly found in thin men and is harmless. Affected individuals acquire a faint yellow colouring in the white of the eyes, particularly when they are hungry, and lab tests show a slight increase of the bilirubin level with otherwise normal liver function test results. (If other lab results are affected in addition to the bilirubin, then this could indicate other and perhaps more serious causes – such as, for example, a viral liver inflammation or biliary stasis due to a stone or even a tumour. Obviously, in such cases, Chelidonium Ferro cultum, described below, should not be used). Many of those affected also experience a mild feeling of faintness and a slight inhibition when it comes to making decisions and taking the initiative. Their 'Mars force' is slightly impaired in this sense.

In such cases, potentised Chelidonium grown on soil fertilised with iron (Chelidonium Ferro cultum) can be of assistance. As described elsewhere in this book with regards to the 'vegetablisation of metals' (see Chapter 4 on dandelion), the first generation of greater celandine grown on this type of soil is composted after harvest. Then more greater celandine is grown on this compost, the plants once more composted – and only the third generation of plants are processed into the remedy (further details are given in Chapter 28). This is available as a rhythmised and alcohol-free Rh preparation as drops at D3. I usually prescribe 5 drops morning and afternoon and find this produces not only an improvement in the lab results, but, more importantly, in how the patient feels. They often experience greater alertness and drive, and sometimes there is even improvement in a prevailing mild depression.

Greater celandine can be of benefit in so many ways that it is a real art to use the right part of the plant, to process it at the correct time or to modify its effect by specific fertilising measures, and to select the correct concentration and potency for treatment. It is also a real art to choose the right type of application (oral administration, eye drops, ointments and injection), as these result in quite different areas of efficacy.

CHAPTER 12

Chamomile

Perhaps chamomile is the most well-known medicinal plant. It might be an exaggeration to say that it is to be found in every home, but this is very often the case. My own relationship to chamomile is clouded by the fact that, as a small child, when I was really ill after being nourished by intravenous drip for several days, I was given rusks soaked in chamomile tea, which I found so appalling that I preferred to go hungry than eat. Perhaps these kind of experiences with chamomile are more widespread, because I have the impression that this medicinal plant arouses both enthusiasm and passionate dislike more often than many others.

The scent of chamomile is so characteristic that almost everyone can recognise it. Smell is an experience that takes place in the air, and this is the element that belongs to chamomile. Its leaves have reduced their surface to a minimum and have so little substance that they seem like needles spreading the air between them. In the centre of the flower, the yellow heart arches strikingly upwards surrounded by the white ray florets, giving an impression of tension. If you open this centre it appears to be filled with air, a feature used to distinguish the medicinal chamomile from all other species.

The plant generally grows on dry, rather sandy soil in warm places. The sun draws out the scent from the chamomile and we notice that the plant is larger than its visible form. The whole atmosphere that it influences is part of it. From this point of view, the use of chamomile in a steam bath is part of its natural tendency. The hot water brings the dried flowers 'back to life' to a certain degree. Transformed into steam, this master at handling the air ensures that our airways are opened up again if the mucous membranes are swollen and the entries to the

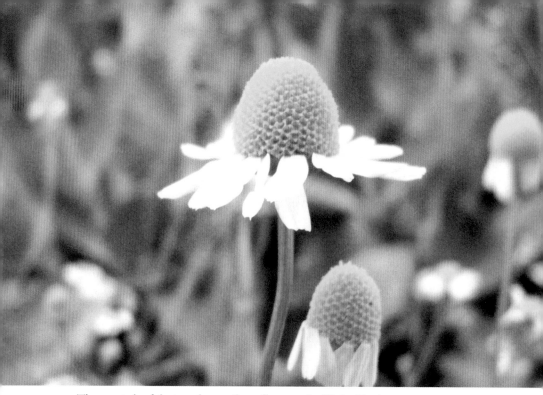

The receptacle of the true chamomile swells upwards, filled with air.

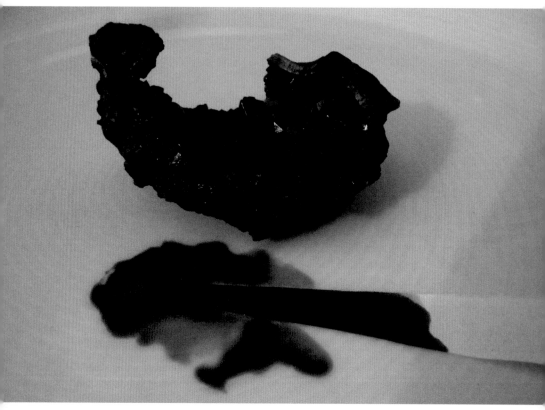

Azurite and chamomile oil dyed blue from azulen.

nasal sinuses have become blocked; for instance due to a *cold*. The air 'trapped' in these is slowly absorbed by the body and the resulting low pressure leads to unpleasant pains. If you put a handful of chamomile flowers into a bowl, pour on boiling water, hold your head over the bowl draping a towel over everything, and breathe in deeply, then you will usually not have to wait long to obtain relief.

In fact, the substances in chamomile oil which vaporise and are breathed in belong to the strongest anti-inflammatories and decongestants that exist. If the oil is pressed from the flowers or extracted with a solvent, then it appears yellow with a pale green tinge. However, if you follow the 'gesture' of the plant and put the flowers into a flask filled with water, boil everything up and then collect the steam, cool it and let the distillate stand, then a deep dark-blue, strong-smelling oil separates out on the surface, which would not exist without this human intervention.

For a long time this 'blue oil' was considered to be the active substance in chamomile. It is now known that it is only one of many important constituents. Those who know something about natural history will be reminded of azurite, a deep blue copper mineral, and of one or two more copper compounds of similar colour. In homeopathy and anthroposophical medicine copper and its compounds are well-known and powerful remedies for alleviating cramps. Chamomile is also well-known for its antispasmodic effect. It can be particularly helpful for *stomach cramps* which are often caused by *flatus* (gas) in the intestine; air bubbles trapped in the intestine around which the strong musculature of the intestinal wall contracts.[1] We are reminded here again of the air contained in the domed receptacle. Chamomile preparations can also be used to alleviate spasms in other hollow organs in the abdomen: *menstruation pains* due to spasms in the uterus and also *cystospasm*. The bladder (whose name actually has a reference to the air – the Old English *blædre* meaning 'to blow') also responds particularly well to chamomile vapour. In this case, the steaming bowl is put in the toilet bowl. The patient sits on it with the legs and stomach wrapped in a warm blanket which keeps the steam where it is needed. Naturally, care must be taken not to get burnt.

A study carried out at the transplant unit of Munich University Hospital showed that chamomile steam baths of this kind could protect patients who had undergone kidney transplants from *urinary tract infections*, which they would otherwise often get after the operation. In a clinical study, 25 women who had just undergone a kidney transplant were given regular chamomile steam baths. Only three of them got urinary tract infections. In the control group, who did not receive any chamomile treatment, fourteen of the twenty-five women contracted urinary tract infections.[2] Chamomile in fact has not only antispasmodic and anti-inflammatory effects, but also germicidal ones.

Thanks to the pharmacist's art we have seen that the effect of the medicinal plant can be extended by the extraction of the 'blue oil'. We also identified a relationship to copper. A particularly complicated but effective means of carrying the plant further than nature itself also exists: metal vegetabilisation. The aim of this is to bring plants and metals closer together. Copper minerals are first transformed into fine fertiliser in the laboratory. This copper fertiliser is added to a bed where chamomile plants are grown, which then absorb the metal. These plants are composted and chamomile is grown on the compost containing copper and chamomile. This process is repeated a total of three times, during which the copper is increasingly raised into the life of the plant – 'refined' as it were, and potentised at the same time. The 'copper chamomile' obtained in this way is processed into a medicine which is then used, for example, for *babies with colic* and also in specific cases (as part of an overall treatment) for spastic conditions affecting the whole body, such as *epilepsy*.

Epilepsy is really the most extensive form of spasm and medically it is also referred to as a *convulsive siezure*. However, spasms can also be less extreme and experienced primarily emotionally or as muscular tension. For all these conditions – from psychological tension (which may be accompanied by anxiety) via muscular tension to an epileptic seizure – conventional medicine commonly uses a group of drugs known as benzodiazepines, the best known of which is Valium (or its active substance, diazepam). These benzodiazepines are bound in the brain at very specific locations, the benzodiazepine receptors, leading to a reduction in agitation and therefore to psychological relaxation and the release of muscular spasm. It has been proved using very complex methods that the ingredients of chamomile do exactly the same. They too activate the benzodiazepine receptors, and so the antispasmodic and psychologically relaxing effect of chamomile now has scientific proof.[3] Because the benzodiazepines were developed about 50 years ago, our organism has certainly not developed a receptor, an organ of perception, for these chemical substances. If you think about the fact that the relation of us to chamomile is much older and deeper than that to the benzodiazepines, we actually should consider a 'chamomile receptor' or an apigenine receptor, the substance of the plant, for which arousal reduction in nerve cells has been demonstrated. If chamomile is used as part of an overall treatment for epileptic spasmodic conditions, this should only be done by a qualified physician.

It is possible to discover how the plant can help us by direct experience of the plant itself, without the need for any instruments. This is what our forebears must have done when they recognised the chamomile as a medicinal plant. It has found its way into almost every household to this day.

Chamomile (*Matricaria recutita,* formerly *M. chamomilla*)

Many species of chamomile that you may find on a walk are not the true medicinal chamomile. The medicinal species, which grows up to half a metre (20 in) in height, can be easily recognised by its yellow receptacle which bulges high above the white collar of its ray florets. You can see by cutting it that it is hollow and filled with air. If you collect chamomile yourself it should be dried quickly in an airy and at least partially shaded place and then kept in an airtight container so that its essential oils are not lost too quickly. As specially bred varieties of medicinal chamomile contain particularly high levels of essential oils, it is usually worth obtaining the dried herb from a pharmacy.

Chamomile tea and phytotherapeutic use

Chamomile tea is prepared by pouring a large cup of boiling water over a heaped teaspoon of the dried flowers. For the 'rolling cure' mentioned below and for local application (mouthwash, compresses etc.), the tea can be made stronger by using a whole tablespoon of flowers per cup. Leave this to stand covered for around 10 minutes and drink 3–4 cups daily for *gastrointestinal complaints*. A rolling cure can be helpful for *stomach problems*. After drinking the tea, lie for a few minutes each on your back, your left side, your stomach, and your right side, so that the tea comes into contact with all the walls of the stomach. As the exit from the stomach is on the right side, it is considered best to lie on this side last of all so that the tea does not run out into the intestine at the beginning of the rolling cure.

In the past this type of rolling cure was often prescribed for *stomach ulcers* as it has actually been demonstrated that chamomile is able to help these to heal more quickly. Nowadays it is unlikely that anyone would dispense with the use of drugs which block the acid production of the stomach and therefore provide a better chance of healing ulcers of this kind. However, it can still be useful to use chamomile preparations to encourage healing. It should be noted that any stomach problems which persist over a longer period require careful investigation, which may include endoscopy.

For *inflammation of the mouth and throat,* for example due to *aphthae* caused by viral infections or *pressure points from dentures,* it can be useful to gargle and rinse out the mouth with cooled chamomile tea. Chamomile tea is also used for compresses and baths for mild *dermatitis.* Both the antibacterial and anti-inflammatory effects of chamomile are involved here. Oversensitivity or allergies to chamomile are very rare; however, if an inflammation does not improve within a few days, then advice should be sought from qualified practitioners and self-treatment should not be continued indefinitely.

For external application there are also concentrated chamomile preparations (for example Kamillosan, etc.), which can be used if making chamomile tea seems too much trouble. Before the advent of medicines which suppress the formation of stomach acids (e.g. Omeprazole, Pantoprozole), Azupanthenol was frequently prescribed for internal administration (for example, as a rolling cure). It contains blue chamomile distillate. This product is no longer produced industrially. However, a corresponding product is still produced in some pharmacies, and is valued by patients who cannot tolerate the so-called 'modern' remedies. The pure blue chamomile distillate is also used in aromatherapy.

It has already been mentioned that chamomile tea can have a calming effect. Chamomile tea can therefore be a good tea to drink in the evening for anyone with a tendency to *stomach troubles*. The relaxing and sleep-promoting effect can be heightened by mixing lemon balm leaves with the chamomile flowers.

Chamomile steam bath

A chamomile steam bath can be very beneficial if the nose is blocked due to an *acute cold* or *inflammation of the sinuses*. Put a handful of chamomile flowers into a bowl with hot water, lean over the bowl and drape a towel over the head and bowl so that the warm steam does not evaporate too quickly and the face and nose can benefit from the heat as well as the effect of the chamomile. It is very important to make sure that the bowl is stable so that there is no risk of scalding due to inadvertently tipping it over. For this reason this application is not suitable for young or restless children.

As chamomile steam not only clears the nose but also dries it, this kind of steam bath should not be done more than once daily. It is therefore also prudent to use Nasenbalsam (nasal balsam, Wala), Schnupfencreme (catarrh cream, Weleda) or Nasenöl (Oleum rhinale, Weleda). The last-named contains an oily extract of chamomile.

Things needed for a chamomile steam bath.

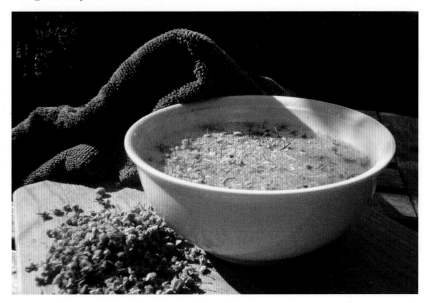

Oil dispersion bath

An oil dispersion unit that combines water and oil without resorting to emulsifiers can be used for a bath (see Chapter 5). There is an oily extract of chamomile flowers for this purpose which goes by the name of Chamomilla e floribus W 10%, Oleum (Wala). During the manufacturing process, gentle heat acts upon the flowers and oil, enabling a particularly efficient transfer of the plant's active agents into the oil.

Oil dispersion baths with chamomile oil are used for *skin inflammations* (for example in *acne*), for *relaxation* and for a tendency to *spasmodic stomach complaints.*

Demeter olive oil with blue chamomile (Dr Heberer Naturheilmittel) is also intended for use in the oil dispersion bath device (again, see Chapter 5). Whilst for the Wala preparation chamomile flowers are extracted with olive oil using gentle heat, here blue essential chamomile oil is dissolved in the olive oil. It is reported that this preparation is particularly beneficial for the elderly and that they value the feeling of its protective effect.

This small piece of glass equipment can be used to mix oil with additives from medicinal plants to such a fine emulsion that it disperses into milky drops, thus creating very close contact with the body of the person taking the bath. Available from www.elixator.de.

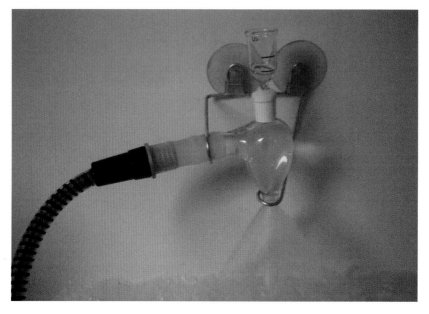

Potentised chamomile

In homeopathy the whole flowering plant is used, while in anthroposophical medicine a distinction is made between different parts of the plant. Besides the whole plant (Chamomilla e planta tota globules, Wala) there are preparations made from chamomile root (Chamomilla e radice, Wala and Chamomilla, Radix, Weleda). In general, preparations from the root have a stronger effect on the nervous system or those disease symptoms related to powerful processes from the nervous system.

A well-known use of chamomile is for *teething*. If the child is very restless and irritable due to the pain, then *Chamomilla e rad.* D6 globules (Wala, 3 globules hourly) is often a great help. Weleda have also begun to produce more globules which are alcohol-free. These are available with Chamomilla as D6, D12 and D30. Wala produce globules from the whole plant as Chamomilla e planta tota in D3, D6 and D12 and from the chamomile root as Chamomilla e radice as ampoules in D6 and D30 and as globules in the potencies D3, D6, D20 and D30. For adults, Chamomilla e radice sometimes helps *facial neuralgia,* for which I tend to administer higher potencies (for example D20, D30).

In order to decide when to use the whole plant and when to use the root, it can be useful to know that the root is of particular relevance either where nerve processes need to be influenced or where nerve processes have become too prominent in the metabolic region. This can be the case, for example, with *intestinal spasm* or *menstrual cramps (dysmenorrhoea),* which are worsened by nervousness, stress or sensory overload. In these cases Chamomilla, Radix 2% tablets (3–6 times daily) can be particularly beneficial.

Chamomile fertilised with copper

It has already been mentioned that chamomile fertilised with copper and composted can be used as a fertiliser sold under the name of Chamomilla Cupro culta, Radix (Weleda). Further details of these kind of 'vegetablised metals' can be found in Chapter 28 on the stinging nettle. The antispasmodic effect of chamomile is enhanced by the copper and sometimes this remedy – which is available in an alcohol-free preparation (Chamomilla Cupro culta, Radix Rh D3 drops) – is particularly good for *stomach colic in babies*.

On one occasion I recommended giving a three and a half month old baby (who initially cried for an hour every evening but then almost the whole night through and could only be calmed by carrying him around) 3 drops of the remedy in question with every breast-feed. He began sleeping peacefully the very next night.

Chamomilla is particularly efficacious for rather strong babies which seem very short-tempered when suffering from stomach pain, while babies which tend to be weaker and appear to suffer more passively can gain relief from the corresponding Melissa preparation Melissa Cupro culta (Weleda) (see Chapter 20 on Lemon balm/Melissa). Chamomilla Cupro culta (Weleda) ampoules (D2 and D3) can give immediate and very effective relief for patients with severe *period pains*. Copper chamomile has also been helpful in cases where all other remedies have failed.

In general, potentised copper preparations appear to be particularly efficacious when those affected feel themselves completely over-

A 29-year-old female patient suffered such severe abdominal cramps during menstruation that she felt completely overwhelmed by the pain and was unable to do anything except lie in bed, curling up with pain every time a new attack of cramps occurred. She was intolerant of conventional analgesics and trials of herbal and potentized remedies had only led to a slight temporary relief. On one occasion the patient managed to come to my practice in this condition, where I injected her subcutaneously with an ampoule of Chamomilla Cupro culta Rh D3. After about ten minutes the pain had almost vanished and the patient felt an enormous sense of relief. Since then she has injected herself with this remedy during menstruation once or twice daily which, although it does not remove the pain completely, helps her so much that she can carry on with her normal activities without difficulty.

whelmed by the pain. However valuable the 'copper chamomile' can be in such situations, it is nevertheless essential that severe pain must first be investigated before self-treatment, in case alternative treatment is needed for a potentially serious illness.

Chamomile in composite remedies

Chamomile is an important component along with other constituents in a series of composite remedies. For example, it is contained in Weleda's Fieber und Zahnungszäpfchen D2 along with caraway and other antispasmodic agents and in Carum carvi children's suppositories (Wala), which can be used for *wind and restlessness in babies*. In contrast, Ammi visnaga comp. suppositories (Wala), where chamomile is combined with such things as Belladonna and the antispasmodic Egyptian Ammi plant tend to be used for adults. *Stomach cramps,* particularly related to *menstruation,* are often greatly relieved by this remedy. Chamomile is also combined with other potentised plant extracts in remedies such as Nicotiana comp. (Wala), which is used for *irritable bowel syndrome,* for example.

CHAPTER 13

Plantain

This plant is familiar to almost everyone. It does not call attention to itself with bright colours but its characteristic shape is very noticeable. In addition, it grows in most meadows and on many paths. This is what gives it its German name of *Wegerich* (from *Weg*, meaning 'path'). There are actually two related species of plantain. They are rather reminiscent of the tall lean knight Don Quixote and his short fat attendant, Sancho Panza: the ribwort plantain and the greater plantain. The latter appears totally relaxed and often a bit untidy and its rounded leaf is usually rather dishevelled. The ribwort plantain, *Plantago lanceolata,* is not called 'lance-like' *(lanceolatus)* for nothing. This applies not only to its leaf shape. The leaves always appear rigid, as though under tension, and often stand upright.

Medicinally, this plantain is the more important one. Its leaves rise up from a single point on the ground forming a rosette, from the middle of which a bare stem stretches upwards. At the tip of this stem is a cylindrical flower head, which bobs forwards in every gentle breeze as though it was bowing politely, only to spring upright again. A little distance from the flower head a ring of white dots appears to float around the flower, giving the plant a comical appearance, similar to a fringe of white hair sticking out around a bald head. The white dots are the stamens of the tiny open flowers that compose the whole flowerhead. To see more requires a magnifying glass. The individual flowers are made up of four sharply pointed, paper-dry and transparent petals. Four stamens emerge from between these, sticking out with amazing strength. The plantain has no colour, scent or sweet nectar to entice insects but is pollinated by wind. The female part of the flower develops long before the stamens, to prevent the flower from self-

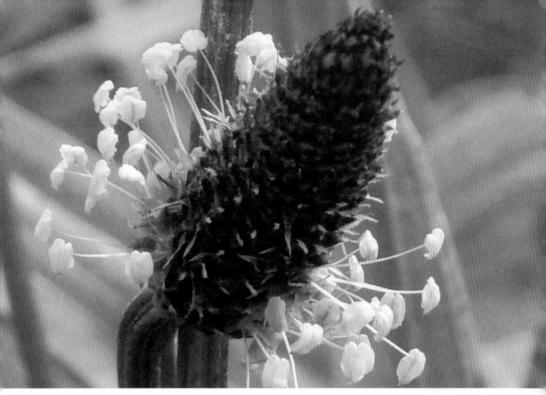

Flower of the ribwort plantain.

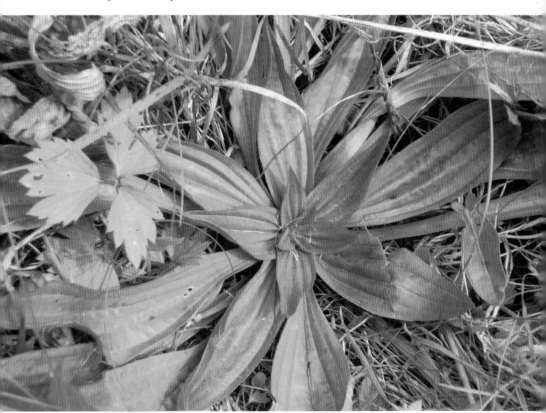

Ribwort plantain leaf rosette.

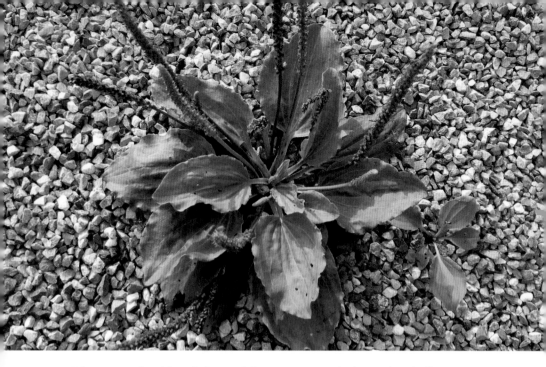

The greater or broad-leaved plantain (Plantago major) *also has medicinal effects. However, in contrast to its narrow-leaved relative, it is not used in composite anthroposophical remedies.*

pollinating. Even before the petals have opened, it pushes out like a straight rod. This is visible in the upper part of the inflorescence above the satellite-like ring of stamens. The oldest parts of the inflorescence are at the bottom. Here, the stamens which have turned dry and brown hang limply while the seeds begin to ripen.

The leaves are also worth a closer look. Veins run almost parallel through these leaves, like those usually found in the grasses surrounding the plantain in the meadow, but these belong to a completely different group of plants. If we tear a leaf, then the tough veins can be pulled out and hang like loose cables from the torn edge. In earlier times these 'vein cables' were described in various countries as a good remedy for toothache, for which they had to be placed in the ears. I have never tried this (particularly as the ear-nose-and-throat doctors always warn us not to put anything into our ears), but there are reports that it was often helpful. This is probably due to the plant's anti-inflammatory properties. Nowadays it is used almost exclusively for *inflammation of the buccal mucosa* and for *coughs*. It must have been different in earlier times as the two species of plantain were considered to be virtually a cure-all. The Swedish name *Läkeblad* ('healing leaf') is still a reference to this.

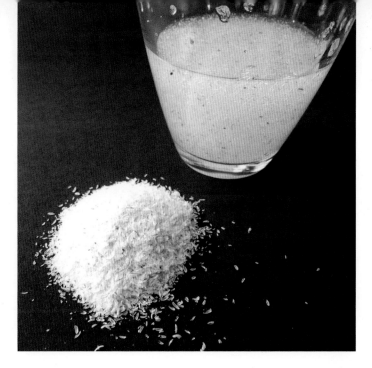

When mixed with liquid, the seed coats of Plantago ovata *swell up to more than 40 times their volume and thus help to regulate stool consistency and cholesterol level.*

The fact that plantain grows on paths has already been mentioned, but meadows have also been created largely by human activity. In earlier times much of the earth was covered by a kind of primeval forest and only by clearing trees did enough light reach the ground so that meadow plants could spread. In Europe it was only in the Middle Ages that this change in the landscape occurred on a large scale. When Parzival passed through regions scarcely touched by man, it could still be said that he rode 'where few plantains grew' – in other words, where not much light reached an uncultivated soil. In Wolfram von Eschenbach's Middle High German account, plantain was *wegerîches*. *Wege* means path, and *rîch* means king or ruler. So the plantain was the ruler of the path. However, this meant not just any path, but primarily the *Hellweg,* the route that led into the realm of Hel; the goddess of death. It is clear that a ruler of this path must be powerful, including against disease. It is fitting that plantain was also known under the name *Herba proserpinacia,* as in 'Proserpina's plant'. This is the Latin name for the Greek Persephone, the daughter of the goddess of the fields, Demeter. Persephone was stolen away by Pluto, the god of the underworld, and taken as his wife. She had to spend half the year in the

141

underworld with him and was then allowed to climb up to the earth again, which covered itself in herbs and flowers for joy. Persephone/Proserpina knew the secrets of the underworld and the earthly world (especially those of plants). She bears a similarity to the god Mercury, who mediated between the gods and human beings and was also the god of physicians. If plantain was quite simply *the* plant of Proserpina, then it would have been an excellent plant for all ills.

Its present-day use is much more modest. However, it is amongst the most reliable cough remedies. Besides its anti-inflammatory action, the mucilage content also helps by laying a protective and healing coating on the sore mucous membranes.

The fact that there is more to the plant than this might be suspected because, as studies have shown, it can protect the liver from the effects of toxins to a certain extent. (Substances which offer protection from poisons were highly rated in times when those in power were afraid of falling victim to a poisoning attack!) Incidentally, the most mucilage is found in the seed coats. The seed coats of a closely related species of plantain (Plantago ovata, psyllium, available as a preparatory medicine such as Mucofalk, Metamucil, etc.) are often used for *constipation* because they soften the stool and can therefore relieve the problems of *irritable bowel syndrome.* In wet weather all plantain seeds coat themselves with mucilage so they are able to stick to the soles of shoes, for example. Because a huge quantity of seeds are produced, the plant can spread far and wide, carried by human feet.

As plantain did not occur in America originally, its appearance shows the presence of European immigrants. To the Indians it was therefore known as the 'footsteps of the white man'. The Latin name *Plantago* also refers to the foot because *planta* means the 'sole of the foot'. Plantain leaves placed in the shoes are actually supposed to prevent *sore feet.*

In anthroposophical medicine plantain is prepared in a specific way, with cowslip flowers amongst others, and used for a remedy for *muscular problems* particularly in the legs, sometimes with astonishing efficacy (see Chapter 7 on the birch). So, there are possibly a considerable variety of therapeutic effects after all. Perhaps in due course the esteem the plant was accorded in past times might turn out to be more appropriate than we might have thought.

Ribwort plantain (*Plantago lanceolata*)

Ribwort plantain is easy and worthwhile to collect. It tends to grow in predominantly dry, grassy places and is almost impossible to confuse with any other plants, poisonous or not. Cut off the narrow leaves and flower stalk just above the ground and dry them quickly. A good way is to tie them into loose bunches and hang them up.

Plantain tea and cold extract

Take 2 teaspoons of the dried roughly cut up herb and pour over 1 cup of boiling water. Pour off the liquid after 10 minutes and drink the tea for *coughs*. It is more usual to use plantain mixed with other herbs for this purpose. Suitable additions are, for example, common mallow flowers, marshmallow root, Iceland moss etc. (The last-named is nowadays unfortunately often contaminated by radioactivity. This plant is not a moss but a lichen; a composite consisting of an alga and a fungus. Like most fungi, it collects radioactive metals.)

A cold extract is best for treating *pharyngitis* and *sores in the mouth* (for example due to *pressure points from dentures*) is prepared by soaking 2 teaspoons of the herb overnight in a cup of cold water and sieving in the morning. This extract can be used several times a day for gargling and rinsing out the mouth and can also be alternated with chamomile tea (see Chapter 12).

Cough mixture

The plantain's capacity to reduce a *tickly throat* and its anti-inflammatory action are also the reason for its use in Plantago-Hustensaft (Wala). It is combined with an extract of young spruce shoots which act as an expectorant and butterbur *(Petasites)* which is an antispasmodic. For the treatment of a cough, take 1–2 teaspoons in some warm water several times a day.

Potentised plantain

Bronchi/Plantago comp. (Wala) is a fairly broad remedy for *colds* with *hoarseness* and *cough*. Besides potentised plantain (in D5) it contains bryony *(Bryonia)*, hemp agrimony *(Eupatorium)*, the iron/ sulfur mineral pyrite and organ preparations which direct the action of the medicine to the bronchial tubes, larynx and nasal mucosa. According to the manufacturer's directions, the dose is 5–10 globules once or twice daily; however, I advise a much more frequent dose of 5 times daily. I rarely use the ampoules of this preparation although these can sometimes be remarkably efficacious if the cough refuses to ease.

A simple cold should pass within a few days. If the symptoms persist for longer or are unusually severe, then a diagnosis should be made, in case there is a more serious illness or further treatment is required.

The prescription-only medicine Plantago-Primula cum Hyoscyamo (Weleda: see also Chapter 8 on the cowslip), is not suitable for self-treatment. Its profound effect is not explained by the individual plants it contains (cowslip and henbane in addition to plantain) but by the particular composition, which was indicated by Rudolf Steiner. The remedy was produced for treating *muscular diseases* to which its earlier name Myodoron refers (which roughly translates as 'gift for the muscles'). The remedy with the difficult name Plantago-Primula cum Hyoscyamo has proved efficacious particularly for conditions accompanied by *muscular spasm (spasticity)*. This can occur in the simplest case in *lumbago* or *a stiff neck*. Conditions of severe muscle spasm such as in *multiple sclerosis* or other serious neurological diseases, after *stroke* or *early childhood brain damage (spastic cerebral palsy, spastic diplegia)* are much more difficult to treat.

After injection of the preparation, many patients experience a considerable improvement in the spasticity lasting several days. A patient who had been dependent on a wheelchair almost her whole life because of a birth trauma and whose joints were badly deformed due to severe spasticity, wrote to thank me: 'These injections have changed my life!' Unfortunately the remedy does not help all those affected and not all for the same length of time. However, it is one of the most important remedies in my practice because it can often offer very pronounced help to people with a great deal of suffering for whom almost nothing else can be done. Patients with rare hereditary muscular diseases – particularly those which cause both muscle weakness and stiffness (such as hereditary spastic paraplegia or myotonic dystrophy) – often experience a distinct relief in their daily lives thanks to this remedy.[1]

Recently, Dr Irene Stiltz reported that she had had considerable success with Plantago-Primula cum Hyoscyamo in treating the illness *amyotrophic lateral sclerosis* (which the famous physicist Stephen Hawking suffers from) which leads to progressive muscle weakness. Besides the weakness, those affected suffer from involuntary movements of the muscle fibres (fasciculation), which often deny them rest and sleep. After the doctor had prescribed her patient this remedy with great success, it spread rapidly amongst the members of a self-help group for this illness. However, its use should be supervised by a doctor in all cases, particularly as it may be contraindicated, for example in case of raised intraocular pressure, enlarged prostate, etc.

Inspired by the scientific name *Plantago*, Dr Johannes Wilkens gave injections of this remedy for persistent *pain in the sole of the foot* and reported that he (and other colleagues) had found this very effective.

CHAPTER 14

Horsetail

In Chapter 7 I talked about the birch, about its relationship to light and its ability to stimulate our kidneys. The horsetail has very similar effects and sometimes both plants are found in close association. We experienced this a couple of years ago. I was with my wife, walking in the Lofoten Islands in the far north of Norway above the Arctic circle. In summer the sun never sets there and for a few weeks you can enjoy a world of light.

In a boggy birch wood we were suddenly standing in a magical world: the ground was covered by a carpet of graceful horsetails as high as our knees, their soft whorls looking like hair. Sunbeams fell on to the delicate green of the horsetails through the birch branches and stripes and patches of light danced above the plants like little fairies. Something of this mood can still be captured from the photograph opposite. You have the feeling that horsetail has a special relationship to water, light and air.

You may remember this plant from childhood games. It is made up of ray-like pale green segments which end in a small fringe of hairs holding the next similar stem segment, rather reminiscent of the way Lego works. You can even separate the segments carefully from one another and then fit them together again to see who can build the longest horsetail without it falling apart. We are familiar with this kind of regular structure from other plants such as ferns. In fact, like horsetail, these belong to the very old and 'primitive' plants from primeval times. Similar plants grew on the earth when coal beds were laid down, and these plants form a significant part of the total coal mass. There were horsetails up to 30 m (100 ft) in height at that time and, even today, there are specimens in South America which can grow to over 8 m (26 ft).

146

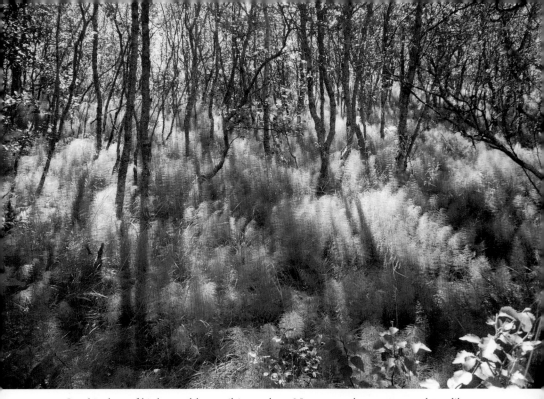

On this slope of birches and horsetail in northern Norway, sunbeams seem to dance like elves.

The green above-ground parts, however, are only a small part of the horsetail plant. Underground, the small 'Christmas trees' we see are connected horizontally. Like the above-ground parts, these connections are fitted together from segments, joining the small 'trees' like water pipes. The necessary water flows through this plant system, often lying more than a metre (3ft) below the surface. There is a hollow channel containing air in the centre of the plant parts, with the water pipes grouped around it. But it is not only water that is transported in this system. The fine roots also dissolve silica (the substance of quartz crystals, for example) from the soil. This silica is then raised up along with the water and excreted at the surface of the plant. In the early morning when the leaves are still covered in dew, we can see little shiny droplets on the 'branches' of the horsetail, which are not dew from the night but active secretions from the water brought up from the ground. When this water evaporates during the day it leaves behind a thin skin of silica on the surface of the plant. This does not form crystals, but an amorphous body of silica which is mineralogically similar to opal. It is also the reason why the horsetail feels rough and is suitable for

147

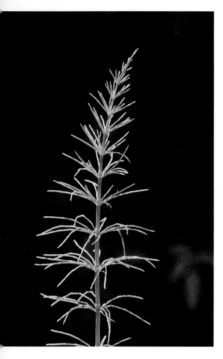

Field horsetail.

polishing pewter articles. This is why it is also called *Zinnkraut* ('tin' or 'pewter' herb) in German. In the Agricultural Course, which we have already mentioned, Rudolf Steiner also talked about horsetail and how, with the help of silica, the plant can 'barricade itself as though in a castle'. This effect can be used to the benefit of other plants if horsetail is boiled and this strong 'tea' is sprayed onto plants which have a tendency to be attacked by fungi like mildew.

The silica secreted on the horsetail is nevertheless not totally formless, nor merely a simple coating. It is not clear why the plant should make this effort to dissolve the silica in the soil, transport it and excrete it if it then serves no purpose for the plant structure. In fact, the silica makes a kind of lens on the surface of the plant, which collects, focuses and transmits light in concentrated form into the plant cells. The silica does not simply produce a 'castle wall' for the plant, but also the 'windows' in it. The plant cells are then able to absorb particularly large amounts of light and can carry out the marvel of producing plant substance through photosynthesis which 'normally' takes place in leaves with a large surface area. Horsetail, however, manages without leaves, really only producing stems.

Besides its high silica content and skilful processing of silica (silicon dioxide), the field horsetail is also characterised by a particularly high sulfur content. While silica has a special connection to light, sulfur has one to heat. Sulfur, which is also found as a mineral (illustrated in Chapter 2 on bulbs), belongs to the few 'combustible rocks'. It actually burns with an amazingly hot flame. It tends to occur where the hot interior of the earth appears on the surface in volcanoes. There is almost always sulfur vapour along with glowing lava and this precipitates as a yellow deposit in cooler places. The combination of 'cool', clearly structured silica and 'fiery' sulfur in one plant is something

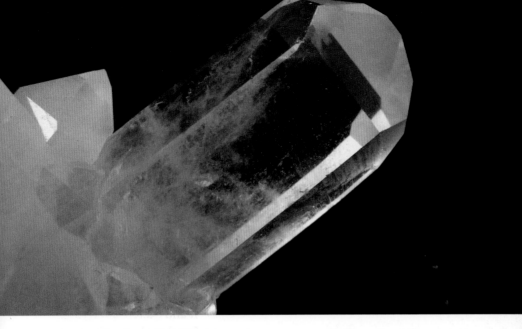

In crystalline form, silica (SiO$_2$) appears as a quartz crystal. Horsetail transforms it into a living skin.

unique to the horsetail. Sulfur is also related to water excretion and the substances most often used in medicine for stimulating urination, the thiazides, also contain sulfur.

We see that horsetail is a master at dealing with water, light and silica. It is therefore no surprise that it is used for treating *skin diseases,* because the skin and its associated organ, the hair, are in fact amongst the most silica-rich substances in our body, as well as containing large amounts of sulfur. Our skin also has to be able to deal with light. When exposed to sunlight it produces vitamin D, which helps to strengthen our bones and also supports our immune system. We can well imagine that horsetail can be beneficial as a tea compress, as oil or in ointments for skin conditions in which the surface of the skin and its barrier function dissolve, and, for example, *weeping eczema* develops. The plant is also used in some anthroposophical medicines which are beneficial for bone and vertebral diseases. Medicinal preparations made from horsetail grown on soil specially fertilised with silica can also be used for some cases of particular *susceptibility to infection* in which the 'outward boundaries' of the mucus membranes are not

149

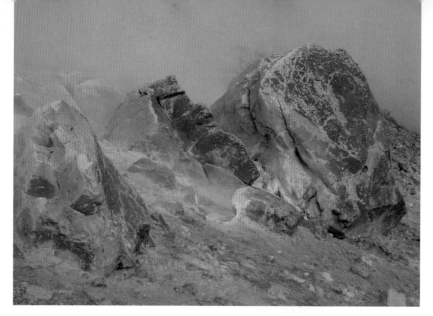

Yellow sulphur coating on the rock beside the fumaroles on a volcano (in Sicily).

stable enough and there is an inner 'lack of light'. Stronger decoctions of horsetail used in agriculture and horticulture (in order to protect plants from fungal diseases) can also be understood in this way.

However, horsetail is most frequently used for *kidney and urinary tract diseases,* and in fact horsetail is a plant which can be regarded in some ways as the kidneys and ureter of nature. The kidneys do not simply filter water to be carried out of the body. Rather, numerous salts are dissolved (like silica in the plant), transported and concentrated and a proportion of them is excreted. Beyond the general relationships between the horsetail and the kidneys, there are amazing connections, which are only visible in the medicinal field. They go beyond the observations in the context of this book.[1]

Field horsetail (*Equisetum arvense*)

As already mentioned, anyone who is not very familiar with the botany of horsetail is advised not to collect it themselves; slightly poisonous and non-poisonous species look very similar. Take expert advice to distinguish the species.

Horsetail tea and decoction

Horsetail tea can be used for a 'flushing-out' therapy when there is a tendency to *kidney stones* and *bladder infections*. Put 1–2 teaspoons into a cup, fill with boiling water and leave to stand for 10 minutes. The effect can be increased by boiling the mixture of water and horsetail for 5 minutes. This allows more silicic acid to be released into the water.[2]

For purging the urinary tract, horsetail is often used in mixtures with other medicinal teas. For instance, field horsetail, birch leaves, stinging nettle and golden rod leaves can be used in equal parts. This mixture should only be prepared by pouring boiling water over it, not by boiling it. Several cups of this kind of tea can be drunk per day. The tea can be sweetened slightly if required.

A decoction of pure horsetail can be used (cooled) for compresses for weeping skin conditions. This will be described in more detail in the section on external application below.

Potentised horsetail

In anthroposophical pharmacy there is horsetail which has been prepared (by a prolonged decoction) as Equisetum arvense, ethanol. Decoctum (Weleda) (D1, D3, D4, D6), as a liquid alcoholic dilution. Due to the increased solubility of silicic acid in heat, the silicic acid and therefore the mineral element is emphasised.

Another type of preparation is rhythmising in which the plant material plus water is rhythmically alternated between 4 °C and 37 °C (39 °F and 99 °F) and also exposed to a rhythm of illumination and darkness, of movement and stillness, of being enclosed and exposed to airing from outside. This process, inaugurated by Rudolf Hauschka, the founder of Wala, aims to transfer the vitality of the plant into the medicine and hence bring it close to the human being through a type of metamorphosis. In the case of horsetail, this rhythmising process is prepared as a particularly time-consuming seven-stage charge in which horsetail is harvested daily before sunrise and added to the charge prepared on previous days. As is the case with other medicines manufactured using this kind of rhythmical process, you get the impression that the high level of effort expended by those making it has a crucial effect on the quality achieved. (In fact we also come across this in daily life where we can experience that a carefully prepared meal – preferably with vegetables picked from the cook's own garden – has a totally different quality to a ready-made meal which is quickly heated up in the oven.) Medicines produced in this way are available as Equisetum ex herba (Wala) as globules (D3, D6, D10, D15) and ampoules (D6, D8, D15, D30) and as similarly prepared (but with less effort) Equisetum arvense Rh (Weleda) as aqueous drops (D3, D6, D15, D30) and ampoules (D3, D6). These remedies are often given for *kidney diseases* and also for *skin conditions* where it appears that kidney function needs to be improved. One reason for this can be that the skin performs 'excretion' by means of a rash if the kidneys are not working properly. This approach has been particularly successful for *weeping eczema.* As it is a complex task to discover the cause of eczema, this field is not suitable for self-treatment.

A 'kidney treatment' with Equisetum can also help other diseases, such as an *inflamed tendon sheath* or *chronic polyarthritis.* Medium (D6 to D12) to high (D30) potencies are often used for this. Anthroposophical gynaecologists have often found that the use of the D6 (as injection, globules or drops) can be helpful in late pregnancy if there is a tendency to water retention or high blood pressure. These can be signs of the onset of *toxaemia* (or *eclampsia)* which can become dangerous if they develop further, which is why careful monitoring and expert supervision are required in such cases.

The experienced Austrian paediatrician Reinhard Schwarz has reported how persistent recurring nappy rash (due to the skin being infected with the yeast *Candida albicans)* can be cleared up by administering the alcohol-free Equisetum arvense Rh D6 drops (Weleda) (5 drops 2–3 times daily). We can recall the picture of the 'fortress' in which horsetail plant defends itself by means of the silica and can therefore ward off fungi. Our skin is also a silica-rich barrier against influences from outside. The skin is subject to particular challenges in the nappy area and the horsetail can help it to defend itself effectively. In addition, for local treatment Dr Schwarz recommends the use of body silk powder (Dr Hauschka).

Horsetail in composite remedies

Horsetail is used in many composite medicines. A special pharmaceutical preparation method is used for Equisetum cum Sulfure tostum (Weleda). The dry horsetail plant is heated and infused with sulfur vapour. As mentioned briefly above, horsetail not only has a relationship to silicic acid but also to sulfur, which is intensified by this method of preparation. One of the consequences of this is to increase its effect in promoting excretion. I often prescribe this remedy as a trituration in D3 for slightly *raised blood pressure* and minor *fluid retention around the ankles* (D1, D4 and D6 are also available). It has also proved beneficial for *rheumatic complaints* where it is used at higher potencies (mostly injection of D15) and for *arthroses* and *joint inflammation* but also for *ankylosing spondylitis* in which a chronic inflammation of the vertebral joints leads to gradual stiffening.

The relationship of horsetail to silicic acid enables it to be helpful in diseases which affect the connective tissue (which is also particularly rich in silica). All the Wala Disci preparations which have proved efficacious for various back and disc problems contain potentised horsetail, for example Disci comp. cum Stanno, Disci comp. cum Nicotiana (which can also be used for ankylosing spondylitis) or Disci comp. cum Pulsatilla. Amongst other things they stimulate strengthening of loose and painful ligaments and disc tissue.

Another remedy which can be helpful for *back pain* is Pancreas/Equisetum (Wala). This remedy often produces a significant increase in excretion. The dose is usually 10 globules 3 times daily, following which many patients experience increased excretion of urine and faeces and an improvement in the back pain. A remedy which has a broad application for *pain in the connective tissue and musculoskeletal system* is Solum (globules and injection; Wala). This is a combination of peat extract, horse chestnut and horsetail. All three of these substances have a connection to the element of water. The peat extract stores and accumulates water in nature, horsetail sets it in active movement and in high summer horse chestnut creates a cool moist shaded area and helps with venous congestion. The medicine as a total composition is particularly efficacious where *pain* arises due to congestion *in the connective tissue* and in the organs which arise from it (tendons, fasciae etc.). For example, it can be effective for *pain caused by bone metastases* in which the growing tumour is restricted by the solid bone, giving rise to severe pain. This makes *Solum* one of the most important remedies in anthroposophical medicine which can contribute to the *palliative medical care* of patients suffering from advanced tumours.

Horsetail is produced along with ant extract as Equisetum/Formica (Wala) which is helpful for areas where a tendency to excessive stiffening in connective tissue needs to be countered. This can happen in the lung in cases of *pulmonary fibrosis* and also in serious *rheumatic diseases*. In the case of these serious illnesses the remedy only forms part of the whole therapeutic treatment. Equisetum/Stannum (Wala), in which the plant is linked to potentised tin (which has a connection to the cartilage) is used particularly for *joint conditions*.

The horsetail's connection to light described earlier can explain why it is included in potentised form in the eye remedy Lens/Viscum comp. (Wala) which us used to treat *cataracts*, a disease in which the lens of the eye slowly becomes cloudy. In this remedy horsetail is combined with an ant extract (Formica). The function performed by ants in the forest is to break down dying material and feed it back into the life cycle. Deposits in us also need to be dissolved from time to time in order to create transparency. This process can be stimulated particularly well by mistletoe (Viscum) which is also contained in this remedy, along with bamboo. Bamboo, like horsetail, has an intensive lively relationship to silica. The eye is one of the most silica-rich organs in our body. This is perhaps not surprising, because in the world of minerals – the world of silica – the greatest lucency and 'clarification' are achieved, which comes to expression in the quartz crystal. This actually allows more light to pass through than normal glass. Lens/Viscum comp. also contains an organ preparation of the lens.

Renes/Equisetum comp. (Wala) once more relates to the 'classical' field of application of the horsetail, the influence on the kidneys and urinary tract. This remedy combines an organ preparation from the kidney with horsetail, potentised bee and false hellebore (Veratrum), which also acts on the circulation and kidneys. This remedy stimulates malfunctioning excretory processes in connection with *kidney diseases*.

In Cantharis Blasen globules and injection (bladder remedy, Wala), however, the effect of the horsetail is directed at the bladder through its preparation along with Spanish fly (Cantharis) – also proven for *bladder infections* in homeopathy – and an organic preparation of the bladder. Potentised yarrow also has a warming and relaxing effect on this area (see also page 40). In paraesthesia and *burning upon urination,* prompt use (5 globules up to hourly, less frequently when improvement sets in, for instance 3–4 times daily) can often prevent development into a serious urinary tract infection. If a significant improvement is not achieved in two days then professional help must be sought. Symptoms of raised temperature or back pain which could point to the kidneys being involved are often signs of a dangerous development indicating that the infection has spread to the kidneys and requires immediate medical attention. The use of this remedy for preventing recurring urinary tract infections is described in Chapter 3.

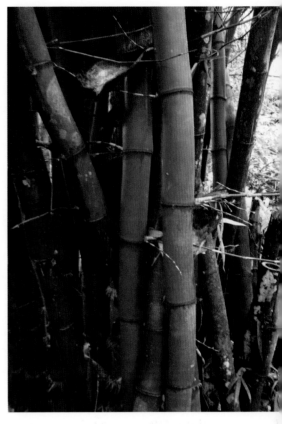

Like horsetail, bamboo has a rhythmically segmented shoot. Some composite remedies for treatment of the spine contain both plants.

Lien comp. (Wala) combines the excretory and therefore detoxifying effect of the horsetail with the digestive stimulating effect of chicory (*Cichorium,* see Chapter 27). Besides the architectural structure and emphasis on form, both plants are characterised by their high content of silicic acid which points to an effect on the connective tissue, that is, to the realm in us which mediates between 'inside' and 'outside', but also to a certain extent between the 'above' of the nerve and senses system and the 'below' of the metabolic limb system. Correspondingly, in embryology, the connective tissue and the tissue which succeeds it arise from the mesoderm of the embryo. This also applies to the spleen, which is a 'home' and 'production unit' for immune cells but also clears old and useless cells from the blood. The remedy contains a potentised organic preparation of the spleen and, like one made from mesenchyme, the primordial connective tissue, contributes to *promoting regeneration* and *stimulating immune function*. Lien comp. can be beneficial for recurring *infections* and it can also stimulate defence mechanisms in *cancer patients*. I usually prescribe 10 globules twice daily.

Horsetail on soil fertilised with silica

We have frequently described how plants are cultivated on soil fertilised with metals. The plants selected for this always have a natural relationship to the specific metal used, and this is intensified by this method. In the case of horsetail it is not a metal but its relationship to silica which is intensified and enlivened in the preparation Equisetum arvense Silicea cultum (Weleda). The soil is fertilised using potentised silica. The horsetail grown on this soil is composted, and horsetail is again grown on the compost. This is again composted and only the third generation of horsetail plants grown on this soil are incorporated in the remedy in question.

This remedy has proved particularly successful for children who are often pale, always cold and with frequent *colds* and *catarrh*. It stimulates warmth, drying, and the shaping and formation of the organism, which often leads to significant stabilisation in their health. This remedy can help with *weeping inflammatory eczema* and also with *rheumatic diseases* with a clear tendency to swelling, indicating that the fluid processes are no longer properly under control. I would not recommend a constitutional treatment like this for self-treatment. However, it may be useful to know how a medicine of this kind is produced and to appreciate the amount of work by the gardeners and pharmacists which lies behind something we can buy relatively cheaply in the pharmacy.

External treatment using horsetail

As already mentioned, horsetail is suitable not only for treating human beings but is also helpful for other plants. Add 2 heaped tablespoons to 1 litre (quart) of water and boil for 20 minutes to produce a decoction which, when sprayed onto other plants, protects them from fungal attack. This method is frequently used in biodynamic agriculture, but can also be used on houseplants and garden plants. Here, both the forming and light force mediating effects of the horsetail are at work. The memorable picture of the plant being able to 'barricade' itself with the help of the silica 'as though in a fortress' was already mentioned. On the other hand, a fungal attack which is already far advanced cannot be cured using horsetail decoction (just as the castle wall is no longer of any help when the attacker has already broken in).

In human beings, it is primarily the skin for which external application of horsetail can be beneficial. A decoction prepared as described above can be efficacious for *weeping skin diseases* (if this preparation is too much trouble, then Equisetum-Essenz (Wala) can also be used at a rate of 2 teaspoons in $\frac{1}{4}$ litre (8 fl oz) lukewarm water). Compresses with this type of horsetail decoction are often recommended in these cases. For larger areas in particular, it is advisable to cover the cotton cloth soaked in the decoction with a piece of cling film (plastic wrap) from the kitchen in order to slow down evaporation and the cooling effect it produces. In particular cases it may be suitable to use a bath to which 1 litre (quart) of the horsetail decoction has been added. These kinds of baths are used for *Parkinson's disease* (and in some cases for other chronic diseases) as part of a complete treatment programme. The use of an oil dispersion bath (see also page 134) which is prepared using Equisetum ex herba W 5% Oleum (Wala) is particularly beneficial. This makes the skin more supple and stimulates heat production as well as helping moisture to penetrate the skin. At the same time, it enhances the excretion of deposits, which is why it achieves an antisclerotic effect similar to the birch. In contrast to its use as a compress, the oil dispersion bath can also be helpful for *dry skin conditions* and *dry itchy neurodermatitis*.

If the skin is irritated and itchy, Rose-Schachtelhalm in Olivenöl (Dr Heberer Naturheilmittel) can also be used instead of pure Equisetum oil. The rose contained in this has an emotionally balancing effect, which can often be beneficial in skin diseases.

Compresses and lavation with horsetail decoction can have a healing effect on *chronic wounds* and *sores*. However, in such cases their use should be reserved for experienced practitioners.

CHAPTER 15

St John's Wort

Summer is the season when we yearn for sunshine, warmth and the countryside in order to 'recharge our batteries', to get energy for everyday life and the coming winter. Perhaps the 'dog days' of August may be the hottest time of the year, but the maximum light lies some time before that. In the northern hemisphere, June 21 is the longest day of the year, with the sun above the horizon for many more hours than in winter. In some places the shortest night of the year is lit up by St John's fires. This plant, likewise named after John the Baptist, whose feast day is three days after midsummer, begins to open its bright starry flowers at this time.

When you see the heads of glowing golden five-petalled St John's Wort flowers swaying above their nondescript shoots and notice the dense bunch of stamens which seem to burst out of the flowers (looking like the rays surrounding the sun on a child's drawing), you have the impression of little 'earthly suns' or the earth's response to the intensity of the sun's power at this time of year. The fact that grazing animals with pale coats can suffer from sunburn if they eat too much St John's Wort shows that this plant increases the effect of the sun. This effect does not seem to be of any great significance for human beings, as no increased light sensitivity could be detected from internal use of concentrated St John's Wort preparations or from using creams containing St John's Wort extracts on the skin.[1]

Ancient writings mentioned St John's Wort as a valuable medicinal plant. Paracelsus (1493-1541) who counts as one of the greatest doctors of all time, wrote at length about this plant. He dedicated himself tirelessly to the patients who had placed their faith in him. At the same time, he was also a conscientious and careful observer who

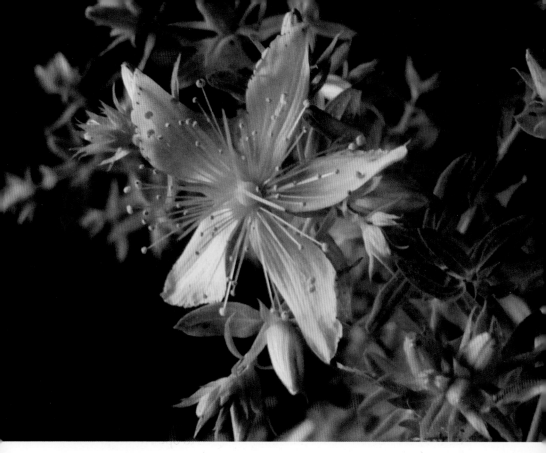

Flowering St John's wort.

did not accept anything he was expected to believe simply because it appeared in heavy tomes or was claimed by authorities, unless he had understood it himself. He was convinced that the cures for all ills could be found in nature.

In a work on St John's Wort he justified his view: God has made the human body from the 'dust' (literally 'mud') of the earth, from a substance containing something from all other forms of creation. Every rock will one day turn to dust, and so will every living being. The human being is therefore related to everything in the world, and when he lacks something, there is always something that can help. The art consists of finding out which power God put in every entity, for then we can know what it is able to heal.

The appearance and the whole nature of each entity tells us about its powers: we can decipher these when we take the trouble to do so. Paracelsus said of St John's Wort that it is a king, a centre around which other things circle. He wrote that it was similar to the sun, 'which

159

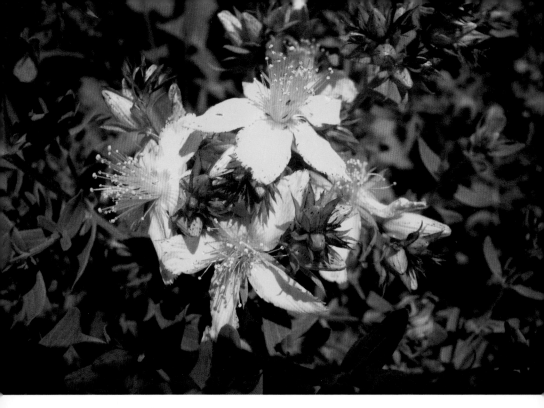

Flowering St John's wort.

shines on everything, good and bad, as does the remedy'. Paracelsus then described how the plant's powers can be recognised in all its details (for example, the small dots on the leaves which shine when you hold them up to the light, or the red colour which remains on your finger when you rub the flower) and mentioned areas of use for the herb which still apply today and are borne out to an increasing degree the more that research progresses.

He described it as almost the only remedy for 'confused fantasies which make people despair', for diseases which cause people 'to leave their senses' and 'compel people to kill themselves,' by which he was referring to depression and its worst outcome. Many people experience this as though the inner sun has disappeared, as though everything is cold, bleak and hopeless. Studies on what now amounts to thousands of patients have confirmed the experience from practice that preparations made from St John's Wort can indeed help mild and moderate *depression* just as well as the standard chemical antidepressants (and in some cases light therapy). Laboratory experiments have shown that St John's Wort extracts have effects on the metabolism of nerve cells

160

similar to those of synthetic antidepressants. These effects could not be achieved using an isolated single substance from the St John's Wort, hypericin, which was believed to be the active ingredient, but were obtained from preparations of the whole plant. When looking for new medicinal substances nowadays, the approach is to manufacture and test innumerable new compounds – first in laboratory experiments – to see whether they have possibly useful effects. This was the other way round with the St John's Wort. The effect was first recognised and applied through a spiritual approach to the plant and this effect was then confirmed in laboratory tests.

Nowadays St John's Wort is better established in orthodox medicine than almost any other medicinal plant. It has very few side effects; however, certain concentrated plant preparations for treating depression require a prescription. This is for the best, as St John's Wort not only stimulates the metabolism of the nerves but also metabolic processes in the liver. This is helpful because depression also involves metabolic disturbances below the diaphragm. However, the increase in metabolism brought about by the St John's Wort can mean that some drugs are broken down and excreted more quickly. Some medicines then have an insufficient effect (for example, those for suppressing the immune system after transplants, those to combat HIV viruses or for reducing the blood's clotting tendency). It is therefore essential that treatment is supervised by an expert, and this is all the more important the more drugs the patient is taking.

In the case of depression, the danger Paracelsus mentioned must be kept in mind: a tendency to want to commit suicide can arise. Simply prescribing a drug is inadequate in this case – as it always is. It is essential to acknowledge the distress of the person affected, to provide a listening ear, support and, if necessary, protection from their own impulses which are no longer under their control. This also requires careful and expert supervision which is not available if you only buy a remedy for yourself. Even Paracelsus was aware of the fact that love – and therefore the relationship between people, which is precisely the issue in the case of depression – is the best medicine.

Paracelsus also recommended this herb for other illnesses. It is 'not possible that a better remedy for wounds could be found.' Apparently this did not apply only to the Middle Ages, because a current study has shown that St John's Wort promotes healing even in wounds

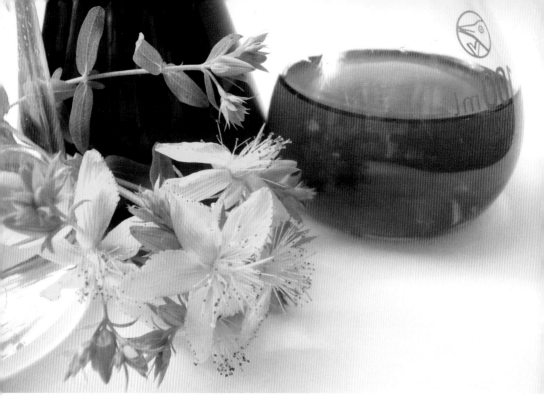

St John's wort oil.

which are as difficult to treat as the chronic *pressure sores* suffered by
the bedridden.[2] St John's Wort oil belongs to the standard therapeutic
agents in the anthroposophical treatment of wounds.[3] Many positive
effects on the skin have been identified – for example by Professor
Dr Christoph Schempp's research at the dermatology department of
the University of Freiburg – including a significant anti-inflammatory
action and a powerful effect against most organisms involved in *wound
infections.*[4] Even bacteria which were resistant to most antibiotics,
could be killed by St John's Wort extracts.[5] The substance hyperforin,
which is particularly effective against these organisms, is light-sensitive,
which is why St John's Wort extracts manufactured in the dark have
particularly high amounts of it. In contrast, St John's Wort oil is
traditionally manufactured in sunlight and the hypericin only becomes
soluble in the oil during the fermentation processes, which occur
during this manufacturing procedure. This is why the oil develops an
increasingly deep red colour when exposed to light. It is interesting to
note that both the constituents mentioned are apparently involved in
the antidepressant effect of St John's Wort.

Paracelsus recommended harvesting the plant at sunrise and exposing it to light for a long period when preparing the extract. The special manufacturing processes at sunrise or sunset – without reference to Paracelsus but due to equally careful observations – are adhered to in the preparation of anthroposophical remedies from St John's Wort. This can be seen, for example, in the rhythmising process used by Wala: it is not only harvested in the early morning, but the plant substance is also exposed to the effects of the morning and evening every day. The power of the sun can be collected in different ways – by spending time outdoors (which can be done to a greater degree during vacations than during normal routine), working in the fields or at the laboratory bench.

St John's Wort (*Hypericum perforatum*)

St John's Wort flowers picked around the time of the summer solstice can then be collected and dried for use as a medicinal tea. Only the wild herb is used, not the various garden varieties of the plant. The St John's Wort which can be used medicinally can be identified by the small dots on the leaves which are transparent when held up to the light and the red-brown colour which appears when you rub the flowers. An observant reader wrote to tell me that there are occasionally other species of St John's Wort to which this applies. The perforate St John's Wort has large spots on the surface of the petals (which can be clearly seen in the illustration on page 160). Officially, only the perforate St John's Wort is used medicinally, although the other species which produce a red-brown colour when rubbed may have at least some of the well-known ingredients. It is presumably not essential for the preparation of an oil for home use (see below) to be totally botanically precise, but if you want to be sure, it is best to compare the plant you have found with an identification guide.

Another important preparation method besides drying the plant is oil extraction. Put the fresh St John's Wort into a transparent container, cover it with olive oil and leave to stand in the light for several weeks. After a while the oil turns a glowing red colour, which is why this is also known as 'red oil'. Unfortunately the olive oil can acquire a rancid smell during this process. Peanut or sesame oil can also be used

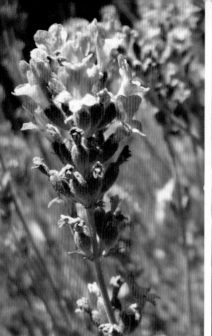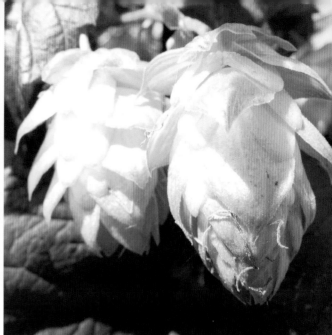

Lavender flowers (left) or hop cones (right) are a good addition to St John's wort in a sleep-inducing tea.

as extraction agents. Industrially, extracts are also produced in the dark – for example by extraction using carbonic acid – which obtains the light sensitive ingredient hyperforin particularly efficiently. It is possible that the creams made from this have particularly good anti-inflammatory properties and extracts of this kind may be particularly efficacious for *neurodermatitis*.

St John's Wort tea

You need 2 heaped teaspoons for 1 cup of hot water. The tea has a mildly relaxing effect and elevates mood slightly. For *insomnia and restlessness* add lemon balm, hop cones and some lavender flowers to the St John's wort.

St John's Wort tea is also traditionally recommended for bed-wetting. However, I find that the Wala Berberis/Hypericum comp. mentioned below is more effective. In any case, this is usually a complex problem, one that cannot be tackled merely with drugs. It needs to be discussed with a paediatrician.

Concentrated herbal preparations made from St John's wort

There are a large number of proprietary remedies intended for the treatment of depression in particular, such as Hyperforat, Felis, Jarsin etc. As already mentioned, these remedies can be relatively effective. Research has shown that, like many chemically produced antidepressants, St John's Wort influences metabolism in the neurotransmitters, that is, the messengers which are involved in the exchange of information between nerve cells. In general, St John's Wort preparations appear to have fewer side effects than synthetic preparations. Even though research results contradict it, the claim that people taking remedies of this kind become significantly more light-sensitive may be true in individual cases, especially amongst very pale-skinned people. (I believe I may have experienced a case of this myself.) What is certain is that concentrated Hypericum preparations affect metabolism and therefore affect the efficacy of other medicines. This is why in many countries they are only available on prescription. It should be noted that, as is the case with chemical antidepressants, the desired effect does not take place quickly, but often only after around two weeks.

Potentised St John's wort

Hypericum has been advocated in homeopathy for nerve and spinal chord damage for a long time. The characteristic for this is particular pain in very localised areas. On several occasions I have been able to achieve an impressive rapid cure of sometimes very severe pain of this type by administering Hypericum ex herba D6 or D12 as injection, even when a long and unsuccessful treatment with other remedies had often preceded this. The unpleasant pain after *damage to the coccyx* can also respond well to this type of treatment.

Mild *depression* can also sometimes be treated with potentised St John's wort. The simultaneous administration of the above-mentioned concentrated extracts and potentised St John's Wort (often D3 or D6) have also proved successful. I have often had the impression that the desired effect also set in more quickly as a result.

Another area of application for potentised Hypericum is for pronounced oversensitivity to light in the form of a 'light allergy' or, more correctly, *polymorphic light eruption*. Those affected develop

A 51-year-old female patient suffered from recurrent sharp punctiform lower back pain. She had already been to numerous doctors about this. The orthopaedic specialist, the surgeon and the neurologist had no explanation for the pain. An MRI scan was carried out without any pathological findings being recorded. Local injections had had just as little sustained effect as physiotherapy and treatment by an osteopath. The patient had therefore been taking strong analgesics for a long time in order to keep the pain down to a bearable level. She nevertheless repeatedly suffered severe pain and her sleep was often disturbed as a result. Due to the nature of the pain she described, I injected Hypericum ex herba D6 (Wala) at the point where the pain was felt. The very next night her sleep was scarcely affected by pain. I repeated this injection a few more times and the patient has been pain free for several years.

itchy tubercles on the skin when exposed to sunlight. Prescribing Hypericum D6 (also prophylactically) has repeatedly been helpful for this condition.

Wala produce Hypericum ex herba ampoules in the potencies D3, D6, D12 and D30 and globules in D2, D3 and D6. Weleda manufacture a Hypericum, Herba mother tincture and Hypericum Rh, which is also made from a rhythmised basic substance. This remedy is available as drops in D3 and as ampoules in D6 and D30.

Hypericum Auro cultum

It was shown that St John's Wort has a special connection to the sun. Gold was also always seen as having a relationship to the power of the sun and in potentised form it is one of the major remedies for the treatment of depression (see also Chapter 38 on gold). This explains why the method developed by anthroposophical pharmacy of growing plants on soil fertilised with metals (which is described in more detail on page 292 of Chapter 28) is also used for St John's Wort and gold. Weleda manufactures Hypericum Auro cultum Rh as a rhythmised aqueous substance in D3 as drops and in D2 and D3 as ampoules (these are prescription only medicines). The remedy is available as alcoholic drops in D2 and D3 under the name of Hypericum Auro cultum, Herba (prescription only). These medicines can be valuable for some forms of depression accompanied by the feeling of an inner loss of light. As previously mentioned, however, depression should not be treated under self-medication.

Hypericum used externally

The (home) production of St John's Wort oil or red oil has already been described. This can also be bought. Weleda supplies a particularly concentrated vivid red oil under the name of Hypericum, Flos 25% oil while Hypericum ex herba 5% Oleum (Wala) is considerably less concentrated. Both are suitable for rubbing in for *muscular* and *back pain*. Good results have also been reported for these remedies for the post-treatment of *mild burns* (also for *sunburn* or *radiotherapy*). The anti-inflammatory effects of St John's Wort and promotion of cell differentiation (and therefore also regeneration in the case of certain skin changes) are well known.[6] If a patient wishes to use St John's Wort oil during radiotherapy, then this should be discussed in advance with the radiotherapist. Another remedy that can be used during radiotherapy is the marigold *(Calendula officinalis)*, which is described in Chapter 23.

Hypericum in composite medicines

The composition Berberis/Hypericum comp. (Wala) has already been mentioned. Apart from St John's Wort and a preparation of Berberis root, this also contains potentised potassium phosphate. This remedy has a long tradition in the treatment of 'conditions of nervous exhaustion'. As part of a holistic treatment it can be helpful for bed-wetting and incontinence at a dosage of 5 globules 3 times daily, something that Rudolf Steiner recommended as an application for St John's Wort.

Levico comp. (Wala) is mentioned in Chapter 33 on blackthorn.

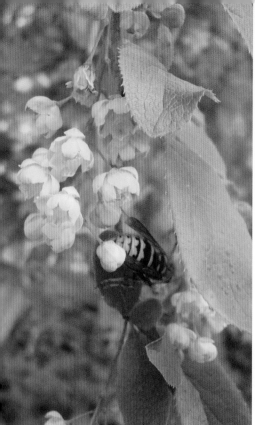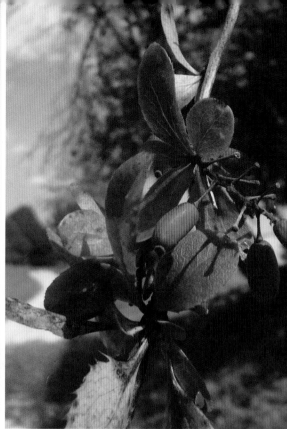

The flowers and fruits of barberry (Berberis vulgaris) *used together with St John's wort in some composite remedies.*

Water from the Levico spring, rich in copper, iron, arsenic and sulfur, is prepared in potentised form with blackthorn flowers and shoot tips as well as St John's wort. This remedy is often very helpful for conditions of exhaustion due to long-term strain from various sources. It can have a restorative effect both for overwork and too much responsibility and also for exhaustion after serious physical illness. The remedy can also help in cases of long-term strain resulting in *chronic thyroiditis* (Hashimoto's thyroiditis).

CHAPTER 16

Starry Elder

In high summer you cannot miss the elder. Its flower heads gleam almost white against the dark green leaves of the tall bush or low tree, seeming to float above the foliage. And something else wafts around it: a cloud of scent, which spreads out on these warm summer days. But what does it smell of? It is difficult to say. There is a rather herby green damp base note, which emanates from the dark leaves even before the flower appears. And on top of this (a perfumist calls this a top note) is the delicate sweet scent of the flower. It is brighter, lighter: far less heavy than the sweet heavy scent of the lime which is also in flower at this time. Anyone who has once smelt the scent of elder will always be able to recognise it. The official pharmacopoeia takes the easy way out: the flowers 'smell peculiar', it says. This does not mean curious or strange but that they are characteristic of their kind, according to their nature.

But what is the nature of the elder? It has two sides, which we have already got to know from the scent. One is dark, full, earthy and the other is light, floating, cosmic. Elder likes to grow on slightly moist rich soil, such as on a compost heap, for which the bush is also useful in giving shade and forming a dark inner space. The flat pale flower heads of the elder open almost exactly at the start of summer in June or July when the sun is highest in the sky, the days are longest and we are urged out into nature. They are composed of masses of tiny five-pointed starry flowers from which the scent emanates. It is almost as though they wanted to stand out from the dark earth from which they came. And they succeed in this to a certain degree when their scent spreads out in the sun-drenched summer air.

We encounter a gesture of dissolving, not only at the periphery

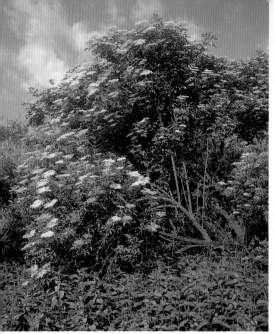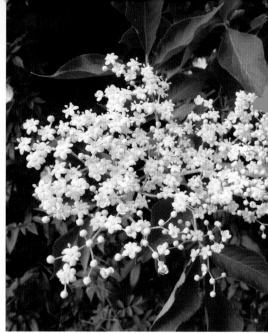

Flowering elder gives off a typical scent.   *Elderflowers.*

of the plant but also at its centre. We can break even the thicker branches surprisingly easily. We find that the older ones are hollow inside, the younger ones are filled with a dry white substance which can be easily dented and is reminiscent of plastic foam. If you cut them into thin slices and put them under the microscope, then you will see that this substance is made of small bubbles of air enclosed by cell walls.

While other trees produce very hard heartwood, in the elder it is as though the wood dissolves into foam. These gestures reveal the plant's therapeutic effect. The 'dissolving power' is also predominant here. The elder is best known for its sudorific (sweat-inducing) property. Tea made from the flowers is commonly used at the *start of a cold*, as it is also able to liquefy viscous secretions which annoyingly block the nose and bronchial tubes. This is actually the main indication in homeopathy, where elder is well known for the treatment of *head colds in babies*. Because a baby's larynx is located even higher than later in life, it is impossible for it to drink with a blocked nose. Globules of potentised elder (*Sambucus* in Latin) often free them quickly from this annoyance.

Despite relatively extensive research, no substance has been found in elder which is responsible for this effect. It was therefore alleged that the sweat-producing and liquefying effects were simply due to

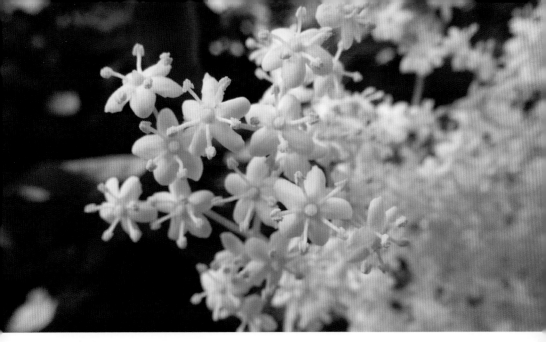

The flower head is made up of a mass of small five-petalled flowers.

the hot water which was used to make the tea. However, to accept this explanation means disregarding a classical experiment carried out by the herbalist Gerhard Madaus (1890–1942) using dried elderflower powder (in other words, with no hot water at all!). Three quarters of the 20 subjects who performed desk work without any physical effort at normal room temperature during the experiment felt not only warmed through but sweated all over their bodies. 'In one case the test subject was really hot and running with sweat, a strong smell of sweat could be noticed even at a distance and the subject complained of palpitations,' the report states.[1]

In addition to the flowers, other parts of the plant also encourage excretion. In the days when there was still no efficacious and safe synthetic agent for the purpose, preparations from the root were famous for *stimulating urination* in cases of pathological fluid retention.

If you remove the external grey-brown bark, you come across the greenish inner bark. Curiously, it is claimed that it produces diarrhoea and therefore has a loosening effect on *persistent constipation* if you scrape the bark off from top to bottom. However, it is said to cause vomiting if you scrape it off the substrate the other way around, from the bottom upwards. I have never tried out whether this is true (and probably neither has anyone who spreads these reports), but it is not only claimed in folk medicine in Germany, Russia and Romania but also in a work by the famous Albertus Magnus (from where it may have come into popular tradition). Eating the berries raw definitely produces a nauseous effect. (This was proved impressively when I was seven and a fellow classmate brought berries into the class for all to try as elder was the subject of the lesson. The consequences were as appalling as they were memorable.) The berries are only palatable after being cooked, in the form of juice, jam or compote. Their strong red-black colour (which can almost never be removed from fabrics) is due to anthocyanins, plant substances which have strongly antioxidant effects and therefore counteract the processes of ageing. (These can also be understood as 'hardening' or 'sclerotic' processes). It is even claimed that elder can prevent cancer. No wonder the elder was viewed as the farmers' pharmacy in earlier times – even being accorded such veneration that it was common to doff your hat to it.

The flowering elder is evoked best by the poet Oda Schaefer: [2]

Sitting in the darkest green
Dreaming by the bark so grey
Rocked to sleep by summer winds –
Your bright flowering I can see
Everywhere in darkest green,
Still I see your wonder,
Starry elder.

Leaves play above my head
Like fingers of light and shade
On the tender beds of phlox,
In the Here and Now I rest
Heat and midday above my head,
Listen to your wonder
Starry elder.

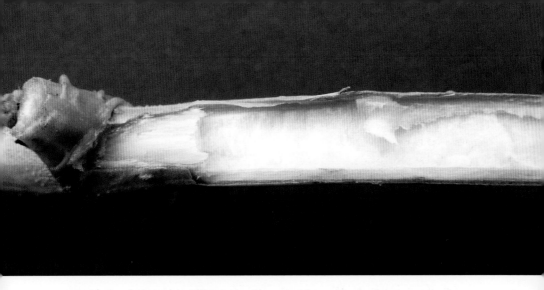

The inside of elder twigs is filled with white pith. This – like the flowers – is used to make a remedy for colds in babies.

Elder (*Sambucus nigra*)

The elder forms a sturdy (3–7 m, or 10–23 ft) bush in many hedgerows, and on slopes and woodland edges in most of Europe, as well as closely related subspecies in North America and Asia. It cannot be missed when it opens its white umbels between the end of May and the beginning of July. Care must be taken not to confuse it with its much smaller relative, the dwarf elder (*Sambucus ebulus*) or the red elderberry (*Sambucus racemosa*) which later on has red berries (in contrast to the black ones of the common elder).

The flowers lend themselves to self-collection in view of the quantities available and the warm days during flowering time, which are suitable for drying the flowers quickly in partial shade. The fresh flowers are also fermented with sugar water to produce elderflower champagne. Boiled up with sugar and water (100–200 g of sugar per litre of water, 4–7 oz per quart) and filled hot into bottles, they produce a delicious elderflower syrup which is later used by diluting and adding a little lemon juice to improve the flavour. In contrast to the champagne, which has to be used straight away, the syrup keeps until the next harvesting opportunity the following year. The diluted syrup is good simply as a tasty drink, or can be drunk hot for a cold.

Elderflowers also make a typical early summer speciality as elderflower fritters when dipped in pancake batter and cooked in hot oil.

The berries cannot be eaten raw as they are mildly poisonous and

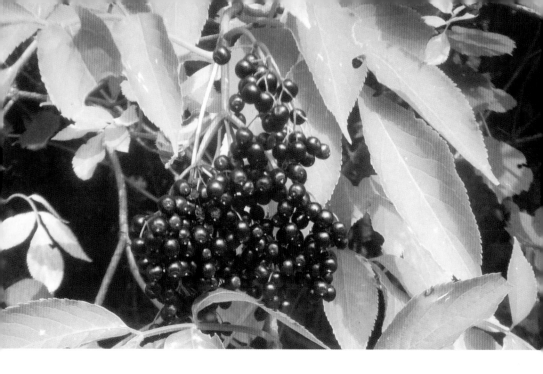

cause nausea. However, they can be processed into a very tart juice if they are prepared hot in a juice steamer. A mixture of elderflower and apple juice tastes better. The berries are also good for making elderberry and apple jelly for which it is best to mix $\frac{1}{3}$ elderberries with $\frac{2}{3}$ apples and add slightly less than equal the quantity of preserving sugar.

Elderflower tea

Allow one heaped teaspoon of dried flowers per cup of boiling water and leave to infuse for 10 minutes, adding a little honey and lemon to taste. The tea has a sweat-producing effect and frees viscous secretions in the nose and bronchial tubes, which is why it is good for *colds*. At the start of a cold you can also add 1 litre of strong elderflower tea (made from 5 heaped teaspoons of the dried flowers) to a full bath. For a tea for treating colds, equal amounts of lime flowers are often added to the elderflowers. If the tea is to be used to alleviate a *dry cough*, then common mallow flowers can also be added to the mixture as their mucilage eases the irritation. The tea turns a greenish-blue due to the mallow. If you then add lemon juice, it turns a bright red. This play of colours is a delight, and not only for children.

If you wish to have a pharmacist make up this tea, the prescription is:

→ *Flor. Sambuci* (elderflowers)
→ *Flor. Tiliae* (lime flowers)
→ *Flor. Malvae* (common mallow flowers) aa ad 50.0.

Sambucus as a potentised remedy

Homeopathically potentised elder as Sambucus D3 or D4 globules can prove beneficial for *colds in babies*. Administer 2 globules several times a day, between the dental ridge and the cheek mucosa. As a (possibly better) alternative, dissolve the globules in a few drops of water or breast milk and administer the solution using a spoon or pipette. This often leads to a rapid improvement, which is initially noticeable from the baby being able to drink more easily again.

An interesting – but as far as I know little-used – recommendation by Rudolf Steiner consists of using Sambucus in medium potency for 'ossification in the ears' (*otosclerosis*). It appears to me that the 'dissolving tendency' of the elder comes into play again here. His recommendation to wash the affected area using 'birch, elder pith and Iceland moss in high potency for rough flaky skin' could be interpreted in the same way. So far, I have not had any experience of this. However, in a case of ichthyosis in which, in extreme cases, the skin can resemble the hardened skin of a reptile, I would try it to see if it may provide relief.

Sambucus in composite medicines

Sambucus comp. globules (Wala) contain elderflowers and elder pith in the final potency of a D6 along with the warming action of larch resin (final potency D8). This composition can be used for colds in babies like the single potency described above. A remedy with a very similar composition goes by the name of Flores Sambuci comp. (Weleda) as drops. Due to the alcohol content of 36%, however, I prefer the globules for babies. For adults the preparation should help stabilise the *late phase of a cold* with nasal congestion symptoms.

This remedy is also suitable for alleviating *sweating attacks as part of the menopause* (and this is what it was originally used for). The normal dose is 5–10 drops of Flores sambuci comp. 3 times daily. Many patients obtain significant relief from this. Here, there appears to be a reverse homeopathic effect compared to the sweat-producing effect of elder in concentrated application. The remedy is reputedly also helpful for unpleasantly itchy eczema of the auditory canal.

Weleda produce the remedy Sambucus/Teucrium comp., which contains potentised Berberis berries, phosphorous and wood sage besides Sambucus D3. Due to the alcohol content, the remedy is not suitable for babies and toddlers in my opinion. However, it can contribute to easing the symptoms of *colds* in children and adults. Take 5–10 drops 3 times daily.

CHAPTER 17

Lime (Linden)

After the winter, doesn't it seem like a miracle when the white gossamer veil of blossom covers the dark thorny blackthorn bushes? Later, the fruit trees are filled with delicate apple blossom like pink foam, 'as though the sky had silently kissed the earth,' as the poet Eichendorff put it. In early summer 'the starry elderflower' sends out its scent and yellow pollen into the air. But then calm returns to the trees and their fruit ripens as autumn approaches. But sometimes, after the middle of June and into July when we seek shelter from the summer heat in a shady avenue, we suddenly notice the steady buzzing of bees and a gentle sweet perfume. Only at second glance, between the heart-shaped leaves shining in the light, do we recognise small yellowish flowers hanging in loose umbels and, where their small stems join, a fan-shaped greenish-yellow bract. We are standing in an avenue of lime trees.

The crowns of the trees form a protected inner space. This is particularly noticeable in certain solitary trees, which form the centre of some village squares or grow as impressive individuals in the countryside. They are often viewed as natural monuments and are named after famous poets. In days gone by – before the time when village discos appeared – the limes were often described as 'dance limes', beneath which the summer parties took place. Their scent, the shady space they form, their soft leaves… everything about the lime appears inviting and friendly, and contributes to a happy mood.

Even though it has completely fallen out of fashion, the German word *lind* ('gentle') describes the atmosphere that radiates from this tree very well. The botanist Jan Albert Rispens has pointed out another word context which illustrates the nature of the lime. Even before limes were an invitation to a celebration, they (and their sisters, the oaks) were

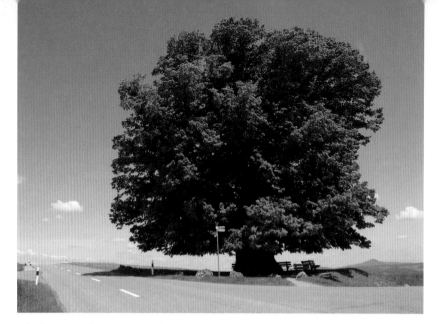

The lime tree of Linn, Switzerland.

places where trials took place. Rispens was of the opinion that the serious criminals tended to be tried under the hard gnarled oaks, while disputes where it was more a case of 'subtle' investigation and wise arbitration took place beneath the softer limes[1]. Indeed the word 'subtle' comes from the Latin name of the tree *Tilia,* so *sub-til* means 'beneath the lime'.

What is more, the wood of the lime is also soft and it is therefore the perfect wood for carving. The most beautiful Gothic statues of Mary by Riemenschneider are made from this wood. Softness does not equal weakness, and this can be seen in the vitality of lime trees, which can live for many hundreds of years. So lime trees can reach a greater age than oaks with their hard wood, for example.

One aspect of the 'mildness' of the lime can be seen in an old remedy. In earlier times, young wood and the bast fibres from the bark were combined with water and then beaten until a fine foam was produced. This was used for relieving eye inflammation in babies, or laid on burns. All these things indicate an inner 'softness' which is unusual in a tree. The ability to create foam is also a sign that this tree produces large quantities of mucilage, which is more usually the case with herbs. The lime flowers not only contain fragrant essential oil but also mucilage which can help to relieve *tussive irritation in colds.* When I prescribe lime flowers for this purpose, I often have them combined with other medicines for treating phlegm, such as marshmallow root or mallow flowers. Surprisingly, the lime is related botanically to the mallow; which can be recognised from this similarity.

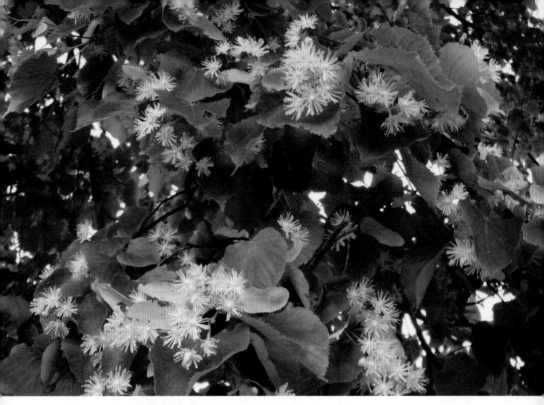

Flowering lime branches give off a sweet perfume.

However, I value lime flowers above all because they are able to take the 'summer forces' from the time when they blossom into the winter where they can be used for a *cold* or also to prevent one. It is therefore not surprising that lime flower tea can make a patient sweat slightly. This is another sign of its warming effect. This action can be enhanced by adding some lime flower honey. It has already been mentioned how the bees swarm about the summer limes. This is due to the enormous amount of nectar that this tree exudes. However, the owners of cars whose vehicles can appear decorated after standing for a while under a lime tree are less delighted. This is probably one of the reasons why this beautiful tree is seen less and less in towns.

If you come across a flowering lime, far away from car exhaust fumes, then you can pick the flowers yourself and dry them as tea for the winter. This must be done each year as the essential oil easily evaporates.

The lime can help healing in another, much more important way: now and again mistletoe grows on it. As is well known, medicines made from mistletoe can play a part in the treatment of cancers (more on this appears in Chapter 35 on mistletoe). Mistletoe is influenced by

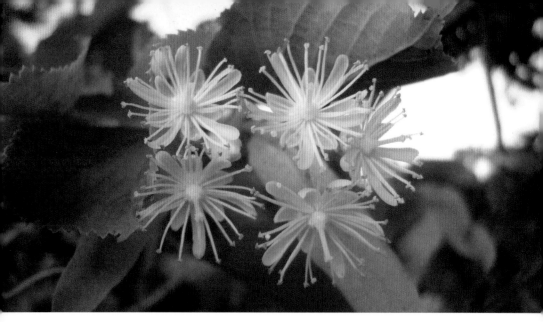

Lime flowers.

the tree on which it grows and this affects the nature of its efficacy. I repeatedly have the impression that the lime mistletoe has a particular ability to warm the patient. It also makes sense that people suffering from cancer who have a soft, giving character and inner wealth can be helped especially well using this mistletoe. What is more, the types of cancer which have a softer consistency tend to respond better to lime mistletoe than hard tumours. Whenever this happens, a special thankfulness arises for the lime, which is so close to human beings and appears so friendly.

Lime (Linden) (*Tilia platyphyllos, Tilia cordata*)

You can easily collect lime flowers for making tea, as long as the trees are not exposed to too much exhaust fumes from traffic or pesticides from agriculture. The flowers are used along with the attached bract. To ensure that the essential oils (which produce the sweet lime flower smell) are not lost, the flowers should be dried quickly in a thin layer in a shaded place, and then stored in sealed containers.

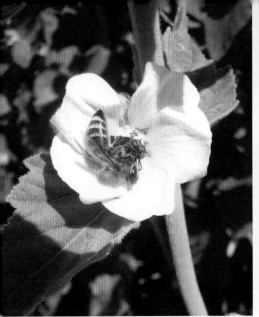

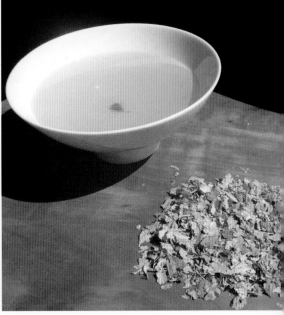

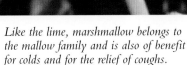

Like the lime, marshmallow belongs to the mallow family and is also of benefit for colds and for the relief of coughs.

Lime flower tea.

Lime flower tea

Pour 1 cup of boiling water over 2 teaspoons of lime flowers, cover, and leave to stand for 10 minutes. The tea can be sweetened with a little honey to taste or mixed with some lemon juice.

Lime flower tea has a warming and mucolytic effect and also encourages sweating. For these reasons it is a popular and effective tea for colds. If lime flowers are used for a dry cough they can be mixed with mallow and elderflowers, plantain leaves and/or marshmallow root.

If it is mainly the warming effect that is desired, then a few slices of ginger can be added to the lime flower tea.

External use

Lindenblüte 5% in Olivenöl (Dr Heberer Naturheilmittel) can achieve a warming and relaxing effect at the start of a cold, when used as an oil dispersion bath. Warm baths can be helpful in the initial phase of a cold when the patient has a tendency to shiver as the body tries to reach a higher temperature in order to combat the cold. It has been shown that cold viruses cannot multiply so fast at higher body temperatures and can be more easily defeated by our immune system. Even if the temperature of the bath is not greater than body temperature, an

181

oil dispersion bath encourages a slightly raised body temperature, especially in the resting phase after the actual (not too prolonged) bath. After a lime flower oil dispersion bath, *muscle pains* and an unpleasant feeling in the body usually give way to a pleasantly relaxed feeling. A feeling of being under pressure (which is often the reason for catching a cold) is easier to transform after this type of application of 'summer forces' from the lime tree.

As an alternative to using the oil (although less efficacious), you can also use an extract from 3 heaped tablespoons of lime flowers to one litre (quart) of boiling water which is added to the bath after leaving to infuse for 10 minutes.

Potentised lime flowers

The lime is very rarely used in potentised form. Occasionally Tilia (for example, D6) is used for a tendency to *excessive sweating* or *hot flushes*.

The lime as a host tree for mistletoe

Mistletoe always grows on trees. The soil on which a plant is grown influences its character and efficacy. For example, the same plant growing on calcareous or siliceous soil can have a different form and effect. Likewise, the tree may influence the sphere of application of the mistletoe that grows on it. If the host tree itself has therapeutic properties, then these can often 'transfer' over to the mistletoe growing on it. Sometimes characteristic substances in the host tree can even be found in the mistletoe. It is therefore not surprising that the mistletoe from lime can stimulate the development of warmth in patients more than mistletoe from other trees. It also appears that the lime mistletoe is especially suitable for treating certain *tumours of the lung* (lime flowers also act on the thoracic cavity). Experience seems to indicate that the hard squamous cell carcinomas in the bronchial tubes linked to smoking respond less to treatment with lime mistletoe than the usually softer and often *mucilaginous adenocarcinomas* which tend to occur in women.[2] I have repeatedly found that the lime mistletoe in higher potency (e.g. Iscucin Tiliae strengths A to C) is excellent at promoting sleep.

CHAPTER 18

Thistle

August. Vacation time – everything dry, baking sun, walking barefoot on dusty paths and in the hay on newly mown meadows. But suddenly we flinch: something has jabbed us in the sole of the foot. Luckily it was not a snake (which, after the fall into sin, was condemned to 'bruise the heel' of man), but one of the annoying thistles with prickles we now have to remove from our skin.

Thistles are not simply unpleasant; you need to know how to handle them. Several animals have thistles as part of their German name, because they belong to their favourite food. The most beautiful one is the *Distelfink* – literally 'thistle finch' (goldfinch) with its blood-red face set off by the contrasting white and black and its yellow and black wing markings. When it lands on a ripening thistle head, then the white parachutes – which enable the thistle seeds to disperse – fly about, while the bird eats the seeds themselves with obvious relish.

Things are more sedate when the *Distelfalter* – 'thistle butterfly' (painted lady butterfly) lowers its proboscis into the predominantly purple flowers or lays its eggs on the leaves that serve as food for the caterpillars. Honey bees and bumble bees also visit the flowers and, if we smell them, then we understand the reason. A seductive sweet scent emanates from them, indicating plentiful nectar.

But did you know that we also eat thistles? Artichokes are some of the tallest thistles, and they have pretty much the largest flower buds found in Europe. They are also prickly and hard and even the pollen is armed with spines if we look at it under the microscope. But after sufficient cooking, the base of the stringy prickly scales and the receptacle are deliciously soft and taste bitter and aromatic.

A bitter taste is often a sign of liver action, indicating that these plants

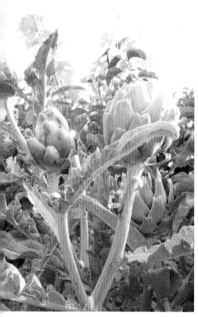

Artichoke plant.

stimulate the – likewise bitter – bile. This is also the case for the artichoke, which is therefore considered to aid digestion and is served as a starter before heavy meals. Increasing the biliary flow can also achieve a slight reduction in the cholesterol level, especially if the resorption of bile acids from the gut is reduced, for example by roughage (which can be found in psyllium or wheat bran) or by using special drugs. The body then needs to produce more bile acids and uses cholesterol to do this (see also chapter 11 on greater celandine).

Another thistle almost as tall as a man is the milk thistle. While most thistles count as weeds, this species is sometimes grown in gardens on account of its attractiveness. Their very large deep green leaves look as though they had been sprinkled with milk and, unlike the other (mostly flat) leaves, have an immense regular three-dimensional form. Like all thistles, it appreciates compacted soil, which its roots are able to break up.

As thistles like sun and warmth, they become rarer in the cool north. It was therefore a minor sensation when a milk thistle appeared in the middle of a cow pasture on a Norwegian island. A fence was put around it to protect the botanical rarity. However, the following year it appeared just outside the fence where the stamping hooves of the cows had dug up the soil. It almost seemed as though this proud plant was ready to defend itself and did not like to be locked in.

The milk thistle has been valued as a liver remedy since ancient times. Like aniseed, caraway or fennel, the seeds of the milk thistle are used medicinally. The former, which are from the fruits of umbellifers, are aromatic. The milk thistle fruits have almost no smell (but taste bitter) and, as far as I know, they are the only seeds from a plant in the daisy family which are used medicinally.

Plant remedies are generally considered to have a relatively mild effect and only a few have found a place in modern medicine. You would therefore not really expect to find a drug that comes from a native plant in an intensive care unit. Apart from this, it is only medicines obtained

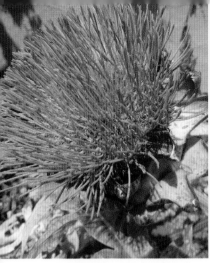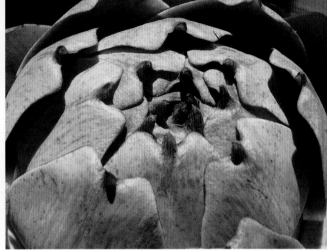

The magnificent purple of flowering artichokes is visible from afar.

The artichoke – bud of a thistle flower.

from the foxglove for treating the heart which have succeeded in penetrating to this centre of technical medicine. However, specialist literature repeatedly recommends using a remedy made from milk thistle fruits for *poisoning by amanita* (an inedible mushroom which causes the greatest number of fatal mushroom poisonings) and this is claimed to reduce the mortality rate significantly. It is more common to use milk thistle preparations for less dramatic liver damage. It has been shown experimentally that it reduces the absorption of some poisons by the liver cells and can stimulate *liver regeneration*. Hundreds of years ago the milk thistle enjoyed a reputation for having a beneficial effect on sclerosis of the liver accompanied by increased development of connective tissue fibres (*cirrhosis of the liver*). It must be pointed out that no large-scale studies have been carried out to conclusively decide how efficacious this remedy is. However, reduced mortality was demonstrated using milk thistle in one study. Moreover, positive experiences have nevertheless been reported in modern times for this disease, which is hard to treat.

An interesting point is that both scientifically based herbal medicine (phytotherapy) and homeopathy and anthroposophical medicine, use this plant in similar ways. Other thistles such as the cotton thistle are also used medicinally. These too often decorate gardens.

In terms of the doctrine of signatures, it is interesting that a plant family which grows so preferentially on hard compacted soils and is itself so characterised by hardening that it makes prickles, can help to counteract excessive hardening processes in us. As so often in life, something which

185

at first appears unappealing and annoying can have unexpected positive sides, which only appear when we have overcome our initial emotional reaction and approach it with attentiveness and interest.

Thistles

Artichoke (Cynara scolymus)

There is a tincture of artichoke by the name of *Cynara scolymus* (Mother Tincture) made by Ceres. I prescribe 5 drops of this 3 times a day to stimulate the production of bile and hence *reduce cholesterol*. The mother tinctures made by Ceres go through a milling process in a granite mill akin to the chewing process of cows. This results in a particularly thorough breakdown of the plant material so that smaller amounts than normal are usually adequate.

More frequently, artichoke preparations are prescribed as sugar-coated tablets, like Cefacynar, Cholagogum, etc.

As the body uses cholesterol to produce bile acids, the cholesterol reducing action can be heightened when, in addition to stimulating bile production with artichoke, the reabsorption of bile acids from the gut is impeded. In orthodox medicine this is achieved, for example, using the synthetic resin cholestyramine. Anyone wishing to find a natural alternative can eat more apples as their pectin (also used to set jams) has a similar effect. You can also make use of the fact that the seed coats of psyllium – a species of plantain – bind bile acids in the intestine. These seed coats are also used to *regulate digestion*. A remedy specifically for lowering raised cholesterol levels is called Mucofalk Fit.

Besides the fact that artichoke preparations stimulate the production of bile and thus lower the *cholesterol* level, they also inhibit the formation of new cholesterol to a certain extent. This means the total cholesterol level can be lowered by about one fifth. Moreover an improvement in the ratio between LDL cholesterol (which is bad for a tendency to arteriosclerosis) and HDL cholesterol (which actually helps reduce deposits in the blood vessels) can be achieved. Artichoke extracts are also thought to be useful for reducing the oxidation of blood lipids. Oxidised fats have an increased tendency to

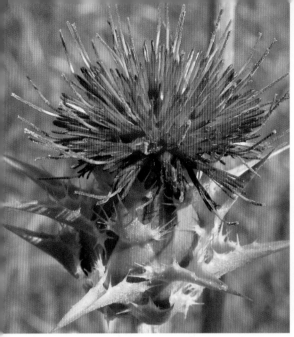
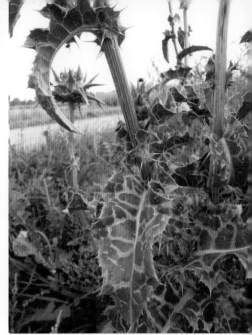

Milk thistle.

A typical characteristic of the milk thistle is its very sculptured white-veined leaves.

form deposits. However, the measures described may be inadequate in cases of serious hereditary lipid metabolism diseases, which is why individual professional advice is always necessary in this case.

Milk thistle

(Called *Carduus marianus* under the old pharmaceutical name; the current *Silybum marianum* corresponds to the botanical nomenclature.)

Like the artichoke, milk thistle is often used as a concentrated phytotherapeutic preparation in the form of sugar-coated tablets. The usual dose is 1 tablet containing at least 150 mg of Silymarin 3 times daily. Trade names for this are Legalon, Silymarin, etc. Carduus marianus capsules (Weleda) are good quality but somewhat less concentrated, so a correspondingly higher quantity (usually 2 capsules 3 times daily) must be taken.

These remedies are used in cases of a *fatty liver* due to excessive consumption of alcohol, the effects of medicines, lipid metabolism disorders and chronic virus infections of the liver (hepatitis B and C). For a fatty liver, besides taking milk thistle, it is usually necessary to reduce the quantity of quickly exploitable carbohydrates (especially

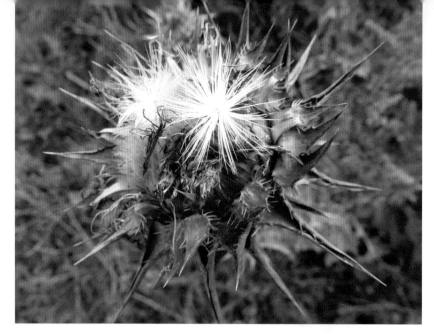

Just like the seeds of the dandelion, those of the milk thistle can be dispersed by the wind with the help of a little umbrella (pappus). These seeds are made into an effective medicine for the liver.

sugar) and to take more exercise, which will usually result in a decrease in the fatty degeneration of the liver.

Serious poisoning involving liver damage – for example the *amanita poisoning* already mentioned – can improve following administration of milk thistle extracts. The remedies may be injected (for example Legalon Sil dry material for making an infusion). As already mentioned, the mortality rate from amanita poisoning has decreased significantly due to this treatment. Naturally a situation as serious as this requires careful supervision, often in intensive care.

A more everyday use of *Carduus marianus capsules* (Weleda) or similar preparations is to improve *liver function* in various diseases such as *acne, inflammatory bowel diseases, chronic rheumatic diseases* and *depression* connected to a malfunction of the liver. In many cases, improving the liver function can bring relief from the diseases mentioned. For mild liver disorders it is worth trying to relieve these by chewing milk thistle seeds which are available in the pharmacy. Chew a small quantity of seeds several times a day.

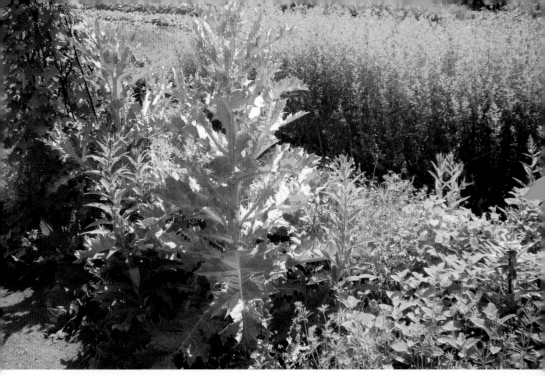

Cotton thistle.

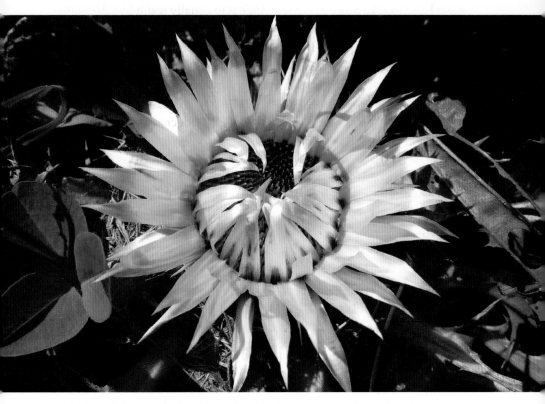

The beautiful carline thistle which is found in the Alps was used in folk medicine in earlier times for influenza, and shepherds ate its receptacles like artichokes. The plant is now protected and the hiker can only enjoy looking at it.

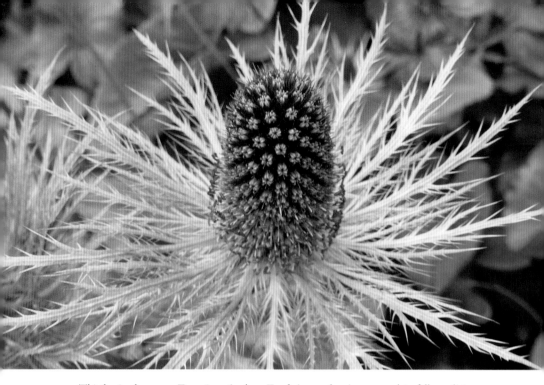

Thistles in the genus Eryngium (such as E. alpinum *here) were used in folk medicine in many regions – for instance, by the native Americans and in Turkey. They tend to be grown nowadays for their attractive appearance.*

Potentised milk thistle

Apart from amanita poisoning, which requires massive doses of the Carduus, for all the other diseases mentioned above it can also be used in potentised form. Milk thistle is available as ampoules and globules as *Carduus marianus e fructibus* D3 (Wala), of which I prescribe 5 globules 3 times daily, occasionally combining this with concentrated phytotherapeutic preparations. I sometimes get the impression that these different types of application can be mutually beneficial.

There is a composite remedy – *Carduus marianus/Oxalis* globuli and ampoules (Wala) – which combines milk thistle and wood sorrel. This remedy has had good results in *heartburn*, which is caused by insufficient closure of the entry to the stomach at the level of the diaphragm (*hiatus hernia*). This remedy may also be helpful for gall stone complaints.

Carduus marianus/Viscum Mali comp. (Wala) as globules or ampoules can be used as a concomitant treatment for patients with cancer (particularly those involving the liver) and also for *chronic*

190

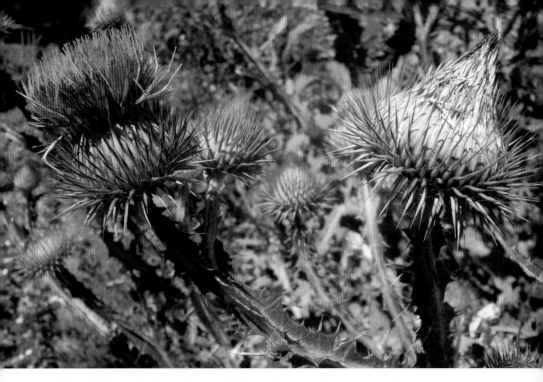

The prickly, purple-flowered cotton thistle is almost as tall as a man and in Cardiodoron *provides the polar ingredient to the cowslip.*

hepatitis (which can turn into liver cancer when prolonged over many years). This remedy combines milk thistle, mistletoe and an organ preparation of the liver in a potentised form.

Reference should also be made in passing to the magnificent cotton thistle *(Onopordum acanthium)* which was mentioned in Chapter 8 on the cowslip, as it is an important component of the heart remedy Cardiodoron (see page 85). The blessed thistle, or St Benedict's thistle *(Carduus* or *Cnicus benedictus)* is recommended in several tea recipes in this book for use in bitter digestive tea mixtures. In contrast to the previously mentioned purple-flowered thistles, the blessed thistle has relatively small yellow flowers. In anthroposophical pharmacy this plant is used in combination with the peony as Carduus benedictus D2/Paeonia officinalis D2 ampoules (Weleda) for symptoms of *congestion around the liver* and portal vein.

191

CHAPTER 19

Coneflower, Echinacea

Most of the plants we have studied so far are common in Central Europe. However, nowadays many medicinal plants are cultivated far from their native homes. Industry puts great efforts into research programmes to unearth buried medicinal treasures from remote cultures in order to extract medicines from them. (This has been done for cancer drugs for a long time. Many substances which originally came from rainforest plants are now synthetically produced). How wise this is has been disputed for hundreds of years. Around 450 years ago, the great physician Paracelsus expressed the opinion that at each place God made everything grow which was needed to treat the diseases which occur at that place. In those days good business was made trading in South American plants which were used for treating syphilis which was spreading at the time. Paracelsus believed that this plague, which destroyed countless lives, had arisen from degenerate behaviour in Europe and therefore had to be combated using local remedies. Nowadays it can be stated with a fair degree of certainty that the organism responsible for this plague was brought to Europe by Christopher Columbus' sailors, where it spread at a terrific speed.[1] In this matter Paracelsus was mistaken. But perhaps he was not entirely wrong, as even back then it was known that the natives of South America possessed herbal remedies for this plague, which helped them to control this dreadful disease. However, these medicinal plants did not appear to have displayed the same efficacy in Europe as in their land of origin and it often appeared to benefit the traders more than the sufferers, something that infuriated the pugnacious Paracelsus.

Just how careful you need to be when transferring medicinal plant knowledge from one culture to another was brought home to me years

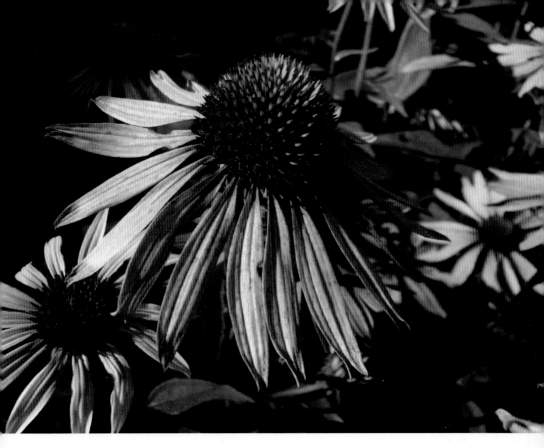

The flower of Echinacea looks like a hedgehog.

ago when I was trekking with a botanist guide in the border region between Nepal and Tibet. He showed me a species of wormwood and explained that in his tribe, the Tamang, this was good for stomach ache, but in the neighbouring Sherpa tribe it was poisonous. Thus, one must ask whether a Tibetan medicinal plant expert should indiscriminantly prescribe medicines which have proven themselves in Tibet to Europeans.

On the other hand, living conditions nowadays are probably more alike in New York and Berlin than they were in regions a few hundred kilometres apart two hundred years ago, which is why we take account of medical research results from other countries.

One medicinal plant whose use has spread with great success across the world is the American coneflower, which tends to be known by its scientific name, Echinacea. If I talk about *one* medicinal plant here, this is not quite correct. At least three species of Echinacea are used medicinally: the purple coneflower *(E. purpurea),* the pale purple coneflower *(E. pallida)* and the narrow-leaved purple coneflower *(E. angustifolia)*. All have stimulating effects on the immune system, although they have rather different constituents. In the older literature it is seldom possible to know which species is being referred to. In what follows I will therefore usually refer simply to 'Echinacea' although I am aware of the lack of distinction this entails.

At the end of the nineteenth century, homeopathy – which had been developed in Germany – was extraordinarily successful in the USA. There were large homeopathic hospitals and it was taught at universities. A homeopath by the name of Joseph Meyer apparently watched a Native American woman rubbing an Echinacea root, who told him that it was a proven remedy for treating wounds. The root was said to be essential for some native tribes when out hunting so as to have immediate help at hand for any injuries to prevent them from becoming infected.

After this encounter, use of the prairie plant spread rapidly, not only for the prevention and treatment of infection after injury but also for many other inflammatory diseases caused by pathogens, for boils and throat infections and even for pelvic infections and appendicitis. In the pre-antibiotic era, Echinacea was actually the most frequently used medicinal plant in North America. Varied research was set up on this plant relatively early on which, due to differing results for closely related species, sometimes produced confusing results.

It was observed that, in the presence of Echinacea extracts, phagocytes (cells that protect the body by ingesting harmful foreign particles) in the blood can absorb more disease pathogens than the could without these extracts. From decade to decade, new effects on the immune system were observed, which were able to explain an improvement in the body's defences. Nevertheless, voices were also raised cautioning against the indiscriminate use of Echinacea, as in cases of autoimmune disease (such as polyarthritis), since existing immune system malfunctions could be exacerbated. There are also isolated allergies to the plant.

No one nowadays would want to use Echinacea to treat a serious appendicitis or go without antibiotics in favour of this plant. All the same, many doctors are convinced that extracts and low potencies of Echinacea can relieve or prevent cold symptoms such as *throat infections*. After the combined evaluations of many studies done years ago gave the impression that this empirical knowledge was not to be trusted, in recent years several meta-analyses of all available studies were published in internationally reputable journals. These provided statistical evidence that taking Echinacea reduces *respiratory tract infections* by 1–2 days; in other words, roughly the amount achieved by modern anti-viral drugs for genuine influenza. Used as a prophylactic, Echinacea more than halves the frequency of *coughs* and *colds*.

In 2010 a new double blind study on the treatment of coughs and colds using tablets containing concentrated Echinacea *(purpurea* und *angustifolia)* was published.[2] This was unable to show a statistically significant difference between the administration of a placebo and the real Echinacea preparation. Technically, there was an 89% probability that Echinacea worked better than the placebo, but only a probability greater than 95% counts as being statistically significant. The length of the cold was on average half a day shorter in patients treated with the 'genuine' medication and they displayed somewhat less severe symptoms. The authors were of the opinion that each patient must decide for themselves whether they wish to use Echinacea preparations or not.

Two years later the results of a further – likewise double blind – study on Echinacea were published (the largest study to be carried out to date).[3] Some 755 subjects were randomly assigned to two groups, the first of which received a liquid extract of *Echinacea purpurea* three times daily for four months while the second was given placebo drops which looked and smelled the same. There were 188 cases of colds in the placebo group but only 149 in the group who actually received Echinacea. The number of days of illness was 850 versus 672. Statistical analysis showed that the combination of frequency and length was significantly reduced by the plant extract by 26%. The number of repeated infections was more than halved. If the participants did get a cold, they increased the dosage from three to five times daily. The subjects in the group receiving the actual medicine subsequently needed far fewer conventional medicines such as paracetamol (acetaminophen) or ibuprofen in order to ease the symptoms of any colds they did catch. There was no difference in the number of undesirable side effects in the placebo and verum groups. Although there are a couple of minor weaknesses in this study (e.g. it seems odd that only three of the five authors state that they have no conflict of interest, that they have not, for example, received payments from pharmaceutical manufacturers), it is nevertheless a credible, high-calibre proof of the efficacy of Echinacea, something of which many doctors and patients have been convinced from their own experience.

Besides looking at international journals, it is worth observing the plant itself as it has long since found its way from the prairie into our gardens. It belongs to the daisy family, like many native European medicinal plants. While the native composites we have talked about so far produce a smooth disc in which the individual flowers are combined into a whole, the individual flowers of Echinacea consist of surprisingly hard pointed floret tubes which point in all directions like prickles. The name 'echinacea' comes from the Greek *echinos* meaning 'hedgehog' or 'sea-urchin'. I wonder whether Native Americans recognised that this plant can boost our own defences against foreign intruders from the similarly to this creature (or possibly, the porcupine and its quills which are native to North America). This would fit very well with the philosophy of Paracelsus, who was convinced that we can recognise the efficacy of a plant from its signs or 'signature'.

Echinacea (*Echinacea angustifolia, Echinacea pallida, Echinacea purpurea*)

Phytotherapy

Phytotherapeutic literature states that you can use ½ a teaspoon of the chopped dried plant per cup of water and allow to infuse for 10 minutes to stimulate the immune system in cases of respiratory tract and urinary tract infections. However, this form of application is very unusual, and I have no experience of it.

It is much more common to use preparatory remedies which contain liquid extracts preserved in alcohol (for example Echinacin liquidum (Madaus), Esberitox mono etc.). The extracted and dried juice is processed into an alcohol-free tablet form (Echinacin tablets, Echinacea Stada, etc.). Refer to the package insert for directions for use of these products. As already mentioned, no concentrated Echinacea preparations should be used by those suffering from autoimmune diseases, HIV and other chronic virus infections, tuberculosis and some other diseases.

To treat the onset of *influenza* or for a high risk situation, adults should usually take around 50 drops of the extracted juice 3 times daily and children less, depending on age. The recommended period for taking this is generally a few weeks.

Side effects can arise, especially in the form of rare allergic reactions which may manifest as rashes on the skin or asthma-like symptoms in the lungs.

Homeopathy

In homeopathy, *Echinacea purpurea* is likewise generally used in the form of a mother tincture or at low potencies to build up resistance against *feverish infections.*

Ceres Echinacea mother tincture has also proven efficacious for this purpose and is used at a dose of 5 drops, 3–4 times daily. Basically, the same exclusions and possible side effects apply as mentioned above.

Echinacea for external application

As already mentioned, Echinacea was used externally by the Native Americans for injuries. We also make use of this application: Weleda produces an ointment containing an extract of purple coneflower, *Echinacea purpurea.* This ointment, which contains 10% of the mother tincture, can be applied to *local infections,* for example for *boils.* This should normally be discussed with your doctor, as there are regions of the body (for example the face) where boils can potentially be dangerous.

Wala make an Echinacea essence from *Echinacea pallida.* This is also recommended for *furuncles* or *wounds which do not heal well,* to activate the local defence system. Add 1 or 2 teaspoons of the essence to ¼ litre (1 cup) of water and use in compresses. As a rule, medical advice should be sought for larger boils and wounds that do not heal of their own accord. Qualified advice should also be sought if there is no significant improvement after two days or if pain, raised temperature, lymph node swellings or a reddened area around the wound indicate an infection. The basic principles for treating wounds (for example in terms of sterile procedure or anti-tetanus measures) must be observed.

Composite remedies containing Echinacea are used more frequently than the individual remedy for external treatment (see below).

Allergies to Echinacea occur occasionally, which should be borne in mind if the symptoms become worse when using it for local application.

Pure Echinacea as a remedy

Echinacea angustifolia is supplied by Weleda as a mother tincture (which also enables it to be used phytotherapeutically), in D3 as aqueous drops and at the same potency as ampoules. Wala manufactures *Echinacea pallida* as D3 and D6 in the form of globules and as D2, D3, D6 and D30 as ampoules. Besides *boils* and *poorly healing wounds*, other indications are *influenza, lymph node inflammation* and *inflammation of the female genital area.*

I have the impression that the globules in D3 are suitable for preventing *coughs and colds* particularly if there is a tendency to being chilled. Take 5 globules, 1–3 times daily during periods when infection is particularly likely. For inflammation of the throat and larynx, it has proved beneficial to inject ampoules of the D6 under the skin of the patient's neck and to also administer the potentised organ preparation Larynx Gl D15 (for *laryngitis*) and Pharynx Gl D15 which further increases the efficacy. Echinacea D15 is likewise injected between the shoulder blades for *bronchitis* (along with Bronchi Gl D15 if required). These applications are usually carried out in the doctor's surgery and may then be continued by giving globules orally.

Echinacea in composite medicinal preparations

Echinacea is often combined with marigold (Calendula), a plant commonly found in gardens and which comes from the same *Compositae* or daisy family. This applies to such remedies as Calcea Wund- und Heilcreme (Wala) which is good for treating *wounds at risk of becoming infected* or for *surface skin inflammation* (including for *pressure sores* and their prevention). Apart from minor injuries, treatment of wounds should also be performed with the advice of an experienced practitioner (usually a doctor or nurse).

The above-mentioned plants are also combined in Wecesin powder

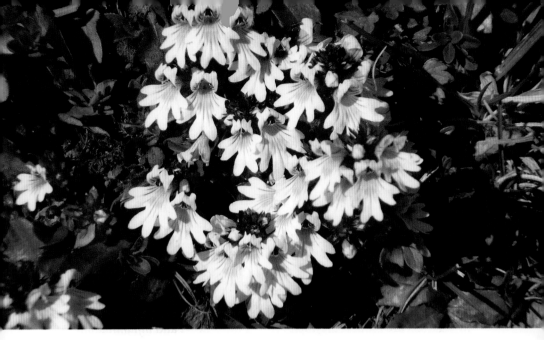

Eyebright (Euphrasia) is suitable for treating non-infectious inflammation of the conjunctiva.

and ointment (Weleda) with the addition of Arnica (a famous plant for wounds and also from the daisy family) and the mineral substances silica and antimony (Stibium metallicum praeparatum) in a finely powdered potentised form. The last-named have a structuring effect on the healing process in wounds. The powder is recommended for drying surface wounds, the ointment is also good for the follow-up care of burns after other acute treatment, for example using Wund- und Brandessenz (Wala) or Combudoron (Weleda). In fact, Echinacea was previously used for treating burns and had an excellent reputation for this.

Wecesin powder also appears to work well time and again for controlling the inflammatory symptoms in the skin during *radiotherapy*. However, the radiotherapist must agree to its use in such cases.

Its use as eye drops is a 'semi-external' one. Due to the sensitivity of the eye, disease symptoms in this area should generally only be self-treated in the short-term. If the symptoms persist (for more than 2 days) or in any case of doubt as to whether it is just a minor condition, a GP or ophthalmologist should always be consulted.

Euphrasia comp. eye ointment (Weleda) has proved effective for *styes* (hordeolum), an inflammation of the small glands at the base of the eyelashes. In addition to eyebright (Euphrasia), this ointment also contains Echinacea and Calendula. *Suppurating conjunctivitis* is often cured by administering Echinacea/Quarz eye drops from Wala (1 drop in the conjunctival sac 2 times daily).

Wala's Mundbalsam flüssig or Mundbalsam Gel are useful as home remedies for local oral mucositis such as *mouth ulcers* or *denture pressure points*. These remedies combine higher potencies of silver nitrate (Argentum nitricum) and deadly nightshade (Belladonna), which have a pain-relieving effect, along with Echinacea to strengthen the body's defences and the structure-forming antimony and silica. The mouth gel should not be used for babies and asthma patients due to the content of potentially irritating essential oils. Denture pressure points often improve quickly if you spread the gel onto the dentures before fitting them; mouth ulcers can be dabbed with the gel. Rinsing with the diluted essence is preferable when larger areas of the oral mucosa are affected. It is very satisfying to see how quickly such annoying conditions can be resolved using this treatment.

In anthroposophical medicine, remedies containing Echinacea are also used in cases of marked symptoms of *inflammation with high fever*. These situations require an experienced therapist who also has to decide when other measures such as surgically lancing an abscess or using an antibiotic are necessary. Examples of medicines which are *not* suitable for self-treatment in my opinion are Argentum D30/Echinacea D6 (Weleda) and Echinacea/Argentum (Wala), and Echinacea/Mercurius suppositories (Wala), all of which often have excellent effects when in the hands of an experienced doctor. They can frequently help to avoid antibiotics. As we now know, they encourage the development of resistant organisms. Moreover, every dose of antibiotics in childhood increases the risk of developing an allergy later in life, or even developing a condition such as asthma.

CHAPTER 20

Lemon balm (Melissa)

After the flush of fruit tree blossom, tulips and dandelions and before roses, delphiniums, phlox and lilies herald the flowery height of summer, there is a pause, a cessation of flowering. For a little while, the world is not all colour and scent – but there is still no need to live without the experience of smell. There is a whole plant family that gives off scent the whole year round; their leaves producing aromas. If we rub the leaves of thyme, sage, marjoram, rosemary or lavender between our fingers and thumb, then scents are set free, the like of which we find only in flowers. All these plants come from the *Labiatae* or *Lamiaceae* family, which includes more medicinal and culinary herbs than all other families. Remarkably, it hardly includes any poisonous plants. It is no surprise that these plants have had a permanent place in monastery and medicinal herb gardens for centuries.

The flowers of most *Labiatae* species are inconspicuous at first. It often takes a magnifying glass to reveal the charm of the flowers which are formed into a tube with complicated pollination organs and lips, giving the family its Latin name *(labia,* meaning 'lips'). In the plant as a whole, the flowers usually disappear totally in the foliage and only in exceptional cases (such as the lavender) do they sit at the end of the shoot. The flowers usually sit close to the stem in the axils of the leaves, which are arranged in regular rhythmical layer upon layer along the shoot.

This can be seen particularly well in the dead nettle, one of the few species with larger and more brightly coloured flowers. In order to 'compensate', so to speak, its leaves are 'dead' and without any characteristic smell. This is in sharp contrast to the stinging nettles: no one would claim that their similarly-shaped leaves lack firepower, although they do not give off much smell.

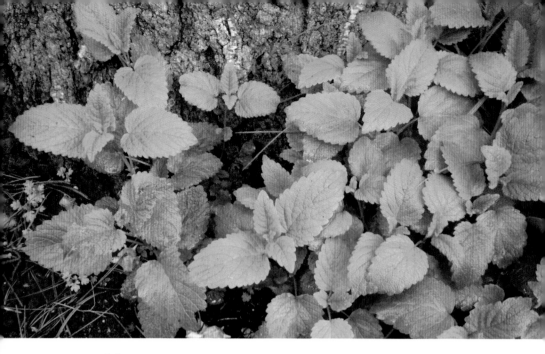

Lemon balm.

The leaf of lemon balm (or melissa) can easily be confused with those of the stinging nettles (which, however, do not belong to the *Labiatae*). It is equally deep green and regularly lobed on the margin. However, while the stinging nettle leaf is sharply serrated, that of the lemon balm is gently wavy. It is worth looking carefully so that you avoid stinging your hand, because you need to rub the foliage between thumb and finger in order to get close to its character.

What a scent is released! On the one hand it is really fresh, like lemon, which is why the plant is called lemon balm. On the other hand, it has a warm undertone that is difficult to describe, something the lemon does not have. While the main experience with the scent of lemon is an awakening light, in melissa warmth and light appear to be in balance with each other. Perhaps this is why it has such an emotionally balancing effect. This is what melissa is famed for: it has always been considered as relaxing as it is enlivening. Anyone who cannot go to sleep at night because too much is going round in their head would do well to drink a cup of melissa tea. Also, if too much stress has upset your stomach, then this kind of tea can help, although it is sometimes useful to add a couple of leaves of peppermint. Lemon balm can also be useful for more serious disorders. Melissa oil (for example in an ointment applied to the lips) can be effective in treating *herpes* and other viruses. A little while ago a study even showed that melissa has a noticeable effect on *Alzheimer's disease.* It can also produce a relaxing effect in this case and reduce the agitation and restiveness which are sometimes such a serious problem with this disease.

In such cases, melissa can help to cut down on the use of neuroleptics, psychotropic drugs which are otherwise used for serious mental illnesses such as schizophrenia. They are often unavoidable for treating the latter but can have serious side effects, especially in older patients. We can only be thankful that a plant like melissa can at least help some patients. Particularly as there are no known side effects from its use to date.

Melissa not only has a relaxing effect, but also appears to have a positive influence on the course of the disease itself by delaying it and producing a degree of improvement in memory and the ability to concentrate.[1] Even if no miracle can be expected from this, I am grateful for any help for those affected and their relatives in such difficult circumstances.

Lemon balm or melissa has enjoyed such a persistently good reputation in medicine for hundreds of years. But why is it that new areas of application are still being discovered, although it does not contain any highly active substances which are poisonous at high doses? Unlike many other medicinal plants, it has so far not been possible to trace the effects of melissa back to an 'active substance' which could be isolated or manufactured synthetically. Perhaps the plant as a whole has a therapeutic effect. It may be possible to get closer to an answer if you look for a 'gesture' characterising the plant. It appears to me as though melissa incorporates flower qualities in its vigorous foliage which seem to be completely connected with the vitality of the leaf. What it means when a plant clearly separates these two principles is shown impressively by the Agave, a member of the lily family, which we usually know only from its fleshy, blue-green thorny-edged leaves (which can withstand drought and strong sunlight). For several years there is nothing to be seen but leaves, until, at some point, a massive shoot grows out of their centre with an ornate scented inflorescence at its end. When this impressive miracle of a flower is over, the leaves appear to be sucked dry and lie withered and dead on the ground. The plant has completely exhausted itself in flowering, which speaks so keenly to our hearts.

The same applies to many herbs, though in a less spectacular

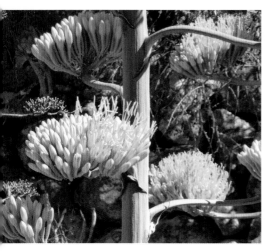

Agave has large flower buds which encapsulate its whole vitality.

manner. They reach the peak of their existence in flowering and then die. In contrast, melissa is perennial, sprouting anew every spring over several decades – and if you split the gradually spreading plant in the garden, you will find that this rejuvenates it.

Even if the flowers of the melissa appear somewhat reduced, they are still of interest to bees. Their very name – which comes from the Greek *mélissa*, ('honeybee') which in turn comes from *méli* ('honey') – shows that they provide a valuable source of nectar for bees. But there again, it seems as though bees are already attracted by the fragrant leaf. In any case, if you rub new beehives with melissa leaves, the bee colony will feel attracted to the new home.

If you want to state very generally what melissa is good for, then you could mention *nervousness*, a condition in which an overexcited psychological state threatens to produce organic breakdown. In this plant a flower-like perfume arises in the luxuriant green foliage. It is as if its fragrant quality and its vital, organic life-forces mutually enhance each other, rather than one being sacrificed to the other. We thus understand how it can help in cases of *nervous exhaustion*.

Melissa/Lemon balm (*Melissa officinalis*)

There is a place for lemon balm in almost every garden (or in a tub or window box). It is one of the oldest medicinal plants cultivated in Europe and no monastery garden has been without it, monks carrying it long distances to newly founded distant monasteries. It flourishes on most soils and likes plenty of sunshine. It is often necessary to cut it back so that it does not spread out too much. The shoots should be harvested in June shortly before flowering, tied together and hung upside down to dry.

Phytotherapy and aromatherapy

To make melissa tea, add 2 teaspoons of the dried leaves to 1 cup of boiling water and allow to infuse for at least 5 minutes. This tea is suitable for slight *restlessness* or *problems with sleep* or *insomnia*. Melissa can be mixed with lavender flowers and hop cones to achieve a sleep-inducing effect. Pure melissa tea is also beneficial for *stomach upset, flatulence* and *mild menstrual pains*. For relieving stomach and intestinal complaints, melissa can be mixed with chamomile and peppermint, while a mixture with yarrow and silverweed is suitable for relieving menstrual cramps.

A relaxing bath additive can be prepared like a strong melissa tea. Pour 1 litre (quart) of boiling water over 20–25 g (1 oz) of dried melissa and leave covered for 10 minutes before adding the strained liquid to a full bath (not above 37°C, 99°F). Oil dispersion baths with melissa oil are discussed later in this chapter.

A relatively large number of ready-made phytotherapeutic products contain extracts of melissa. For example, Iberogast – which contains melissa along with chamomile flowers, milk thistle, caraway, angelica root and other herbs – has proved beneficial for *stomach complaints* and *irritable bowel syndrome*. A pure melissa preparation for the treatment of 'nervous' gastrointestinal conditions goes under the name of Gastrovegetalin, and is available as capsules or a solution. Naturally, in all cases where symptoms do not resolve within a few days or are unusually severe, a medical diagnosis is essential.

Spirit of Melissa is widely used for ordinary *digestive complaints* and as a mildly relaxing remedy. As my experience is primarily with the Melissa comp. (Weleda), this will be discussed on page 209.

Finally, aromatherapy can be seen as a variation of phytotherapy. Melissa can help greatly with the difficult problem of treating restless patients suffering from dementia. A double blind study showed that local application of melissa oil in a skin lotion produced a significant improvement for symptoms of restlessness in patients suffering from advanced *dementia*. In this study the care-givers rubbed the face and arms of restless patients with a small quantity of a lotion containing 10% melissa oil several times daily, so that around 200 mg of the essential oil was applied per day. There were no observed side effects from the

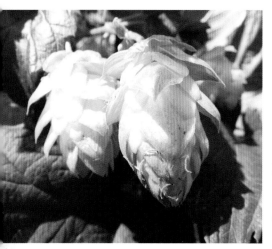

Hop cones, which are often used along with Melissa for sleep disturbances.

application of melissa oil (besides one patient suffering from diarrhoea for two days, which in my opinion may not have been a specific effect of melissa), in contrast to the customary treatment with sedative suppressant drugs which increase the risk of falling, and in older patients may also have a secondary action on the heart and circulation.[2]

A further double blind study with 114 participants who had 10% melissa oil rubbed into their arms and legs twice daily confirms this result. A significant improvement in quality of life took place in the group treated with aromatherapy, which was higher in those patients treated with melissa than in the group who received a chemical medication for dementia (Donepezil). However, in this study there were no observable specific effects on a series of parameters due to melissa, although it obviously did the patients good to be regularly massaged with the oil.[3] The data supporting the possibility of treating restlessness and behavioural disturbances in patients with dementia with aromatherapy has now been confirmed by meta-analysis.[4] This has now led to the specific recommendation by Professor Alexander Kurz, one of the best-known researchers in dementia in Germany, for the 'calming effect of aromatic distillates of lavender, lemon balm, rose and other plants for patients with advanced dementia.'[5]

Homeopathy

Melissa is used very rarely in homeopathy and then exclusively as mother tincture or in low potencies. The areas of application do not differ from those mentioned above (for phytotherapy). It should be mentioned, however, that Ceres Melissa mother tincture officially counts as a homeopathic preparation. I use this remedy from time to time with good effect for dementia patients, particularly when they or the people around them are suffering due to their symptoms of restlessness. In this remedy a particularly good extraction is achieved by a type of grinding process in a granite mill, so that often low doses (for example 3– 5 drops several times a day) are adequate.

In connection with this I would again like to point out the work of the group around Professor Akhondzadeh which, in a clinically controlled study, showed that a daily dose of 60 drops of a melissa extract significantly decreased restlessness in patients suffering from *Alzheimer dementia* and a slight improvement in memory function took place.[6]

Anthroposophical medicine

Naturally all the previously mentioned applications of lemon balm or melissa are used by anthroposophical doctors. In addition to these there is a series of specifically anthroposophical melissa preparations.

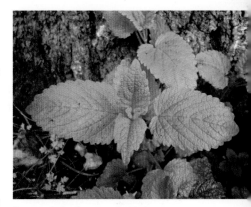

Lemon balm leaves are rich in copper and display a 'feminine' signature.

Melissa grown on soil fertilised with copper

Looking at the gently lobed melissa leaf we get the impression of a 'feminine' gesture – more so if we compare the leaf with the sharply serrated stinging nettle. Whilst the stinging nettle shows a relationship to iron (see Chapter 28 on the stinging nettle), melissa is related to copper, the metal which has been seen as 'feminine' since ancient times. There is actually a measurably higher proportion of copper in the blood of women than men, whilst this is the other way round for iron. Therapeutically, copper has a warming, relaxing

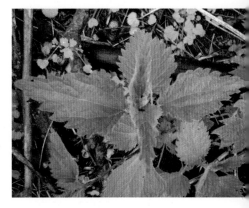

Stinging nettle leaves contain a lot of iron and appear 'masculine'.

207

antispasmodic effect, as does melissa. If this plant is grown on soil fertilised with copper, Melissa Cupro culta (Weleda) is obtained. The manufacturing process is described in more detail in Chapter 28. This remedy is available as an alcoholic drop preparation in D2 and D3 and as a rhythmised aqueous medicine in D3 as drops and in D2 and D3 as ampoules.

Melissa Cupro culta Rh D3 has proved very efficacious for *stomach colics*, which afflict both babies and those around them in their first three months of life ('three-month colic'). Besides administering medication, if babies cannot stop crying it is often helpful to pay attention to whether they are overtired or simply stressed because you believe that you have to do something to calm them down, while it would actually be more helpful to behave calmly yourself. The 'copper melissa' is particularly helpful for babies who do not produce much warmth, are delicate and not very forceful. They give the impression of passively enduring things that happen to them. It is different with babies whose colic responds to Chamomilla or Chamomilla Cupro culta (see Chapter 12 on chamomile). These children appear strong and forceful, often cry shrilly and persistently and tend to appear angry. The gentler 'melissa children' usually quickly obtain relief if they are given 3–5 drops of the non-alcoholic Melissa Cupro culta Rh D3 3 times daily.

In adult life *cramping pains in the abdomen*, particularly *menstrual pains* (dysmenorrhoea) and *flatulence*, can be relieved with Melissa Cupro culta D3 or Rh D3 (10–15 drops 3 times daily). Again, those patients who suffer passively tend to be helped by melissa, while those who are irritable and demanding obtain relief from the corresponding chamomile preparation.

Other anthroposophical melissa preparations

Colic and *flatulence* also benefit from Melissa Oil (Weleda) which, in addition to melissa, contains an oil extract of marjoram and essential oils of caraway and fennel. All these plants are known to reduce flatulence and relieve spasm. It has proved efficacious to rub the oil onto the stomach slowly and gently in a clockwise direction (the same direction in which the contents of the gut are transported).

Olive oil to which pure melissa has been added (Melissa ex herba W

5% Oleum, Wala) is used for oil dispersion baths. When finely dispersed in the bath water using an oil dispersion device (see page 134), the oil settles on the immersed skin like a coat. It has been shown that significant quantities of the essential plant oil are absorbed into the bloodstream through the skin. A melissa oil bath like this has a relaxing and sleep-inducing effect. It can be helpful for difficulty in falling asleep and inner restlessness. It has also been reported that this remedy is good for pelvic complaints in women (e.g. during *menstruation*) and for mild digestive problems, something I have not yet tested myself. Based on the above-mentioned research results (endnotes 3–5) it seems worthwhile using a bath of this kind for dementia patients. I have no personal experience of this to date, although there are very good reports of these type of baths for restless children, for example, those with *ADHD* (attention deficit hyperactivity disorder), or also in cases of handicap (for example due to *infantile cerebral damage* or *autism*).

A composite remedy containing melissa is Melissa/Phosphorus comp. (Weleda). This is used for menstrual disorders and is described in more detail in Chapter 9 on the pasque flower.

Finally I should mention the Melissa comp. (Weleda). This comprises a distillate of melissa leaves, nutmeg, cinnamon bark and small amounts of angelica root, cloves and lemon oil. Melissengeist or Spirit of Melissa is a common home remedy for such varied symptoms as *gastrointestinal complaints* after a heavy meal, a *tendency to faint*, *menstrual problems* and even *toothache*. The relaxing effect of melissa is as effective as the regulating and stimulating effect of the other ingredients on the digestive system. In an emergency situation this remedy is in fact often a good and proven first measure. 10–15 drops should be taken in a little water or on sugar. However, it must be noted that this preparation contains 63% alcohol, which can soon lead to problems with repeated use. I would therefore advise against using it for a prolonged period.

CHAPTER 21

Rosemary

Rosemary entered my life when I was seven years old. Until then my mother's cooking had been defined by the herbs of the north: dill came with cucumber salad, caraway on the potatoes, lovage in soup. But then we travelled to Italy for the first time. It was an overwhelming experience. A superabundance of sun, heat and salty sea, but above all an ever-present scent from the maquis – the aromatic dry shrub heath made up of Cistus, bay, cork oak and rosemary – which surrounded our little holiday house.

It was an experience for me as a small boy simply to go out and pick a handful of rosemary leaves from the bush with pale blue flowers and bring these back to the kitchen where they were chopped up and added to the tomato sauce. I have to admit that the 'pine needles' in the food took a bit of getting used to. But from the start I welcomed the new, aromatic and slightly bitter taste, which then became irrevocably linked to the memory of the holiday – and opened my heart to the south for all time.

By the way, rosemary was not the only bitter plant that expanded my diet from that time onwards. The bittersweet lettuce also became one of my favourite foods, something that surprised me, because up until then I had found it revolting and inedible. But I quickly worked out the explanation: it was a sure sign that I was now grown up – after all, I was already going to school.

Incidentally, rosemary could be very useful in the classroom. A study showed that the scent of rosemary increases the powers of recall (in contrast to lavender, which is actually not so surprising, as the latter is supposed to promote sleep).[1] Maybe Shakespeare also knew about the memory enhancing effect of this plant, because towards

210

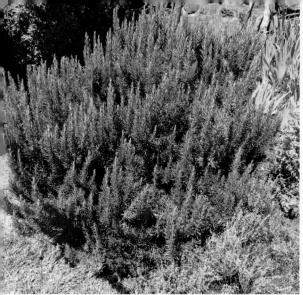
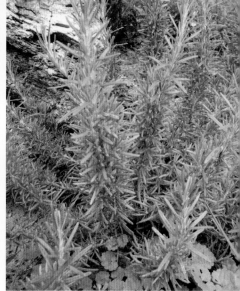

Rosemary plant.

the end of Hamlet he has Ophelia say: 'There's rosemary, that's for remembrance... and there is pansies, that's for thoughts.'

Whether rosemary really protects against *Alzheimer's dementia*, as has been reported in the press from time to time, definitely needs further research before it can be viewed as fact. However, it is well documented that the constituents of rosemary combat the development of 'free radicals', which appear to be involved in this and a number of other brain diseases.

A better established link is the one between a culinary pleasure and a medicinal effect. When barbecuing meat, the formation of carcinogenic nitrosamines is prevented if the meat is first rubbed with rosemary. This is also related to the binding of free radicals, something that helps fats mixed with rosemary to be kept longer without going rancid. This knowledge has been used in hot countries for centuries.

Other effects can be experienced directly and can be recognised without a chemistry laboratory and painstaking research. You only need to rub a few of the aromatic, contracted needle-like leaves between finger and thumb and then breathe in to find what a stimulating and awakening effect rosemary has. A quick rosemary bath or washing with an extract of rosemary can help to get going better in the morning. It is repeatedly reported that people with *low blood pressure* and constant *tiredness* find rosemary helpful. On the other hand, used as an oil extract or additive to an ointment it has a warming and circulatory enhancing effect on the areas treated. It is as though it absorbs some

211

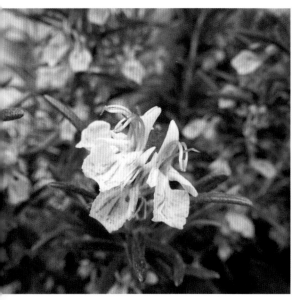

Rosemary flower.

of the sun's power and makes it available again, providing relief for *muscle pain and tension*. The germicidal effect of rosemary oil, which was one of the reasons that rosemary water used to be used for treating wounds, can also be seen as conveying the powers of the sunlight, which is able to kill many pathogens. A number of plants from the same family to which rosemary belongs, the *Labiatae* or *Lamiaceae* – such as sage, but above all thyme – contain similar disinfectant essential oils. There are even laboratories which can determine which essential oils the bacteria present in a wound or the urinary tract are particularly sensitive to in individual patients, similar to what is done for individual antibiotics. If the latter is known as an 'antibiogramme', then the efficacy of essential oils can be studied in an 'aromagramme'. Rosemary oil is frequently found to be one of the most efficacious essential oils.

However, rosemary has a completely different effect, which is not so easy to guess. Almost a century ago Rudolf Steiner mentioned in a lecture that rosemary can help in relieving *diabetes*.[2] It would appear that this applies primarily to what is known as adult-onset diabetes. It has now been repeatedly shown that rosemary can actually delay the uptake of carbohydrates from the intestine and therefore results in a slower rise in blood sugar levels after eating, which can help with this disease, which is becoming more and more common. The pungent rosemary further 'activates' the patient – it stimulates an interest in activities and movement – and this can be an additional help. In any case, anthroposophical doctors (including myself) repeatedly observe perceptible improvements using rosemary extract if the diabetes is not too serious. Naturally an attempt of this kind must be carefully supervised. However, you can only marvel on the one hand at what a useful aid an apparently simple culinary herb can be. At the same time, I am always impressed at how much Rudolf Steiner recognised from his own perception and without complex laboratory tests.

Rosemary (*Rosmarinus officinalis*)

Rosemary growing in a sunny spot in your own garden or a few twigs brought back from holidays in the Mediterranean is suitable as a culinary herb, but the dried leaves can also be used medicinally.

Rosemary tea

Allow 1–2 teaspoons of rosemary to one cup of boiling water and leave to infuse covered for 10 minutes. The bitter aromatic tea can be drunk for *digestive problems* (particularly after a heavy meal) or for *low blood pressure*.

Rosemary used internally

Rosmarinus, Infusum 5%, D3 and D4 are available from Weleda as ampoules. They are a potentised form of rosemary tea and are used as a complementary therapy for *diabetes*. I have found that a strong alcohol extract of 10 % rosemary gives better results for this indication. This can be obtained as Rosmarinus recens D1 from the Weleda pharmacy or made yourself by mixing 25 g (1 oz) rosemary leaves which have been crushed in a mortar with 250 ml (1 fl oz) 45% alcohol from the pharmacy or a good brandy. Shake the liquid several times a day for 2 weeks and then strain it through a clean cloth. Wring out the leaves left in the cloth to increase the rosemary content. I generally prescribe 10 drops of the solution before each meal. Do not expect miracles for *diabetes*, but I often observe a distinctly improved and better stabilised metabolism if rosemary is taken in addition to other therapeutic measures. It is always recommended to discuss this with the attending doctor and monitor blood sugar regularly.

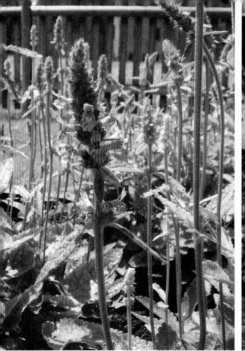
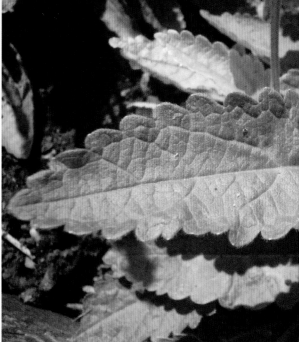

Wood betony (Stachys officinalis) *is found in many monastery gardens. Prepared in combination with rosemary, this upright plant is helpful for treating spinal complaints.*

The leaves of betony are strikingly regularly sinuate.

An antidiabetic effect using rosemary extracts has also been shown in laboratory animals (diabetic rabbits).[3]

One of the many remedies indicated by Rudolf Steiner (which at first seem difficult to understand, because there are no examples of such use in orthodox medicine, but are nevertheless of astonishing efficacy) is Betonica D3/Rosmarinus D3 (Weleda) normally only available as ampoules, but can be purchased as drops direct from Weleda. Steiner stated that this remedy can be helpful for *neuroparalyses* due to the displacement of vertebrae. Indeed, rosemary is sometime successfully used for adjunctive treatment of paralysis and for treating *muscular complaints*. *Betonica officinalis,* betony or wood betony, has almost disappeared from modern books on herbal medicine. This was not always the case; in the Middle Ages it was a highly esteemed plant to which a variety of healing properties were ascribed. So this is obviously a case of our knowledge declining over time. In the ancient world, Musa, the personal physician to Caesar Augustus, wrote a whole book entitled *De Herba Betonica*. I can only comment here that betony comes from the same *Labiatae* family as rosemary and is

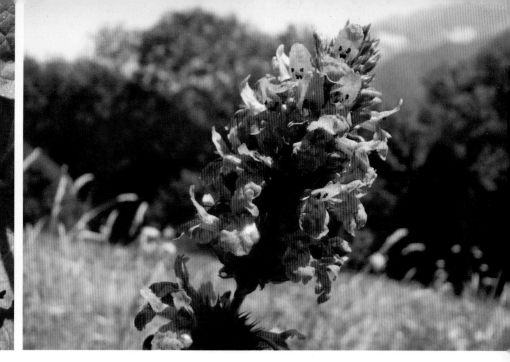

If you look closely at the flowers you will see that betony comes from the same family (the Labiatae) as rosemary.

noticeable due to is marked uprightness and the regularity of its lobed leaves. Betony is also frequently found in monastery gardens. I have repeatedly been able to alleviate or even completely cure longstanding back pain using the combination of Betonica and rosemary, if the condition was caused by 'displacements' e.g. after an earlier *whiplash* or other *back injury.* The experienced orthopaedic specialists Dr Michael Hübner and Dr Reinhard Jeserschek have also observed good effects using this remedy for conditions arising from *poor posture* in children and adolescents and for rotation of the spinal column (*torsion scoliosis*).

Rosemary in external application

Rosemary is used in a great variety of ways externally. These range from oil dispersion baths, to a pure aroma treatments (for example using aroma lamps), to rosemary ointments and oils which are applied to the skin.

Many remedies contain rosemary oil because it stabilises the preparation and prevents microbial contamination or actually creates an antibacterial effect in the area of application. This applies to Rosmarinus/Prunus comp. Gel (Wala), for example, which is used for *chronic inflammation and itching in the genital and anal areas.*

A young man once came to me for treatment who had been to see many specialists and attended several clinics. He was suffering from severe pain which had had an adverse affect on his life for a number of years. The pain was located in the lower back and at times radiated down into the legs. The patient's last treatment had involved morphine and antidepressants which had made him unable to work due to being unfit to drive. At first I too was unsuccessful in achieving any substantial improvement, and it was only after I had noticed a slight rotation of the spinal column and given daily subcutaneous injections of Betonica D3/Rosmarinus D3 that a relatively rapid improvement began. Analgesics were no longer required and the patient was able to return to work after a few weeks. The remedy was then administered only twice a week and finally the man became completely pain free.

The awakening effect of rosemary and its ability to stimulate the circulation and improve memory can be used therapeutically by adding a few drops of Rosemary Invigorating Bath Milk (Weleda) or Rosemary Bath (Dr Hauschka) to the washing water. Although it requires more effort, taking an oil dispersion bath with Rosmarinus Ol. aetherol. 10% (Wala) has more lasting effects. These kinds of rosemary baths can also help to improve the state of mind in chronic muscular diseases and also for exhaustion symptoms. Rosemary baths and washes have also helped to reduce various types of paralysis.

A longer-lasting effect from the scent of rosemary can be achieved by adding a few drops of essential oil to the water in an aroma lamp. However, care should be taken not to let the water evaporate completely because unpleasant oxidation products from the essential oil are then produced. Another way to have a continuous effect of the smell of rosemary is to rub in Rosmarinus Ol. aetherol. 10% (Wala) diluted with olive oil in equal to double parts. Even adding a few drops of essential oil of rosemary to the conditioner compartment in the washing machine makes the rosemary scent in the clothes have a more lasting effect during the day. This can be helpful for a tendency to tiredness and poor memory.

It has already been mentioned that healthy people show better powers of recall when exposed to the smell of rosemary. A Japanese research team studying a large number of *Alzheimer* patients has now demonstrated that their orientation and memory improved when they were given aromatherapy treatments with rosemary and lemon in the morning and lavender and orange in the evening.[4] It is probable that, besides the effect of the aroma, the regular application had helped to stabilise their sense of time in the rhythm of the day.

The antidiabetic effect mentioned is also achieved by external application. The development of these oil dispersion baths originated in the 1920s based on a recommendation by Rudolf Steiner who suggested using a fine dispersion of rosemary oil in water for *diabetes*.[5] At the time nothing was known about the antidiabetic effect of rosemary, but an extensive scientific database has now been built up. Generally the oil dispersion baths are carried out 1–2 times per week using Rosmarinus, Ol. aetherol. 10% (Wala), after which it is very important to rest for about half an hour.

In *gestational diabetes* good results have been found (in the gynaecological department of the Richterswil hospital near Zurich, for example) by putting some rosemary bath milk (Weleda) on a damp facecloth and using this to rub in in the mornings. It should be mentioned that, due to possible negative effects of ongoing hyperglycaemia on the unborn child, diabetes in a pregnant mother needs to be very carefully monitored.

Essential oil of rosemary has a stimulating effect on the circulation if it is applied directly to the skin. This effect is used when Rosmarin-Salbe (Weleda) is rubbed over *tight muscles* (for example round the neck and shoulders). Cuprum/Quarz comp. ointment (Wala) also contains a large quantity of rosemary oil, which has a warming effect and stimulates the blood flow and can therefore disperse *haematomas*. It often provides rapid relief for *pulled muscles and tendons*.

The stimulating effect on circulation and therefore a local strengthening effect on mucus membranes can help prevent the vaginal mucosa from becoming thin and sensitive during the *menopause* if a thin layer of Rosmarin-Salbe (Weleda) or Rosmarinus/Prunus Gel (Wala) is applied in the genital area.

Rosmarin-Salbe (Weleda) has also proved effective for mild forms of *fungal infections between the toes*, particularly as fungal infections in general tend to occur in cool parts of the body with poor circulation. However, rosemary also has a direct antifungal effect, which is apparently responsible for the good efficacy of Rosmarin-Salbe for nappy rash. Rubbing the ointment into the affected area twice daily should produce a significant improvement after a week and complete healing after two weeks. Alternatively, I have found that ointments containing preparations of birch bark (see page 80) are also good for both these indications.

CHAPTER 22

Rose

Although it has its main flowering period around Midsummer's Day, the rose is close to us throughout the year. On Christmas Eve in the bitter cold the old carol, *Es ist ein Ros entsprungen* ('A Rose has Come to Blossom') is sung in most German churches in order to celebrate the appearance of the saviour on earth. Then another German carol, *Maria durch ein Dornwald ging* ('Mary Walked Through a Forest of Thorns') will often be sung, telling of the thorn thicket which, after a long drought, is once again covered in leaves and roses. The picture of a blossoming rose appears to be particularly appropriate as a symbol of the fulfilment of our deepest striving. But this picture was never used to depict purely outer, material fulfilment. No one would link the successful conclusion of a contract or a win in the lottery with a rose, but rather the fulfilment of a deep love. The rose always appears to indicate a spiritual aspect. Love poetry is full of roses, but they also seem to be at home where we try to connect with the origin of our soul.

If we observe someone smelling a scented rose, we notice that almost always at least the trace of a smile plays around their features when the experience of the scent spreads through them. If we do this ourselves, we notice that a peaceful harmonious mood is awakened for a moment, making whatever we had been preoccupied with just a little less important. It may well be this effect of the rose which made Hildegard of Bingen advise 'those prone to anger' to smell dried rose petals at the moment when their wrath was aroused.

Wherever roses grow, there appears to be a knowledge that, when we experience their scent, we come closer to the divine world and our 'higher self', that we should actually be or will one day become. Many years ago, my future wife and I entered a most holy temple in a remote

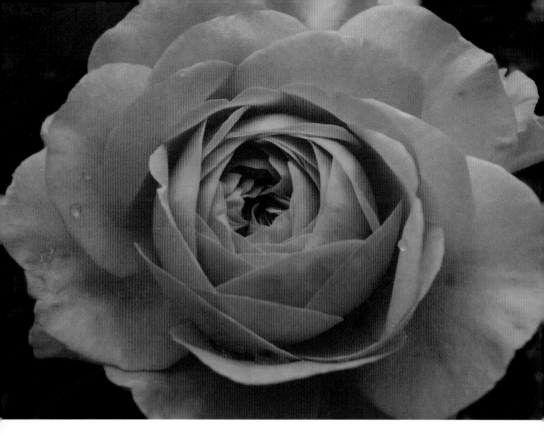

Rose flowers radiate a particular harmony.

place in India, and we were overwhelmed by the mesmerising scent of roses drifting through the temple. One courtyard of the ancient building was completely covered in delicate pink rose flowers.

Another time I entered a mosque in Turkey where a ritual was taking place for someone who had died. At the moment when it was said that the soul was now rising up to Allah, the nieces and nephew of the person who had passed away distributed rosewater to all the participants, pouring it into their hands, and a delicate perfume, which swelled the hearts of those present and eased their sadness, pervaded the mosque.

The rose whose flower emerges from the thorny shrub was present in every monastery garden in earlier times and the care and grafting of a rose bush can be taken as an outer picture of the inner work which those living in the monastery performed on their souls. The Islamic poets and mystics also knew about the relationship of the rose to the soul. The great founder of Sufism, Jalal ad-Din Muhammad Rumi, knew that 'The rose is a messenger from the garden of the soul.'[1] The

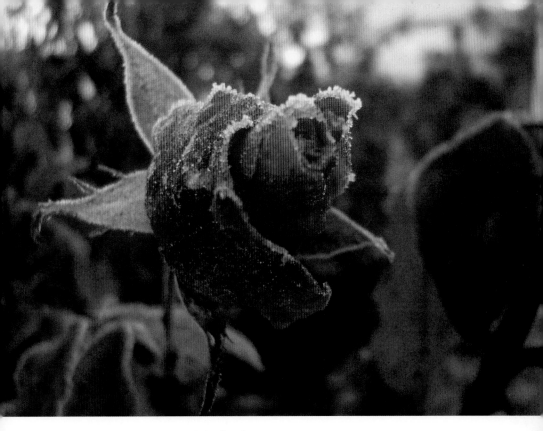

Some rose flowers persist until the first frosts

fourteenth century Persian poet, Hafez – whom Goethe and Emerson admired so highly – sees its surrender to the sky with its roots firmly in the earth as an example which requires no further teaching.

> The rose should become your example! ...
> It needs not the wisdom of the prophet,
> Because it lives just as he speaks.[2]

The rose is not a powerful medicinal plant as such. But it can become a wonderful support through its restorative effect on the soul when you are at risk of being lost in the daily round or you feel tense and exhausted. It can also help after a draining illness or difficult experiences. To quote Rumi again:

> New life will lend the spirit wings
> Whenever it smells the sweet scent of the rose.[3]

221

Many years ago, Wala produced an elixir made from rose petals which was rhythmically exposed to sunrise and sunset during preparation and which proved particularly successful in bringing those suffering from exhaustion back in touch with the 'rose forces'. This remedy is no longer available. However, an ointment made from rose and lavender oils, combined with potentised gold (this and its relationship to the sun forces will be discussed in Chapter 38 on gold) can have similar effects, improving sleep and restoring calm in *anxiety states with palpitations*. The use of rose oil in cosmetics is not only due to the fact that it has an anti-microbial and mildly anti-inflammatory action, but mainly because of its emotional effects which can act on our 'aura' and therefore on our skin.

However, nowadays not everything that seems to smell of roses is made with real rose oil. It requires a large basket of rose petals to make one drop of the precious oil, which is why cheap substitutes are often used. The anthroposophical medicine companies Wala and Weleda are now the largest purchasers of genuine rose oil in the world and have set up projects for cultivating organic and fair trade roses in several countries.

Something 'regal' emanates from the scent of roses. And in fact the rose is called the queen of flowers, a title first used by the ancient poet Sappho almost three thousand years ago. It is not so easy to explain what the regency of the rose is based on. There are flowers that are larger, smell stronger (just think of lilies) and are more brightly coloured. But the rose possesses a distinct harmony, which really gives it a unique position. There is another aspect as well. The rose combines a heavenly scent with being deeply anchored in the earth with its woody rootstock (which survives for decades). It forms a harmonious synthesis between a fleeting appearance and a solidification striving for permanence, between delicate evanescence and gnarled strength. Perhaps the rose can be a companion to human beings who also have to find a balance between the extremes again and again. It can help to preserve hope of a new flowering, when life has for too long been only a thorny thicket. Anthroposophical medicine not only uses medicines in the healing process but also makes use of external measures such as massage, the patient's own activity such as in curative eurythmy or art therapy and sometimes a purely mental action such as meditation, which the doctor can recommend for a patient.

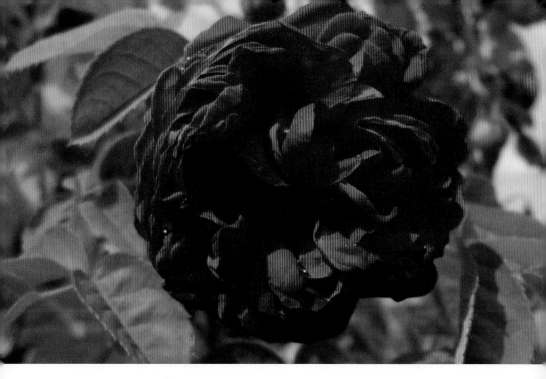

The highly aromatic rose de Rescht is particularly good for making scented rose jam.

One of the patients for whom the first anthroposophical doctors called in Rudolf Steiner was given a rose medicine and the additional advice to meditate on roses (I know of another case where the patient had to imagine her medicinal plant and the ground where it grew). In fact we can feel that even our memory of a rose flower, of its appearance and its perfume, can change us and bring harmony to our mood. Without having a direct relationship to physical health, one of the basic meditations offered by anthroposophy for the development of the soul contains a picture of seven roses. There are many ways in which the rose can be a companion for life.

Rose (*Rosa centifolia, Rosa damascena*)

The petals of scented garden roses can be collected (if they have not been treated with pesticides) in the early morning when they smell the strongest and dried in a shady spot. They can be used as tea or for flavouring other teas or tea mixtures. They can also be sprinkled into a bath or filled into a container in layers alternating with salt to make bath salts.

Rose petal jam is common in Turkey but can easily be made at home. Add the petals from 15–20 roses which have been harvested early in the morning to 1 litre (quart) of water, bring to the boil, add the juice of 3 lemons and 1 kg (2 lb) of gelling (jelly) sugar (2:1) – now the colour will deepen – cover and leave to simmer gently for 10 minutes, and then pour into clean jars. Some varieties of rose are particularly good for making rose petal jam. The flowers of rose de Rescht produce particularly tasty jam.

Rose oil and rose water for the cosmetic industry are obtained by steam distillation. Rose oil is very precious and a litre of good quality oil can cost £8,400 ($14,000), which is not so surprising when you realise that this requires 5–6 *tonnes* of rose petals. Rose water, which accumulates during the production of rose oil, is much cheaper. It is used both cosmetically and for cooking (for example, for making marzipan).

Roses in phytotherapy

The rose is no longer used in official phytotherapy, except as rosehips. Nevertheless, a tea made from dried rose petals (2 teaspoons to 1 cup of boiling water, covered and left to stand for 10 minutes) has a relaxing 'harmonising' effect. To obtain a sleep-inducing effect, mix the rose petals with lavender flowers and lemon balm leaves in equal parts. Incidentally, these plants go well together in the garden and are said to encourage each other's growth.

The rose in homeopathy

The rose (*Rosa centifolia*) is used very occasionally in homeopathy for hay fever and asthma. I have no personal experience of this.

The rose in anthroposophical medicine

It has already been mentioned that there used to be a very good Rose Elixir from Wala, which was extremely useful for many symptoms of *nervous exhaustion*. While on this subject, it may be of interest that the founder of Wala, Rudolf Hauschka, used the rose to develop the process which Wala now employs for making all the basic herbal substances.

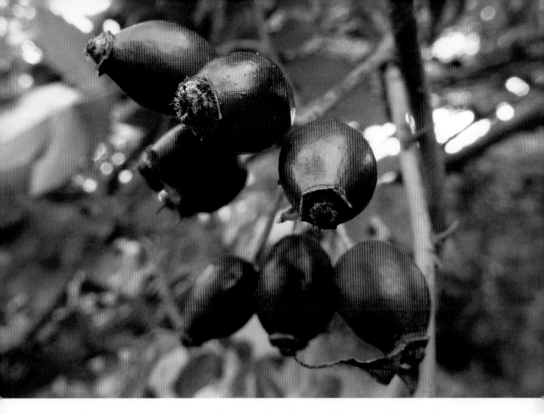

Rosehips contain a large amount of vitamin C and are used for tea and for spreading on bread, but apart from this they are no longer of much importance medicinally.

Hauschka's aim was to increase the 'vitality' of the harvested plants to such a degree that they could be kept without alcohol or other preservatives. By using rhythms – cooling to 4°C (39°F), exposure to light, movement and exposure to the air around sunrise and sunset, heating to 37°C (99°F), excluding light and air and stillness in the intervening period – he succeeded for the first time in producing a strongly scented extract from rose flowers which could be kept for decades. This process, which is aimed at enlivening the substance, brings about a lactic acid fermentation similar to that occurring in our metabolism. The suggestion which Rudolf Hauschka used for developing this process were the words and task from Rudolf Steiner, 'Rhythm carries life. Study rhythms!' The pharmaceutical process described here reminds us a little of the process of breathing and of what the blood goes through when it flows into the lungs, where it meets air which has been drawn in from outside. This cools it, before it then flows into the warm and enclosed interior of the body in order to release oxygen and absorb metabolic products such as lactic acid.

225

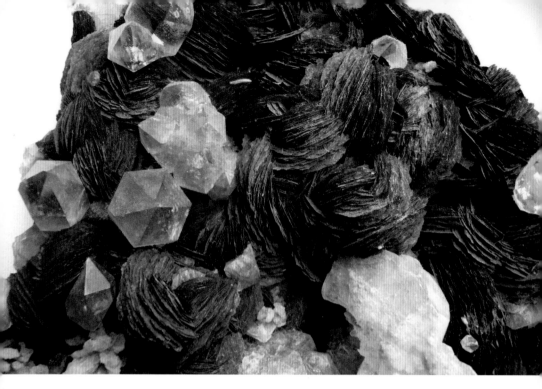

Haematite is added to a rose petal extract to produce Roseneisen.

Nowadays a rose petal extract is manufactured adding the iron oxide haematite as a kind of catalyst, which is removed again afterwards. The rose petal extract is then used to produce Roseneisen D3 globules which have a strengthening effect after *long-term illness* and in particular stimulate and strengthen breathing. Rose iron (Roseneisen) along with potentised graphite (D14) is used to manufacture Roseneisen/Graphit which has proved very successful for *appetite disturbances* but above all as a complementary treatment for *chronic lung diseases,* including *tuberculosis.* I have given rose iron/graphite in addition to other treatments to several patients suffering from this serious disease and have gained the impression that it brought a distinct improvement in their state of health and overall progress. In some cases the usual treatment using antibiotics which are effective against tuberculosis could not be carried out for particular reasons (like intolerance of the medicines) and I am convinced that the rose remedy played a significant role in the eventual recovery. However, Roseneisen/Graphit is used much more frequently for the often beneficial treatment of a *persistent dry cough,* e.g. after measles or other depleting illnesses.

Weleda make a very similar remedy under the name of Ferrum rosatum/Graphit. In this remedy rose petals are not processed with the haematite mined from the earth, but with meteoric iron from the cosmos. There is also no rhythmical alternation between heating and cooling as in the process used by Wala, but a type of fermentation process of the hybrid tea rose flowers is used. The hybrid tea rose flowers are mixed with the meteoric iron powder while cold before the process is completed by adding alcohol. I do not have any experience with this remedy, which, due to the particular origin of the iron used in it, may also have a special effect – something which would need more detailed research.

Oil dispersion baths with Rosa e floribus 10% Oleum are also used for *exhaustion* conditions and for building up after serious illness. Many people who feel drained by work and family tensions experience an effect of relaxation and regeneration from this type of external use of rose. There are now a range of oil compositions in which either the warming, enveloping and protective effects of peat or the reviving effect of potentised gold (see Chapter 38) are combined with the action of the rose (e.g. Torf-Rosenöl, Gold-Rosenblüten-Öl Dr Heberer Naturheilmittel).

Essential rose oil is contained in all the Wala eye drops where its gently warming and soothing effects are beneficial. This oil is also part of the Rosatum-Heilsalbe, which has proved successful for the treatment of *cracked chapped skin*.

The Aurum/Lavandula comp. cream (Weleda) which contains potentised gold (D4), lavender oil and rose extract is also particularly to be recommended. If this is rubbed in over the heart it often has a surprisingly good effect for emotionally linked *heart complaints (feeling of pressure, palpitations* etc.). *Sleep disturbances* and agitation also frequently improve significantly if the cream is applied to the area over the heart. The same substances are combined in Gold-Rosenblüten-Lavendel Öl (Dr Heberer Naturheilmittel) which is used for both rubbing in and for oil dispersion baths, although I have no experience of this.

CHAPTER 23

Arnica and Calendula

If you could have only one plant in your home pharmacy, I would suggest arnica. While this bright golden-yellow mountain flower may not be able to replace an entire pharmacy, it is capable of such powerful healing effects that I would not like to be without it.

Almost everyone knows that arnica is an effective remedy for all kinds of injuries. If you have a bump, sprain or pulled muscle, or even if a bone is broken, you can always use compresses with diluted arnica tincture or arnica gel or cream as long as the skin is not broken. A decrease in the swelling, pain and bruising can soon be detected. Anyone who has experienced this will not be surprised that laboratory studies have shown the anti-inflammatory and analgesic effects to be stronger than those from standard painkillers and anti-inflammatory drugs.

The fact that arnica can also be beneficial for more serious illnesses has become known all over the world due to Eckermann's discussions with Goethe. *Faust II* and many of Goethe's later scientific works might not have been written without arnica. Almost ten years before his death, Goethe had a serious health crisis; many believe that he suffered a heart attack. Not only the doctors thought he was going to die. According to Eckermann's notes dated February 24, 1823, Goethe said to his daughter-in-law: 'I feel that the moment has come in which the struggle in me between life and death begins.' A cup of arnica tea was beneficial 'at the most crucial moment,' and finally 'brought about a happy outcome.' The notes relate that, 'Goethe wrote an elegant description of this plant and praised its powerful effects to the skies.'[1]

Arnica tea is not generally used nowadays. Although compounds have in fact been found in the plant which act on the heart, improving its strength and relieving exhaustion, these can be dangerous in only

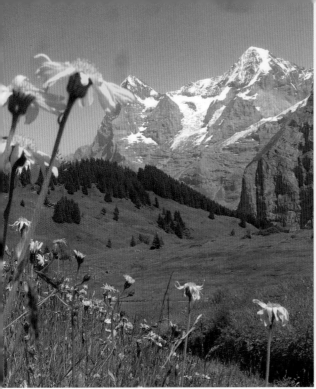

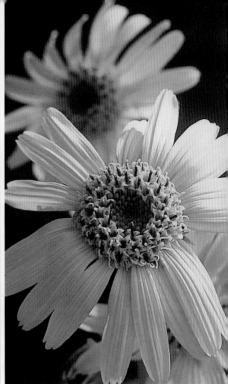

Arnica growing in the Dolomites.   *Arnica flower.*

slightly excessive doses. Harmful effects of this kind are naturally not an issue when using potentised arnica and it is likely than no other potentised remedy in the form of globules or drops is used more widely than this one. It is to be found in household medicine cabinets, travel bags and the medical stores of university hospitals alike, and justifiably so. For instance, in a recent study on patients who had undergone an operation due to a deformation of the basal joint of the big toe (Hallux valgus), the use of Diclofenac, the standard analgesic for treating post-operative pain, was compared with that of Arnica D4. The study showed that patients who took arnica were able to walk again sooner and this group had less swelling and irritation than the group who were given Diclofenac. At the very least, patients given Arnica did not need any additional strong analgesics compared to those who took the standard chemical medication.[2] Most importantly, side effects were experienced by one in five patients taking the standard drug but less than one in twenty of those taking arnica.

Many homeopathic and anthroposophical doctors prescribe potentised arnica and arnica applied externally in addition to other treatment measures for such serious conditions as *cardiac infarction*

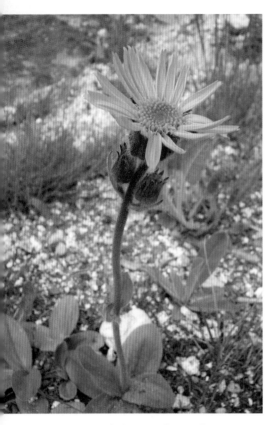

Beneath the main flower of Arnica montana *there are often two lateral flowers — here still at the bud stage. The flower stem arises from a basal rosette of four or six leaves.*

and *stroke*. Besides the objective improvement, it often appears that – just as in Goethe's case – the patient feels better again and even in critical situations takes heart and starts to feel certain that things will 'turn out well'.

Rudolf Steiner once described very graphically and amusingly how this important medicinal plant works. When the body has been injured so that the power of action of the self, or I, has been weakened, the use of arnica summons the soul: 'Hey, get over here! You have work to do. You need to help!'[3] This sounds like a good and trustworthy friend who can be relied on in times of need. This is exactly the feeling you get about arnica when you have used it many times and often been amazed by its good effects.

A very similar feeling arises when you come across arnica in a mountain meadow. It does not appear noble or graceful like a rose or a lily. The flower always seems rather dishevelled, like someone who has run a sweaty hand through their hair. Its glowing orange-yellow appears cheerful, vibrant and almost cheeky; and the more tired he is after a long mountain hike, the more the walker is encouraged by the feeling of cheerfulness when they come across this plant.

I have no idea whether it is true that chewing one of the bitter-tasting arnica flowers refreshes you if you are exhausted. You should refrain from this experiment, not only because internal use of the concentrated plant is inadvisable, but because of the plant's protected status. It is unfortunately becoming rarer, as it does not like fertilised soil. However, it has no problem with exposed, windy and

230

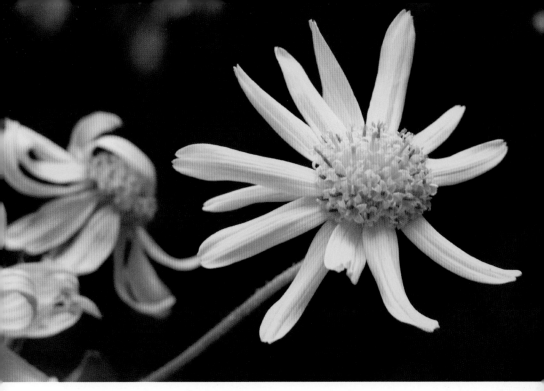

Arnica flowers usually look rather 'dishevelled'.

often somewhat marshy sites where you get the impression that its aromatic-smelling rhizome brings 'inner light' and order into its musty surroundings. It may be a similar ability that makes it so useful for injured humans and animals. Besides the pain relief, it is important that dead material or anything that does not belong at the site is replaced by the patient's own self-regenerating tissue. For instance, arnica helps to dissipate *bruising* and *reduce swellings* and in cases of *local (including bacterial) inflammation* it helps to restore order.

Interestingly, many plants belonging to this same daisy family, the Compositae, have a similar effect. For instance, marigold *(Calendula)* is also a well-known plant for treating *wounds,* as are coneflower *(Echinacea)* and chamomile for *inflamed injuries,* daisy *(Bellis)* for *bruises* and dandelion which is beneficial for *scars* (see chapters 23, 19 and 6).

While arnica is primarily useful where the body surface is still intact, marigold is particularly helpful if the skin is broken or damaged, if a 'hole' has been left which now needs to heal over. In such situations calendula encourages processes of growth and order.

Real order is perhaps the greatest strength of the members of the

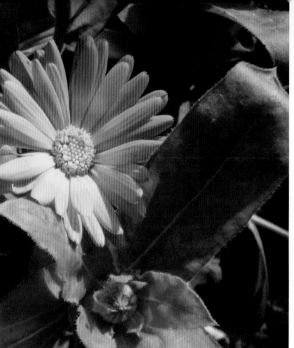
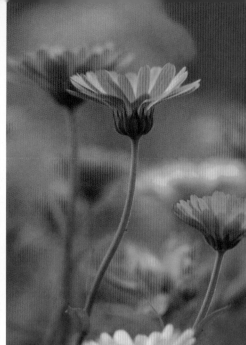

Flower and leaf of calendula.

daisy family. What appears to us as a large flower is to the botanist a collection of many individual flowers in a community. Only the outermost flowers develop beautiful showy petals which attract bees and butterflies; the flowers nearer the centre are often more concerned with reproduction. It is as though each flower 'knew' what was required at the appropriate place. It is still a miracle of every healing process that cell growth must first be initiated, but then each new cell has to find its 'place' and, once there, has to settle down and not simply go on multiplying but adopt the function which corresponds to the place. Maybe it is a particular ability of the Compositae to help with this and is one reason why they are particularly suited to healing injuries and to inspiring trust in the successful outcome of the healing process.

Arnica (*Arnica montana*)

As *Arnica montana* is an endangered species and protected in many countries, it is not suitable for collecting yourself, but it is well worth visiting this splendid plant in its natural habitat in the mountains. However, you quite often think you have found it – and then it turns

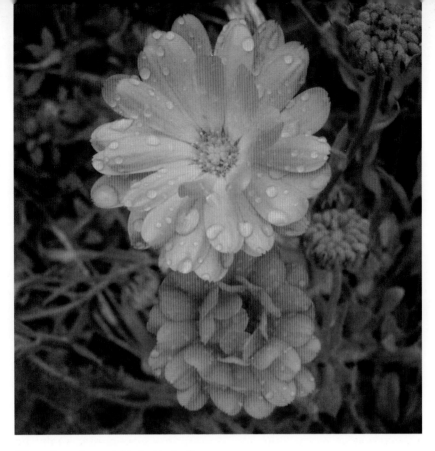

The curly seeds are visible beside the flower.

out to be a leopard's bane *(Doronicum)*, a western salsify *(Tragopodon)*, a hawksbeard *(Hieracium)* or even elecampane *(Inula)*, species which also have large, more or less yellow-orange flowers. Besides the dishevelled appearance of the flower, a characteristic of arnica is that it often has one large flower on each stem and a good bit below this, two smaller flowers branching from the main stem (very symmetrically), so that the entire plant is a little reminiscent of a candelabra. At the base it has a leaf rosette of usually four (sometimes six) relatively large entire leaves with a distinct vein running up the centre.

The range of applications for arnica is so varied and the number of remedies containing arnica so numerous that only a selection can be presented in the following section. It should be pointed out that in homeopathy a remedy by the name of 'Arnica' is generally made from the root of the plant, while in anthroposophical pharmacy it is made from the whole plant (from root to flower). The founder of homeopathy, Samuel Hahnemann, wrote that he would like to have

233

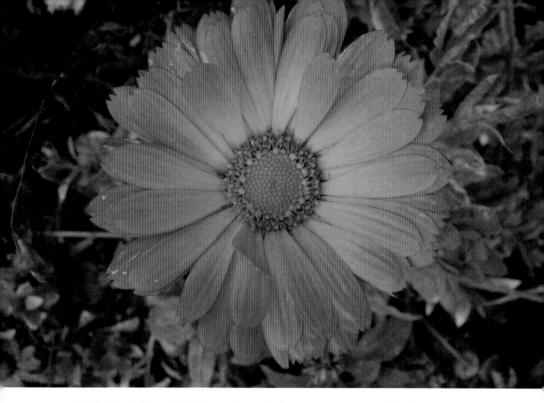

The inside of this marigold flower shows the harmonious structure of the Compositae *family.*

used the whole fresh plant but only the dried root was available. Since his experience was based on preparations made from the root, this tradition has remained in homeopathy.

External use

It has already been mentioned that the use of arnica tea is no longer recommended, however, the external use of the plant is very common. For this purpose there is arnica tincture (which is normally made from the flower) as a pharmaceutical product or proprietary medicine, arnica essence which is obtained by Wala from the flower and by Weleda from the whole plant, and also gels and ointments.

Use 1 tablespoon of the essence or tincture to 250 ml (1 cup) of water for compresses to treat *sprains and bruises*. A small number of people are allergic to arnica and should avoid using it externally. However, a skin irritation is almost always due to incorrect use, such as applying it to broken skin, or applying an airtight covering (occlusion) to the skin and thus making the action too strong. However, if correctly applied, it is usually very beneficial for *swelling* and pain following *blunt injuries*. The arnica wound wipes (Wala) which – similar to wet wipes – are already packaged with the correct concentration of arnica essence, are very handy for using on a walk. All you need to do is take one from its sachet and lay it on the painful area. When they dry out, they can be moistened again with a little water. Another reason why it should not be used on broken skin is that the alcohol content causes an unpleasant burning sensation.

The fresher the injury and the greater the degree of overheating and swelling, the more a moist form of application such as a compress or gel is to be recommended. On the other hand, for somewhat older injuries it is better to use ointments which tend to warm the injured area, helping to dissipate the bruise and stimulate the healing processes. Arnica gel or Arnica Planta tota 30% gelat. (Weleda) is a tried and tested remedy; Arnica ointment 30% (Weleda) contains a high concentration of the medicinal plant while Arnica ointment 10% (Weleda) is weaker. These ointments are particularly suitable if only soft tissue is involved (for example a *bruise* or *pulled muscle*). The Arnica ointment from Wala contains 5% of the rhythmised basic substance from the whole plant along with a small amount of a warming extract of red wood ant (which helps to mobilise and remove 'waste material') and rhythmised basic substance of comfrey. The latter is indicated particularly if the periosteum, joint capsule and tendons are involved.

If there is a great deal of swelling and heat (but no external injury to the skin), then quark compresses to which arnica has been added can be particularly beneficial. I generally recommend stirring ½ teaspoon of arnica essence into 3 tablespoons of quark and applying this to the affected area. When the quark becomes dry and crumbly the coating can be renewed.

Even if you would not nowadays give a cup of arnica tea for a *heart attack*, warm arnica compresses are often an appreciable additional help along with all the other necessary medically prescribed measures for this serious condition, and also for the less serious condition angina pectoris, which is why they are regularly used in anthroposophical hospitals. This requires diluted arnica – 1 tbsp to 250 ml (1 cup) of water – as described above, but using hot water. A cloth soaked in this is wrapped around the wrist at the pulse position and is then covered

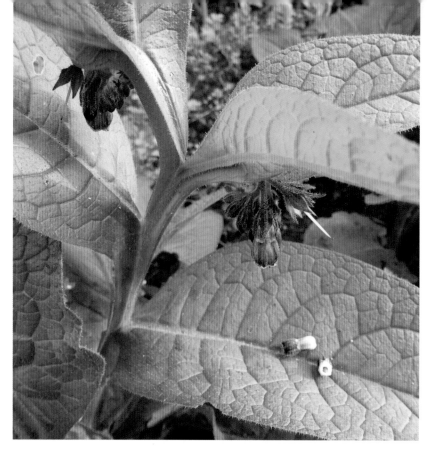

Comfrey (Symphytum officinale) *is often used along with Arnica for bone and ligament injuries.*

with a dry cloth (arnica pulse compress). Less commonly, a hot arnica compress can be applied directly above the heart.

In cases of *concussion* and also *stroke*, some hospitals apply an 'arnica hood' by wrapping cloths with diluted arnica essence round the head. It is simpler and more practical to put diluted arnica essence into a small spray bottle (for example an empty nose spray) and spray the head with this several times a day, so that it is covered by a very thin layer of the essence. Naturally care must be taken that the skin has an adequate tolerance to this. Patients have often told me that they find this form of application particularly pleasant and helpful. Obviously this is also a complementary therapy and does not replace any other required treatment.

Potentised arnica

Potentised arnica globules and drops are perhaps the most common form of homeopathic and anthroposophical medicine. Potentised arnica is often very helpful for *blunt injuries* and also *after operations* for treating pain and overcoming the effects of injury. Arnica e planta tota made from rhythmised basic substance is available from Wala as globuli and ampoules in D2, D3, D4, D6, D10, D12, D15, D20 and D30 and from Weleda as alcoholic drops in D3, D4, D6, D12, D20 and D30; as an aqueous rhythmised substance it is available as drops in Rh D3, D6 and D20 and as ampoules in D3, D20 and D30 and also as globules in D6, D12 and D30. For new injuries I usually prescribe 5 globules of the D6 4–5 times daily. The D6 or D12 can also be given after operations, while in my opinion it is not worth taking arnica before an operation. The higher potencies (D20 and D30) are suitable either for less recent injuries or for treating neurological disturbances (for example in the case of *stroke, multiple sclerosis* etc.), but this generally requires specialist advice.

A completely different area of application for arnica which is perfectly acceptable for self treatment is *flu-like infections* with severe muscle pain (particularly in the back) along with a feeling of total exhaustion, where the patient may feel that the mattress is too hard. Taking Arnica D12 or D30 can often be of greater help than any standard analgesic (dissolve 15 globules in a quarter glass of water and take 1 teaspoon every half hour to begin with).

Arnica in composite preparations

Arnica is used in a very large number of composite preparations. Amongst these, the combinations with stinging nettle – Combudoron (Weleda) and Burns lotion (Brandessenz, Wala), are particularly important and will be described in more detail in Chapter 28 on the stinging nettle. One of these remedies – which appear indispensible to me for first aid for *burns* and *scalds* – should be kept in every household.

A large proportion of the medicines for internal use which contain arnica are beneficial for *musculoskeletal disorders*. For example, for patients with *broken bones*, in addition to the surgical treatment I always prescribe Symphytum comp. to relieve the pain and improve healing.

There are two remedies from Wala and Weleda with the same name but differing composition. My impression is that Symphytum comp. N drops (Weleda) is particularly beneficial in the first two weeks because, besides Arnica Cepa and Symphytum (comfrey) which are contained in both remedies, this one includes Ruta (D3) which has a pain-relieving effect and Bellis (D3), Calendula (D2) and Hamamelis (D2) which are of particular importance during the first phase of healing. I generally prescribe 10 drops 3 times daily. From the third week I prescribe Symphytum comp. globuli (Wala) which, besides Arnica, Symphytum und Cepa, contains Stannum metallicum D14 which encourages the formation of callus tissue which bridges the fracture.

The (mostly) prescription-only remedy, Mandragora comp., (Weleda) is composed particularly for treating *degenerative conditions of the knee* and contains arnica, birch, horsetail (Equisetum), ants and mandrake (Mandragora) in addition to an organ preparation of the knee joint meniscus. Articulatio talocruralis comp. (globuli and ampoules, Wala), on the other hand, is used for *arthroses of the ankle joint*. In addition to potentised arnica and onion (Cepa), comfrey (Symphytum) and tin (Stannum), this remedy contains potentised organ preparations of various sections of the anatomically complicated ankle joint, the periosteum, tendons and the sciatic nerve. To my own and the patients' delight, I have found that this remedy can achieve a largely pain-free state, even in patients who have already been recommended surgical arthrodesis.

Arnica, birch leaves and bark, ants, silver and sulfur in potentised form are contained in Betula/Arnica comp. (globuli and ampoules) which is effective for *arthroses* and *pain around the shoulder joint*.

Lastly, arnica is contained in most of the Disci comp. preparations (Wala) which are used for *back pain* and *intervertebral disc problems*. These medicines contain a complex range of substances which need to be selected to suit the individual situation. However, arnica is always an important component of these very helpful medicines.

Arnica/Levisticum comp. D3 and D6 (Weleda) is also used for back pain (particularly *lumbago* with sciatic nerve pain). The potentised bee venom, in this remedy helps to reduce swelling in the trapped nerve. However, it also precludes giving this remedy to patients with an oversensitivity to bee poison.

Magnesium phosphoricum comp. (globuli and ampoules, Wala) is also effective for the *musculoskeletal* system and often relieves *muscular spasm* remarkably quickly. However, to achieve such fast effects it usually needs to be injected close to the affected muscles. Besides Arnica D2 and Formica (ant) D7, this remedy contains Magnesium phosphoricum D5 (well known as Schüssler salt No. 7 for its ability to relieve cramps). However, in the case of Magnesium phosphoricum comp. (Wala), the magnesium phosphate is not made synthetically but derived from the ash of burned grains of oats. In other words, it comes from plants. It may be significant in this context that oats (Avena) in potentised form are themselves a relaxing remedy in homeopathy or anthroposophical medicine. The globules (5 hourly to several times a day) can be used for less serious problems or to continue treatment after an injection.

Arnica, Planta tota D15/Aurum D10 aa ampoules (Weleda) and Arnica/Aurum I (Arnica D5, Aurum D9) and Arnica/Aurum II (Arnica D19, Aurum D29) from Wala are used for the support and treatment of heart disease. These medicines are indicated in cases of *angina pectoris* (*stenocardia*), *high blood pressure, heart attack* and other diseases affecting the cardiovascular system, which also applies to Arnica, Planta tota D10/Cor D10 aa (Weleda). However, as these conditions are not suitable for self treatment, I only mention these remedies here in order to point out that arnica can also be a helpful support in cases of serious illness. This also applies to the final area of application and preparations mentioned here. Arnica/Plumbum comp. A and B (Wala) can be used for *circulatory problems of the brain*, even including a *stroke* and its consequences. The A remedy primarily contains a potentised organ preparation which is related to the sense of sight, while the B remedy contains an organ preparation which is linked to the sense of hearing. The Weleda Arnica/Betula comp. preparation has a similar composition which, like the above-mentioned remedy by Wala, also contains arnica and birch (Betula) plus a preparation from potentised lead, honey and cane sugar (the antisclerotic Plumbum mellitum), but no additional potentised organ preparation.

The remedies and range of uses of this important medicinal plant presented here are by no means exhaustive. From everyday injuries to serious life-threatening diseases in our core organs, arnica is one of the most potent medicinal plants, providing help for which we can feel deep gratitude if we have experienced this for ourselves.

Marigold (Calendula officinalis)

The marigold is a rewarding flower to grow in the garden, with bright flowers in many shades from light yellow to dark orange. New flowers open every day and close again in the evening. Its large curved seeds are responsible for its German name of 'ringlet flower' and by self-seeding it appears year after year, mostly without any help from the gardener. To make a tea, harvest the flowers and dry them whole, or first remove the green sepals.

Calendula tea

To make 1 cup, pour boiling water over 2 teaspoons of the chopped up flowers or 1–2 whole ones. Strain after 5 minutes. The cooled tea is normally used for rinsing the mouth after dental treatment, for soreness caused by *denture pressure points* or for *mouth ulcers*. It can also be used for *inflammation of the mucosa during chemotherapy*. Dried Calendula flowers are often added to other tea mixtures because they look so attractive.

External application

Calendula has proved very successful for the treatment of *wounds* as a compress, irrigation or ointment. Calendula is particularly beneficial for skin injuries which cannot be remedied simply by sewing up but require a gradual 'closing' of the wound. The same applies to damage and sores which arise when an abscess is opened, from *venal congestion in the lower leg* or after *radiation therapy*. A large randomised study in France showed that the application of a Calendula ointment markedly reduced the side effects of radiotherapy of the breast in comparison to the standard treatment.[4] A large number of studies have demonstrated significant decongestant, anti-inflammatory and immunostimulant effects, promotion of skin cell growth and strengthening of connective tissue.

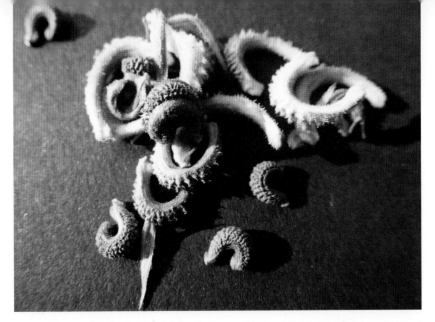

Calendula seeds form 'ringlets' which is why the plant is called Ringelblume *(ringlet flower) in German.*

There are a large number of good Calendula preparations in the form of ointments or essences from different manufacturers. Both Wala and Weleda manufacture a 10% oil and Weleda also makes pure Calendula ointment while Wala produces Calcea Wund– und Heilcreme or Healing Cream (from roughly equal parts of Calendula and Echinacea) and Mercurialis ointment (Wala) which contains extracts of dog's mercury *(Mercurialis)* and onion in addition to marigold. All these greasy preparations are used primarily where the skin's surface is still intact and an underlying inflammation (for example a *boil* or *abscess,* a *nail bed inflammation* or an *inflammation around an embedded splinter*) needs to be alleviated or suppuration needs to mature so that a foreign body can be expelled. After checking with the doctor, Calendula can also be used on an open wound by spreading one of these ointments or creams thinly on a sterile dressing and laying it on the wound. This can stimulate both cleaning of the wound and the formation of new tissue from the base of the wound. A moist wound treatment using soaked compresses and wound irrigation can be carried out using Wala Calendula essence (2 teaspoons to 250 ml / 1 cup of boiled water or physiological saline solution – the latter does not burn) or Calendula 20% / Echinacea 1% tincture (Weleda). Irrigation is particularly suitable for *wound cavities* and narrow entrances

241

(especially *fistulas*) and should generally be carried out by a doctor or nurse. I have repeatedly found that this type of treatment can heal long-standing wounds.[5]

Internal use

Diluted Calendula essence – 1 tablespoon to 125 ml (½ cup) of water – can be used for the same indications specified for Calendula tea. If this is used after having a *tooth extracted*, for example, then the solution should not be swirled too vigorously between the teeth as this can lead to renewed bleeding. But it can ease the pain and encourage healing if moved gently around the mouth. It also helps to ease pain and induce healing in *mouth ulcers* and is beneficial for various kinds of *throat infections*. Patients undergoing *chemotherapy* or *radiotherapy* often suffer from *inflammation of the mucous membranes of the mouth, stomach and intestine*. Prophylactic administration of potentised Calendula in the form of Calendula ex herba D3 ampoules (Wala) has proved beneficial in this case. This application – which has since been repeatedly proven elsewhere – was first reported by the paediatrician Georg Soldner who has considerable experience in treating children suffering from tumours. These ampoules are injected subcutaneously but can also be taken orally (with the help of a drinking straw). Sometimes an aggressive treatment like this, which is necessary for some types of tumour, can only be made bearable by this type of complementary therapy. It is likely that in such cases both the proven activation of the immune system and the anti-inflammatory and healing power of this valuable medicinal plant are at work.

In addition, in cases of *glandular fever*, Calendula ex herba D3 (also available as drops or globuli in D3: 10 drops or globules 3 times daily) can often quickly heal up a significant and long-lasting involvement of the tonsils.[6]

CHAPTER 24

What Bees Tell Us

Strictly speaking, a chapter on bees has no business in a book on medicinal plants. On the other hand, there would be very few medicinal plants if their ancestors had not been pollinated by bees. The animal and plant kingdoms regularly come into very close contact for the benefit of both in this context. In addition, remedies acquired from bees are amongst the most important in the animal kingdom, when we consider their use in anthroposophical medicine and homeopathy.

Perhaps this is why an extraordinary number of my medical colleagues keep bees in their spare time. They love to talk about their experiences and when I listen to them, it soon becomes clear why a bee-keeper is also known in German as *Bienenvater* ('bee father'). Just as a real father is proud of the achievements of his offspring, beekeepers enthuse about the amazing abilities of their bees.

The longer you listen, the more you are convinced that the beekeeper has a very personal relationship to his insects. He knows which colony is doing well and which is not. He even knows the colony's mood and can distinguish whether it is busily collecting nectar or is getting into an excited 'swarming mood', whether the nuptial flight of a young queen is imminent, a new queen is hatching or whether the colony is 'mourning' because its queen has died. If I then ask how he knows all this, my beekeeping colleague says (with a secretive smile) that he hears it. Depending on its mood, the hive emits very different sounds. It seems to me that an experienced beekeeper almost feels the bee colony to be an innate entity; it is as though he is on friendly terms with it. But how is such a thing possible? Is a bee not simply an insect like a mosquito or a ladybird? (Hopefully none of my beekeeping friends are reading this.)

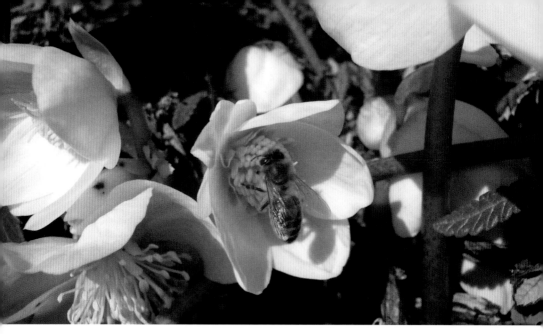

A bee looks for nectar in a Christmas rose flower.

After all, don't they only have a couple of nerve cells, which cannot produce more than a few reflex reactions? This assessment may well do an injustice to mosquitoes and ladybugs, but for bees it is completely mistaken. You may feel attraction or repulsion at the sight of a ladybird or a mosquito, but their activity can generally be understood as the action of single creature. In contrast, the beehive as a totality behaves like one organism. If you look at a single bee, it may indeed be 'just an insect', but it is connected to something greater. The totality of the members of a bee colony really does reveal something like a 'unified being', which influences every single bee.

Bees taken by surprise by cold and rain when out on a flight become motionless and inactive like all other insects and even much more highly evolved cold-blooded animals such as lizards and snakes. And yet bees succeed in producing and maintaining a uniform warmth with a temperature of 35°C (95°F) inside their hive; roughly the value of our own body temperature. They even managed this when the ambient temperature was increased to 70°C (160°F) in an experiment.

In winter the bees crowd together into a group with the queen sitting in the centre. She is surrounded by bees who produce warmth by a kind of muscular trembling. To prevent any bees from freezing, those individuals which have warmed themselves and their surroundings gradually move outwards while 'cool bees' move inwards from outside,

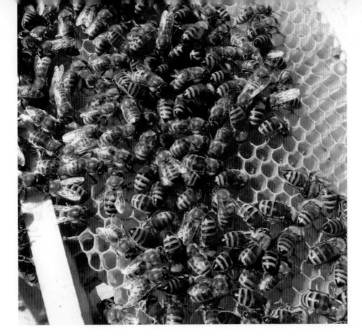

Bees on a rectangular wax comb.

start to tremble and thus warm themselves and their neighbours before then crawling outwards again. In this way the inside of the sphere with the queen always stays warm while around there are shell-like zones with lower temperatures. The warmth reserves stored in the honey and released through the muscular trembling are therefore used as economically as possible so that the summer reserves will last right through the winter. This circulating current of warmth is like our bloodstream, which carries warmth through the entire body. In this picture, the queen bee corresponds to our heart.

The bees' management of warmth goes even further. If a strange, potentially threatening animal which could be a danger to them (such as a hornet) comes into the hive, then a crowd of bees surround it like a thick coat and immediately begin buzzing with their wings which creates so much warmth that the intruder is heated to as much as 45°C (115°F) and dies. This is reminiscent of how a fever develops in us; an active process that serves the purpose of killing pathogens which have gained entry.

Each bee behaves in a way that is beneficial for the whole. The bee's entire life is organised on this principle. It has different tasks at each stage and all bees that fulfil a particular task are known as a caste. Unlike the Indian caste system where a person remains unalterably destined to be a priest, a soldier or a street sweeper throughout life,

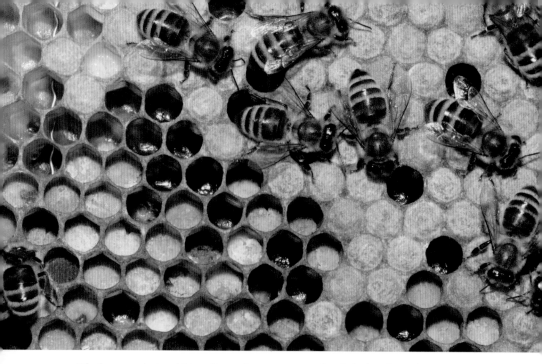

The honeycombs in which pollen and nectar are stored and the brood raised are constructed with astonishing precision.

a bee progresses through different tasks in a set pattern. When first hatched it is assigned to caring for, feeding and cleaning the larvae. Later, it produces wax and builds the honeycomb. (What perfect architecture is revealed in the regular six-sided cells!) Its next task is defence – though at the beginning of its life, it does not even produce venom. Finally it leaves the hive and starts to collect nectar.

It is then able to achieve something that I find utterly amazing: it starts to talk. You might point out that the dog's wagging tail and the position of a horse's ears are also a kind of speech. But these usually express nothing more than the animal's current mood. A bee returning to the hive, however, can communicate the direction and distance from the hive and the amount of nectar-bearing flowers. It can indicate something, and not just by pointing at it with a finger (or wingtip) but by presenting all the information in an abstract way by elements of a dance performed in the dark of the hive. The bee has command of a proper language at a level that is unique in the animal world and is really unbelievable for an insect. You will notice that I have become infected with the beekeeper's enthusiasm. And how much more could be said about bees!

I shall now at least mention the reason why a doctor might be so

246

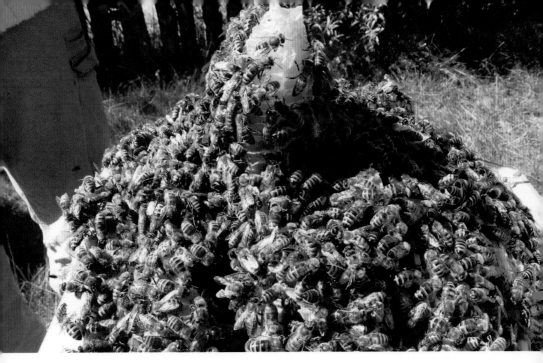

A strong colony is simply swarming with bees.

interested in bees. The effects of bee venom are painfully familiar. In the case of an allergy it can even be quite dangerous. Nevertheless, it has been known since olden times to be beneficial for joint problems.

A beekeeping friend who is a specialist in joint diseases himself had a long-standing problem with his knee. One day a bee stung him in the back of the knee – and the problem eased significantly. Since then he catches a bee from time to time to let it sting him.

It is less unpleasant to use homeopathic preparations made from bees. They have proved very beneficial for insect bites and inflammation similar to that caused by bee stings. In anthroposophical medicine, remedies made from bees are also used where the immune system incorrectly perceives the body's own organs. This results in the organs being attacked like a foreign body or disease pathogen and, in the worst case, being destroyed.

A sentence about bees in a zoological encyclopaedia reads: 'the successful cooperation of the animals or castes within a colony is comparable to the interaction of the organs of an organism and is therefore crucial for survival.'[1] Thus, when treating disorders on the level of the relationship of the organs to one another, the bee can have a healing effect.

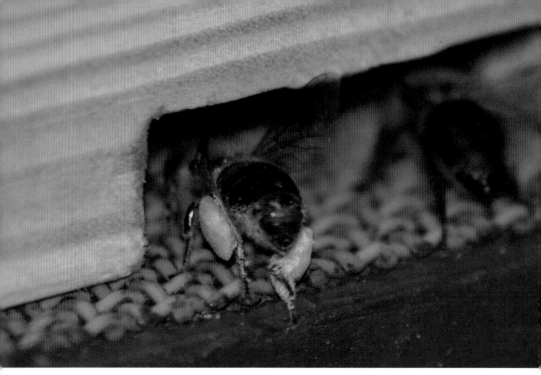

When bees bring pollen into the hive this can be seen from their fat pollen sacs.

Even *disorders in speech development* can be successfully treated by anthroposophical doctors with medicines made from bees. Wax and honey also possess healing properties. If you study the habits of the bee you cannot fail to be amazed. Perhaps the best way to understand bees is to care for them like a beekeeper.

Bee (*Apis mellifica*)

I would tend to discourage the form of self-treatment consisting of purposely allowing the bee to sting you, as practised by my intrepid medical colleague mentioned above. On the one hand the bee loses its life, for the sting and the attached venom sac remain stuck in the skin of the person who has been stung and the bee dies from its injury. But on the other hand (and more importantly), you can never be completely certain whether or not you suffer from a dangerous bee venom allergy or whether this may have developed as a result of previous stings. An allergy of this kind can go beyond a simple skin reaction to swelling of the mucus membranes in the respiratory tract and spasm of the bronchial musculature. It can also result in dangerous circulatory

248

reactions, including complete circulatory failure. In the case of a critical reaction of this kind, first aid measures must be performed immediately, which is why patients with a known bee allergy are equipped with an emergency kit. Desensitisation is also possible. This is a gradual process of reducing the sensitivity to bee venom, but it is not without risk and can only be done where emergency treatment is available.

Using concentrated bee venom

Treatment using concentrated bee venom has a certain similarity to the use of concentrated herbal medicines. Special techniques have been developed to avoid killing the animals. For example, one method consists of letting the bees crawl over moistened filter paper whilst applying a gentle electrical current. The bees sting into the paper and secrete a drop of venom. However, the sting does not remain in the paper as it does in the skin and can be withdrawn without injury. The venom obtained in this way is processed into such things as ointments, which are used for relieving joint and muscle pain. Ointments of this kind have largely disappeared from the market as proprietary remedies, which is due in part to the indisputable possibility of serious allergic reactions. It is also due to issues of regulatory drug approval: the costs of applying for and obtaining approval would be far higher than the expected profits for many pharmaceutical producers.

There is an Apis 1% ointment made by Weleda. It can cause an intensive warming of the skin and can therefore be used, for example, for relieving joint pain and also to produce a beneficial effect in organs at a deeper level through reflex relationships. This ointment must not be used if there is an oversensitivity to bee venom or to the ingredients sesame oil and lanolin. In general it is best kept in experienced hands.

Potentised bee preparations

Homeopathy

Apis is used in homeopathy for various types of *inflammation* which display symptoms of bee poisoning or a *bee sting*. The key symptoms

249

are swelling (often with a shiny surface due to the high tension in the bulging skin), reddening, stinging pain and relief when it is not touched or if kept cool. Apis in various potencies (recommended potencies are usually between D6 and D30) can therefore help in cases of bee or other insect stings and also for such things as an *inflamed nail bed* (paronychia). If it worsens it should be looked at by a doctor because it can lead to suppuration, which can spread to the hand and cause damage. *Sunburn* or an *allergic skin reaction* can also be indications for using potentised Apis. I generally prescribe 20 globules or drops of Apis D6 or D12 in a quarter glass of water from which a teaspoon is taken every 15 minutes to start with, then less frequently.

Homeopathic drug proving has also brought to light a relationship between Apis and internal diseases. For instance, bee extract in potentised form can be beneficial for certain forms of *kidney inflammation* with proteinuria, for *tonsil or ear infections* which display the above-mentioned key symptoms and even for *irritation of the meninges*. In such cases, however, treatment belongs in the hands of a suitably experienced doctor.

Potentised bee in anthroposophical medicine

The anthroposophical manufacturers Wala and Weleda use different methods to produce the starting substance, which is then potentised. Weleda kills the bees using alcohol and then produces an alcoholic extract from them to make the Apis preparation which is available in the potency levels D3, D4, D6, D12, D20 and D30 as drops, D3, D6, D10, D20 and D30 as ampoules and D6, D12 and D30 as globules. At Wala, carbon dioxide is used, which causes anaesthesia at low doses but leads to death at higher concentrations. Fortunately, relatively few animals have to be used for making the potentised preparations. About 8 bees can produce 10 kg of a D4 or 1000 kg of a D6 preparation. Wala uses glycerine instead of alcohol for the extraction medium, which is why their bee preparation is called Apis ex animale Gl (for Glycerine extract).

Pure Apis preparations from Wala are only available as ampoules. (They can also be taken orally by sucking out the contents with a small drinking straw and then holding them for about one minute under the tongue where the remedy is absorbed into the blood particularly well.) Ampoules are available in the potency levels D5, D6, D8, D12, D15,

D20 and D30 under the name of Apis ex animale. Wala only supplies globules for composite remedies which contain Apis.

Anthroposophical Apis preparations are also used for all the areas of application; they have already been mentioned in the section about their homeopathic use. However, they are also often given for autoimmune diseases in which immune processes which should actually protect the body from attack by foreign material go out of control and lead to chronic inflammatory processes of the body's own organs. Examples of such diseases are chronic *rheumatoid arthritis, multiple sclerosis and Lupus erythematodes*. In all these diseases there is a fundamental disruption of the immune system in one way or another, but often also to the general relationship between the body and soul. On closer examination you often find that in these kind of illnesses there are not enough 'sun forces' available. This might suggest why a creature like the bee, which itself displays a high degree of organisation, a connection to the sun and an effective handling of 'immune processes' can be of help. (Just consider the defeat of enemies by local production of warmth, the use of propolis, etc.)

The diseases mentioned are not only complex in both their causes and treatment but they can also be dangerous. They should therefore never be the subject of self treatment, but must always be supervised by an experienced doctor.

Composite medicines containing Apis

Many anthroposophical remedies include potentised Apis. Only a few examples can be given here. Potentised bee is often used in compositions for the relief of pain or swelling in inflammatory diseases. For example, this applies to Wala Apis/Belladonna globules (Apis D4, Atropa belladonna D3) or Weleda Erysidoron (Apis D2, Belladonna D2) and Bolus Eucalypti (this also contains Eucalyptus and purified clay) which are used, for example, for *acute inflammation of the pharynx* or for *inflammation of the skin*. As there is often a need to differentiate between diseases which require special treatment (for example, due to streptococci which are involved in scarlet fever), I do not want to do more here than mention this. Once a disease of this kind has been excluded, then the remedies mentioned are suitable for providing fast relief from the symptoms of pharyngitis.

If a significant *hoarseness* during a cold indicates that the vocal folds in the larynx are also involved in the inflammatory process, then Larynx/Apis comp. globules are often very beneficial. These contain the addition of potentised bryony (Bryonia) and various organ preparations from nerves which supply the larynx. I generally prescribe 5 globules 4 times a day while in very acute cases you can also take 5 globules hourly to start with. If the symptoms do not improve significantly within a few days the larynx needs to be examined by an ENT specialist.

During colds and infections of the upper respiratory tract, the air supply and pressure of the middle ear can become affected. The middle ear is connected to the nose/larynx area by the Eustachian tube. If the mucus membranes become inflamed, the exchange of air is prevented and pressure can develop in the middle ear (which can sometimes be uncomfortable, for example when landing in an aircraft). Hearing is affected and fluid can even collect (tympanic effusion) or an inflammation can develop. A combination of bee and lovage (Apis/Levisticum) can often help in this case. I usually prescribe Wala Apis/Levisticum II (Apis D4, Levisticum D3), 5 globules several times daily. Naturally earache or persistent hearing impairment need to be investigated and treated by a doctor.

The combination of Apis and Levisticum (produced by Weleda as Apis cum Levistico D3) as an injection is also used for acute tension of the musculature (*lumbago*). These type of injections can even help with disc prolapses where the remedy produces intense warmth and muscle relaxation and also reduces inflammation of the irritated nerves. However, this application – despite its reliability – belongs in the hands of the expert. Among other reasons, this is because injections of concentrated bee venom preparations require the careful exclusion of a potential allergy and the ability to treat an allergic reaction immediately if necessary.

Queen bee as a remedy

The queen bee forms the vital inner centre of a beehive. In contrast to a normal worker who lives to a maximum of 6 weeks, the queen can reach 5 years of age. She alone is able to lay eggs and thus preserve the continuity of her colony. She also secretes hormone-like substances whose scent ensures that the individual bees have a feeling of

A 43-year-old patient reported that, after a long period of trying to conceive children, an examination of his seminal fluid was performed. He was told that he could never become a father by natural means because he had too few sperm cells and they were not vigorous enough. Subsequently, the family had had a child by *in vitro* fertilisation, which involved the injection of a sperm cell into the egg under a microscope (ICSI). The patient wondered whether there might not be 'another, less intrusive way using anthroposophical medicine'. After all, *in vitro* fertilisation requires a stressful hormone treatment and surgical removal of egg cells from the mother. It also makes a great difference whether you 'produce' a child using considerable technical effort or whether you 'conceive' one where it is announced itself. I prescribed 10 globules of Testes comp. in the evening. Around a year later the family had had a child without any further intervention. The patient also mentioned – somewhat whimsically – that this treatment had been much less expensive. In the meantime, yet another child has been born without any kind of medical intervention.

belonging together. They also ensure that the workers – which are genetically identical to the queen – do not become sexually active. For a bee larva to develop into a queen it must, essentially, be fed for longer than the ordinary bees with queen substance, the famous royal jelly. It must also be reared in a special queen cell.

Wala supply Apis regina as a single remedy in ampoules of D5, D8, D12, D15 and D30. This remedy is not made solely from the queen bee but also from the royal jelly in the queen cell. One of the uses of this preparation is to stimulate inadequate or declining activity in the gonads. The remedy Testes comp. contains an organ preparation of animal testicle, potentised silver (which is related to the reproductive organs) and Apis regina Gl D4. Ovaria comp. is similar, but contains an organ preparation of ovary. These remedies have repeatedly helped couples to conceive a child in cases where they were unable to do so without assistance.

Ovaria comp. (which can be taken as a dose of 10 globules in the evenings) can be used to ease menopausal symptoms and, at least in the initial phase after *menopause,* this remedy often leads to renewed menstruation or causes a period which has become irregular to occur regularly again.

Apis regina comp., in contrast, makes use of the invigorating effect of the queen bee. A higher potency (D16) of the substance is combined with an organ preparation of the brain stem and is used for symptoms after brain damage and for *degenerative diseases of the nervous system.* Generally Apis regina comp. is prescribed for these serious types of illness as part of a treatment plan along with other medicines and in this sense is not a remedy for self medication.

The situation is different in the case of Aurum/Apis regina comp. which has proved beneficial for symptoms of exhaustion. Particularly when this is the result of nervous overstrain brought on by difficult circumstances, this remedy can help to draw on new strength. Besides Apis regina in D5, potentised gold in the form of soluble gold chloride and potentised St John's Wort (Hypericum) contribute to energising the inner light forces. Phosphate is involved in our metabolism in all transfers of energy, which is why phosphoric acid (the source of all phosphates) in potentised form is an important remedy for treating exhaustion. Oat *(Avena),* which it also contains, has a slightly calming and 'nourishing' effect and encourages sleep when it is harvested in the milk-ripe stage (when the grain oozes a white juice when squeezed). If you are feeling constantly overstrained, then Aurum/Apis regina comp. often helps and also usually relieves *'psychosomatic' problems* such as *headaches* and *digestive disorders* which often ensue. I often recommend taking 7 globules 3 times daily. However, it goes without saying that in such situations a remedy can be a help but is not a solution. It is always worth looking into how a more stable balance between work and relaxation can be found in the long term. It is also appropriate – often as part of a therapeutic discussion – to find out how imbalanced or one-sided emotions contribute to your exhaustion and how these can be transformed. Consciously cultivating your own powers of regeneration through regular sleep, sensible eating, rejuvenating excursions outdoors in nature or satisfying encounters can be as helpful in the long term as external measures. Examples of these are liver compresses with yarrow (see Chapter 3), rhythmical massage, oil massages (for example with lavender oil) or creative activity through art therapy. However, in order to get some initial strength back and to make a start in achieving fundamental changes to an exhausting life style, Aurum/Apis regina comp. can be a good beginning. It is often a help for *children who feel overstrained by school* and react by getting *headaches*. However, in such cases it is recommended to discuss the situation with your doctor.

Wax and honey

Beeswax packs, in which thin sheets of wax laid on silk are warmed using salt packs, often achieve good results for *muscle cramps, back pain* and *fibromyalgia*. They are also used in cases of *bronchitis* where they ease the coughing up of phlegm. They can be obtained from beekeepers or from some beekeeping organisations. Instructions for making them yourself can be found on the internet.

Honey has strong antibacterial properties and promotes wound healing. After the advent of modern antibiotics, the standard wound treatment using honey, which had been used for centuries, disappeared from most hospitals. Since the spread of antibiotic resistance in harmful bacteria, treatment using honey – for which special sterilised honey is often used – has become reestablished. This honey is available commercially, for example, as Medihoney. The treatment with honey has proved especially successful for *pressure sores* in bed-ridden patients. Taking honey after each dose of radiation treatment has been found to prevent serious inflammation of the *mucous membranes of the mouth during radiation treatment to the head and neck.*

In cases of *fungal infections* of the skin, studies have shown surprisingly high healing rates after regular applications of a mixture of honey, beeswax and olive oil. It is astonishing how much help bees can give us.

CHAPTER 25

Yellow Gentian

If we climb a mountain, we will have a variety of experiences. We have to exert ourselves, but gradually we gain altitude and when we look back, everything has grown smaller: trees, houses, cars, people – and, if we are lucky, also one or two of the problems which have occupied us for a long time. When we have climbed high enough, to a region where the sky seems to be clearer and the light stronger, this diminution even applies to plants. However, this is no longer an optical illusion because the flora at our feet has indeed changed. While down in the valley walking through a meadow the dandelions might come up to our knees; up here, they sometimes scarcely reach above our big toe. The expert will say: 'But these are not the same species of dandelion!' This is true, but to our eyes they are very similar.

Many plants have low-growing relatives, which appear high in the mountains where they often seem to be more powerful than down in the valley. The tall thistles of the valley that often tower above us have disappeared, to be replaced by the low but shining silver thistle (*Carlina acaulis*) – in the Pyrenees there is even a golden-coloured one. Instead of tall firs, there are low aromatic mountain pines. While the large rhododendrons seen in gardens would not grow here, they have a worthy representative in the small-flowered, small-leaved azaleas; the alpenrose which spreads across entire hillsides.

But totally new plants also appear. Amongst the most well known are the gentians. Like shining deep blue eyes the low-growing spring gentians look up at us, all very similar – always blue or purple – the 'purple gentian', the 'stemless gentian' and several other species.

And then, on a sunny but not too dry slope or in a clearing there

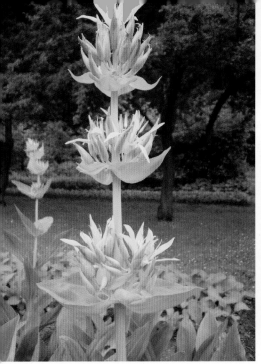

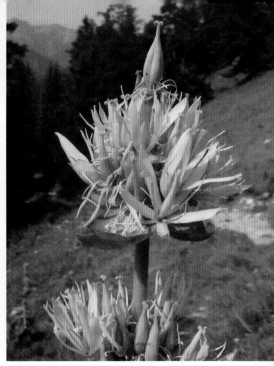

The tiers of flowers of the yellow gentian are arranged at right angles.

You may come across the yellow gentian – of which a flower detail is shown here – beside many paths in the Alps.

is an exception. Coming closer, we see large numbers of tall shapes. Are these statues of people that someone has set up there? No, they are actually plants. They stand there looking immensely powerful. Their structure is strictly organised with pairs of large – up to approximately 20 x 30 cm (8 x 12 in) – leaves arranged as though in tiers, their entire oval blue-green surfaces covered with strong parallel veins. Every level is at right angles to the others and at the top of the plant we see glowing yellow flowers.

This is the famous yellow gentian, which is evidently an exception to the miniaturising rule. It can be a good 1½ m (5 ft) tall and so assume the dimensions of a person. The part of the gentian used medicinally, the root, is enormous: it can reach up to 7 kg (15 lb) in weight. The colour of its flower is also a contrast to most of its relatives. However, it resembles its relatives in its bitter taste, which is characteristic of all species of gentian. The yellow gentian's mighty form is equalled by this intense bitterness. Even a one in ten thousand dilution of the root extract is still distinctly bitter. The characteristic bitter constituent of the yellow gentian, amarogentin, can still be

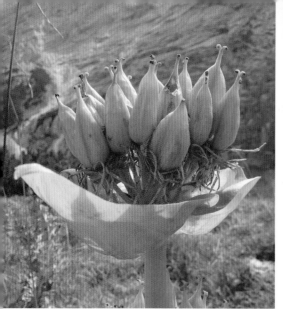

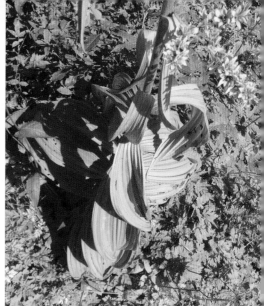

Yellow gentian: fruit detail.

The poisonous white hellebore (Veratrum album) *has spirally arranged leaves – those of the yellow gentian are decussate.*

detected as being bitter when it is diluted by a factor of 1:58,000,000 (which is 1 g in 300 bath-fulls of liquid).

This makes the gentian a veritable giant amongst the bitter herbal substances. Like all these substances, it strengthens the digestion. It has been demonstrated that it increases the flow of almost all the digestive fluids – from the gastric fluids containing hydrochloric acid to the bile which is itself bitter. This is the reason why gentian preparations were always seen as a good accompaniment to a greasy meal. The most well known of these is gentian schnapps. It is prepared from the fermented root because the latter also contains a large quantity of sugar and, since time immemorial, almost everything containing sugar has been turned into alcohol. This is not actually good for the gentian as shown by the fact that a large proportion of the bitter substances decomposes in the fermenting process. If you want to obtain as much of the healing power as possible, then the root should be dried quickly and later decocted and made into medicines (or nutritional supplements).

However, do not harvest this plant in the wild, as it is an endangered species and protected in many countries. In addition, it can easily be confused with the highly poisonous white hellebore *(Veratrum album)*, which has a similar general appearance but whose leaves are not decussate but arranged spirally around the shoot. Yellow gentian and white hellebore sometimes even grow side by side.

As many diseases can be partly caused by poor digestion, bitter agents can also be used in the treatment of *skin diseases, anaemia, headache, sinus problems* and even *colds* and *flu.* This is why gentian is contained in many remedies for *respiratory tract infections* and why the view has developed that good medicine should taste bitter.

At times the gentian was almost viewed as something like a cure-all. This gives it a similar degree of fame to another impressive mountain plant: arnica (Chapter 23).

Just as taking some gentian can help you to feel a little better after eating a rich meal, it can also sometimes help in very hot weather if you are feeling weak and drained. Bitter substances can pull us together and give us strength. This can be done equally well with bitter tea that you can prepare yourself (from gentian root, for example) or using elixirs or tonics to which other bitter and aromatic plants can be added, such as wormwood or ginger. On a strenuous mountain hike a taste of bitterness like this can also give us a feeling of new strength in order to climb up beyond the area where the gentian grows to the rocky peak. From here we can look down on the countryside spread out below and have the feeling that we have come a little nearer to the sky.

Yellow Gentian (*Gentiana lutea*)

It has already been mentioned that the yellow gentian is not suitable for collecting yourself, as it is an endangered species. The dried root drug can be obtained in a pharmacy as can a number of proprietary medicines. However, it is particularly impressive to see the magnificent plant in its natural habitat

Gentian tea

Gentian tea can be useful for a feeling of fullness after an excessively rich meal and also for a generally weak digestion or for a tendency to constipation. You can either brew 1 teaspoon of the root in 1 cup of boiling water and leave it to simmer for 10 minutes as usual, or add

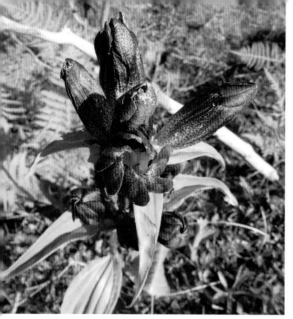

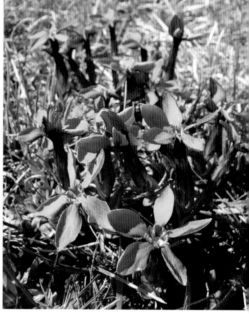

Gentiana pannonica – *a species of gentian with a purple flower.*

*The spring gentian (*Gentiana verna*) is one of the especially vivid blue gentians.*

1 teaspoon to 1 cup of cold water, soak it overnight and then bring it to a boil for a moment. The latter method gives an even more bitter extract.

To *stimulate the appetite* and *strengthen digestion,* a rather more aromatic tea mixture can be prepared from plants such as gentian root, ginger root, angelica and bitter orange peel to which peppermint leaf can be added according to taste.

The Clusius' gentian, Gentiana clusii *(left) is one of the particularly magnificent species of blue gentians, which also includes the willow gentian,* Gentiana asclepiadea *(centre), while the German gentian,* Genianella germanica *(right) tends more towards a purple colour.*

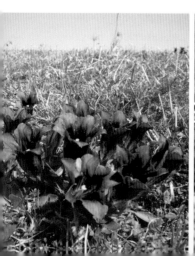

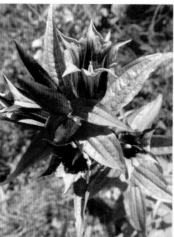

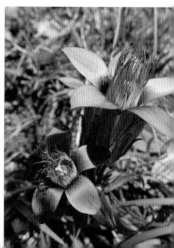

Gentian in phytotherapeutic and concentrated anthroposophical proprietary medicines

Gentian is usually made into aqueous proprietary remedies (which makes the taste very noticeable) along with other bitter and aromatic medicinal plants. They all stimulate the flow of digestive juices and the rhythmical gastro-intestinal movements and help to treat digestive weakness, a feeling of fullness and a tendency to constipation. They can be used as a complement to the treatment of chronic diseases that are improved by stimulating the digestion. This applies, for example, to many *skin diseases* (*eczema, acne* and others), *rheumatic diseases,* some *kidney diseases, bronchial asthma* etc. The uptake of iron is improved by gentian and bitter substances through stimulation of the stomach's activity (production of hydrochloric acid). However, because of the increased acid production, remedies of this kind should not be given when gastric or duodenal ulcers are present. In case of doubt, this should be discussed with your doctor. Aside from other effects, all these bitter substance preparations also have an 'awakening' effect. They likewise promote the body's formative forces. These are the forces which both break down foreign substances – such as those in our food – and also build up new substances in the body's own form. Bitter substances particularly stimulate the breakdown processes in the gastrointestinal tract.

Abdomilon N Liquidum is a preparation of gentian, sweet flag root, angelica, lemon balm and wormwood leaves, which often helps to reduce stomach pain in patients with *irritable bowel syndrome.* Amara-Pascoe drops are used for similar complaints also contain wormwood leaves and gentian. Cinchona bark and cinnamon are also included as bitter substances which stimulate the appetite. There are many other preparations with similar ingredients.

In the case of gentian, the demarcation between general phytotherapeutic and anthroposophical preparations with concentrated plant extracts is, practically speaking, scarcely possible. So I will make an exception here and deal with them together.

Amara drops (Weleda) contain wormwood, common centaury, chicory, juniper, yarrow, masterwort, sage and dandelion in addition to gentian. The usual dose for *loss of appetite* or a *bloated feeling after eating* and also for strengthening the digestion in various chronic diseases (such as skin complaints) is 10–15 drops 3 times daily before meals (for loss of appetite) or after (for bloating).

In contrast to all the remedies mentioned so far, Gentian stomach tonic (Wala) has the advantage of being non-alcoholic. It is obtained using an aqueous extraction of gentian root, wormwood, ginger root, a small amount of aromatic sweet flag root and a trace of pepper fruits. The usual dose is ½ to 1 teaspoon of the very bitter substance diluted in a little water 3 times daily. Like most strong bitter remedies it is suitable for teenagers and adults but is too strong for children. I also prescribe this sugar-free remedy as a complement to the treatment of *fungal infections of the intestine* (candidiasis). These can occur after taking antibiotics (when it is often associated with infection of the vaginal mucosa), in association with a diet containing too much sugar and also due to weakness of the immune system.

In cases where it is not necessary to make a large reduction in sugar consumption and if the taste of the Gentian stomach tonic is difficult to tolerate, Bitter-Elixir (syrup, Wala) is also an option (1 teaspoon 3 times daily). It is also suitable for preparing a refreshing and stimulating bitter drink (for example with carbonated water dilute to taste). This quenches the thirst but also instils new strength (according to many) in cases of *exhaustion* – for example on a mountain hike – and can also alleviate *fatigue.*

Gentian as an anthroposophical medicine

As a single substance, gentian is available from Weleda as an alcoholic decoction by the name of Gentiana lutea, ethanol Decoctum D1 (corresponding to 10%) and also as more dilute 5% drops. Wala produce the non-alcoholic Gentiana lutea Rh 5% drops and Gentiana lutea e radice 5% globules, globules in D2 (corresponding to 1%) and D4. The globules are the least bitter of these and can be given to children to stimulate the appetite. They are also used for *promoting digestion.* For example, in cases of neurodermatitis, they stimulate the digestion to break down and overcome the food – to strip it of its form and nature as a foreign substance – so that it has a less allergenic effect. This likewise prepares the way for building up and shaping substances according to the body's own individual form. Apart from this, all these pure gentian preparations can be prescribed for all the indications mentioned above. The normal dose for the Weleda drops is 5–10 drops 3 times daily before meals or alternatively the same number of the Wala globules (usually 5%).

I like to mix Gentiana lutea D1 (Weleda) with equal parts of Anaemodoron drops (a remedy made from wild strawberry fruits and stinging nettle) when trying to achieve a long-term cure for *iron deficiency in women* who generally feel cold and have other symptoms of iron deficiency. (These symptoms include a tendency to poor circulation, catching colds, cracks in the mucus membranes at the corners of the mouth etc.) I generally prescribe 20 drops of the mixture 3 times daily. One aspect of the efficacy of this mixture is that the digestion must work well to achieve a good uptake of iron (from which haemoglobin is produced) from the food. Gentian stimulates and strengthens the digestion.

It should be mentioned in passing that gentian in low potencies or as mother tincture was used in olden times for a *fever* remedy (one of its names in German also translates as 'fever root'). It is therefore contained in some remedies for *colds and flu* and has been shown to improve the defensive power of the mucous membranes.

In more recent times it has been demonstrated that bitter substances are not only detected by the body in the mouth, stomach and intestinal tract by what are known as bitter receptors but also in the respiratory tract. When these are activated by bitter substances, the respiratory tubes expand and the musculature of the bronchia relax three times more effectively than by using conventional asthma sprays.[1] Rudolf Steiner recommended the use of bitter remedies for *bronchial asthma* almost a century ago, and this therapeutic use has now been confirmed by current research. While bitter remedies were previously mainly swallowed there are now initial good results with inhaling them (for example Gentiana Magen injection, stomach remedy, which is the ampoule form of the globules described below). No conclusive opinion can yet be given on this form of application, but it does seem to be very promising.

Gentian in anthroposophical composite remedies

One medicine containing gentian which is particularly important to me is Gentiana Magen globules (stomach remedy, Wala). In addition to aqueous extracts of gentian and wormwood, which make these globules taste distinctly bitter, they contain extract of dandelion and seeds from the Indian poison nut *(Nux vomica)* in potentised form. This remedy has a broad application for *digestive disorders*, particularly if these are made worse by stress. This is also the reason why the remedy is suitable as a basic treatment for many men in the middle of life. The remedy is also suitable for detoxifying from alcohol or medication. It can also be prescribed for digestive disturbances after infections, when a dose of 10 globules should be taken 3 times daily. The similar Gentiana Magen injection (stomach remedy) in ampoule form is (as mentioned above) also used by some doctors for inhalation.

Vein problems have been successfully treated using Achillea comp. (Weleda) (see also Chapter 3). In this remedy, gentian in D3, along with an extract of horse chestnut, acts to tone the vascular system. Yarrow has an anti-inflammatory relaxing effect and stimulates the liver, and the potentised mineral antimonite (a compound of antimony and sulfur which forms radiating crystals) has a structuring effect on the mucus membranes. The remedy is particularly well known for *haemorrhoids* and *fissures in the mucus membranes* around the anus accompanied by itchiness.

CHAPTER 26

Monkshood

As a small child I could never understand how one and the same thing could have different names, and I argued fiercely with my cousin (who came from the city) about whether the sausages in the local corner shop were called *Schinkenwurst* or *Bierschinken*. What was almost worse was that the shiny yellow 'buttercup' which opened its flowers so innocently to the sky should be called 'crowfoot' according to her. Well, I must admit, if you did not look at the flowers but at the five divided lobes of the leaves, then you might admit with a bit of imagination that it bore a distant resemblance to a crow's foot. When an aunt later gave me an encyclopaedia I started to read it at the letter 'A', and under the heading 'Apple' I came across the unbelievable claim that it belonged to the rose family. The mere fact that it did not have any thorns left me feeling this to be quite impossible. However, now and again one does see roses without thorns ... and if I compared a wild rose flower (instead of a cultivated one) with the flower of an apple tree, then I had to admit that they were really quite similar.

I gradually got to know the principle of the formation of plant families. I could appreciate that many spring flowers which shone yellow in the meadows also belonged to the buttercup family: the lesser celandine, marsh marigold and globe flower. But the idea that the highly poisonous monkshood, which I had always been warned against, should also be part of the buttercup family seemed to me even stranger than the relationship between the rose and the apple.

While the flowers of the buttercups seem like little bowls that catch and reflect the light, the dark violet (sometimes almost black) flowers of the monkshood are quite hidden. They do not face the sky but look into the observer's face. In fact, they resemble a face themselves,

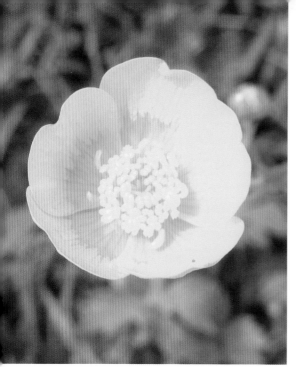
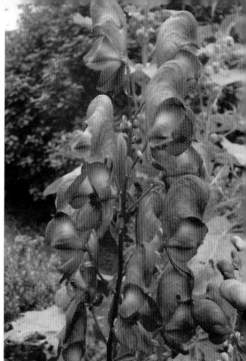

The yellow flower of the meadow buttercup opens wide to the sky, while the monkshood is darkened and turns away from the sun.

or rather the helmet of a knight's armour with the visor down, or a monk's hood, because the upper petal arches over and covers the inside of the flower. This seems to have lost all connection to the light, forming a dark internal space. What has happened to this relative of the shining buttercup species, that it has undergone such a change? In a fairy tale it would be said that a wicked fairy had touched it and cast a spell on it, so that it had now become wicked itself. In fact it is the most poisonous plant known in Central Europe and only a few are said to be able to kill a horse. Even coming into contact with the sap of the plant can cause poisoning. The area that has come into contact with the sap first burns and then goes numb. This reveals the basic nature of the action of the poison: an excessive stimulus is produced and then numbness or paralysis. This applies not only to the skin and tongue, but also to the heart and circulation. In the case of serious poisoning, initial palpitations and a raised pulse are followed by a decline in the pulse rate until the heart stops. Experiments in modern cell biology show that monkshood poison opens the sodium channels in the cell membranes, leading to a constant stimulus until the point of exhaustion.[1]

266

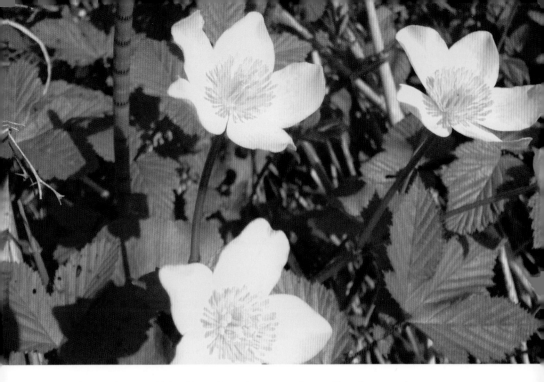

The marsh marigold (Caltha palustris) opens its shiny yellow flower to the sun.

Homeopathic doctors experimented on themselves by using highly diluted monkshood sap, which shows a more detailed picture. The blood vessels in the skin and limbs contract so that hardly any warm blood reaches them, the experimenter turns pale and feels cold, 'as though icy water was running in his veins or he had ice in his bones'. At the same time the experimenter starts to tremble as though having a shivering fit. The entire picture resembles a serious infectious disease, like the start of flu with a high fever. In fact diluted and potentised and therefore harmless monkshood juice – under the botanical name of *Aconitum* – is amongst the most important homeopathic remedies at the beginning of *flu*.

The picture described also resembles a state of great fear and shock, and these psychological feelings are indeed described in the proving of remedies. Highly potentised Aconitum is one of the most effective remedies for the disturbing consequences of a severe fright or *shock* in which, after an initial excitement, a state of numbness can ensue in which the soul is unable to open to the world but apparently becomes insensitive to the light around it and closes off, becoming dark and inaccessible. Because of the overwhelming intrusion into

267

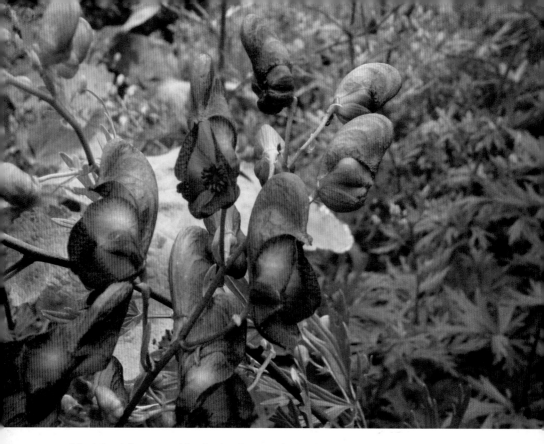

Monkshood flowers are like the closed visors of a knight's armour.

the inner world, the soul can become numb to a certain degree towards new aspects of the outer world. If we bear in mind that monkshood poisoning, accompanied by feelings of severe fright, lead via a 'salinisation' (excess sodium in the cells) to paralysis, we may get the impression that the biblical figure of Lot's wife, who was turned to a pillar of salt when she saw the catastrophic destruction of her native city, might symbolise a comparable paralysis through fright.

I have repeatedly found in practice – and also from the reports of colleagues – that patients who had found themselves in this kind of situation (which corresponds under certain circumstances to the picture of what is known as *post-traumatic stress disorder*) have felt as though warmed through and filled with new light after being given potentised Aconitum. This was also the case with patients with a physical illness attributable to a scare or shock they had experienced. Sometimes this shock lay years or decades in the past before it was treated in this way. As a rule, the longer ago the experience, the

Aconitum napellus *occurs in alpine meadows.*

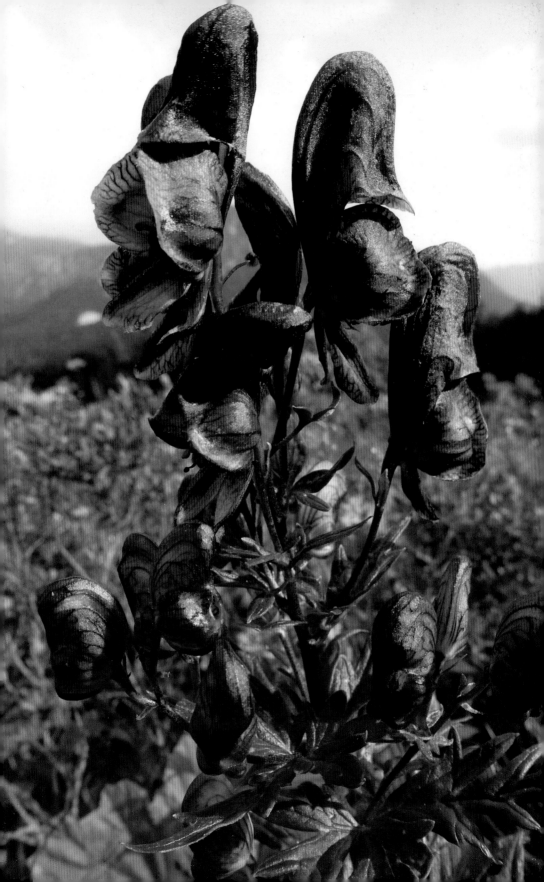

higher the potency required; in other words, the more the pharmacist preparing the remedy needs to work on it in order to transform the poison into a beneficial medicine. A patient, to whom I gave Aconitum C200 decades after a traumatic childhood experience, told me at her following consultation: 'After I took this remedy, it was the first time that I could sleep so deeply and for the first time I felt really connected with the world. My husband, who didn't know that I got a new medicine, said to me, "You look so well, so rosy and glowing!"'

I believe that it is no mere coincidence that medicinal preparations of monkshood from anthroposophical pharmaceutical practice – in which the macerated plant has been exposed rhythmically to the morning and evening sun in a carefully controlled process and therefore placed in a relationship to the light – have often been particularly successful. You have the impression that something has been 'healed' in the plant itself, which is then able to stimulate healing in the person. I have been very pleased to see how, after using this type of remedy, patients have gradually been able to open themselves again and have sometimes later mentioned a feeling as though the curse of a bad fairy had been removed from them.

Monkshood (*Aconitum napellus*)

Obviously this, the most poisonous plant in Europe, is not suitable for collecting yourself. As little as a gram of the root can be fatal. It is primarily in potentised form that the monkshood is made harmless and beneficial.

Potentised monkshood

Aconitum is considered to be non-toxic only above D4. Low potencies are often used at the start of *fevers* when the patient feels very shivery and has a raised pulse, usually looking pale and appearing anxious. Rapid relief of the symptoms and a warming effect can usually be obtained by dissolving 10 drops or globules of Aconitum D6 in half a glass of water and taking a sip every 30 minutes.

As already mentioned, in conditions of *shock* after very traumatic experiences, Aconitum can release feelings that appear to be paralysed. In such cases I usually prescribe 5 globules of Aconitum e tub. D20 or D30 as soon as possible after the event, continuing before going to bed for a few days. For traumatic events in the distant past, which are still having an effect, I sometimes prescribe Aconitum C200 from Gudjons, a company which – like the anthroposophical manufacturers – produce their potentised medicines by hand. This type of treatment often forms a helpful beginning to a long-term cure. (Such high potencies should only be prescribed by an experienced doctor, because they can be harmful if used wrongly. James T. Kent, one of the most famous homeopathic physicians wrote that 'They should be used as carefully as razor-blades.')

Aconitum (D30, as globules or injection) is also an option for *panic attacks* and for high levels of *anxiety* (for example, before operations). Many cases of sleep disturbance, if accompanied by feelings of anxiety, also respond well to taking Aconitum e tub. D30 (5 globules before going to bed or when required).

Aconitum is available in potentised form from all manufacturers of homeopathic medicines. Amongst the anthroposophical medical companies, Weleda supply alcoholic drops of Aconitum napellus D3, D4, D6, D10, D12, D20 and D30 plus a rhythmised aqueous preparation of Aconitum napellus Rh D6 and the same remedy as ampoules in D3, D6, D20 and D30 (the low potency ones may be prescription only in some countries). Weleda has recently also begun providing Aconitum globules in potencies D6, D12 and D30. The preparations by Wala of Aconitum e tubere globules D4, D6, D10, D20 and D30 and ampoules D6, D10, D20 and D30 are thoroughly rhythmised, in other words manufactured with light and warmth rhythms. My good experience with the consequences of shock conditions refers primarily to these rhythmised preparations.

Potentised Aconitum in composite remedies

Due to the characteristics described, Aconitum is contained in many remedies for treating *acute infections with fever*. This applies, for example, to Infludo (Weleda) for which a dose of 5 drops per hour is given for a cold with acute fever. During a sever flu epidemic in the 1920s, the rate of complications was significantly reduced using this remedy. Nowadays the milder but similarly composed Ferrum phosphoricum comp. globules (Weleda) seem to be better as a rule because they do not contain such low potencies of phosphorus which, in stressed patients, often intensifies their level of nervousness. In addition the globules do not contain alcohol.

Like the previous remedy, in addition to potentised Aconitum, Aconitum/China comp. (Wala) contains bryony (*Bryonia*) – which in potentised form helps painful dry mucous membranes – and Eucalyptus. It also contains hemp agrimony *(Eupatorium)* which counteracts muscle pain and strengthening extracts of cinchona bark. This remedy can be used as globules (dissolve 20–30 in a quarter glass of water and sip every half hour) or as suppositories (one at night). It has proved successful especially for *virus infections* accompanied by high fever that have a severe effect on general health.

It goes without saying that a serious disease such as *pneumonia* requires supervision by an experienced physician. However, it is not always appropriate or necessary to prescribe an antibiotic (for example if the infection is caused by a virus). If the doctor decides to do without one, he may often prescribe an external treatment such as mustard compresses, but for some patients a remedy like Pneumodoron 1 (Weleda) which contains low potencies of Bryonia and Aconitum is also helpful. Experienced doctors often find that this remedy can be of real benefit for *pneumonia* and *severe bronchitis*.

Salix/Rhus tox. comp. (Wala), which likewise contains potentised Aconitum, is often very efficacious for *febrile intestinal infections* (irrespective of whether these are caused by viruses or by Salmonella bacteria, for example, both of which require expert treatment including maintaining a balance due to fluid and salt losses). I also prefer to prescribe the remedy in soluble form here (20 globules in half a glass of water) to be taken in sips. The occurrence of fever along with digestive symptoms is always a reason to consult a doctor. Such cases require careful diagnosis as other diseases may also be involved (for example appendicitis or diverticulitis) which may require a different treatment.

The pain-relieving effect of Aconitum is one reason why it is contained in Disci/Rhus toxicodendron comp. (Wala) which, given in injection form, often improves *sciatica*. It is contained in Aconitum comp. (along with Rhus toxicodendron and Atropa belladonna) for similar reasons, and this remedy can sometimes (but not always) relieve *trigeminal neuralgia.*

Aconitum for external application

Wala's Aconite pain-relief oil has a very broad range of application for *neuralgia and muscular pain.* It is especially effective where the pain symptoms have been triggered by the effects of cold such as around the neck and shoulders and also in facial neuralgia. This can be a reminder that monkshood has a tendency to grow in places in the mountains which are totally exposed to the cold wind. Apart from potentised monkshood, the oil contains potentised silica, which is also beneficial for the effects of being chilled. In addition, it contains camphor, which has a direct warming effect and improves the circulation, and essential oil of lavender. The remedy should be applied several times a day to the painful areas.

Aconite ear drops (Aconit Ohrentropfen, Wala) have a very similar composition. They often give rapid pain relief at the start of an *ear infection.* When I worked at a children's hospital twenty years ago, children with a middle ear infection were still routinely prescribed antibiotics at the time. It is nowadays known that this is ineffective in most cases, damages the gut flora and considerably increases the risk of developing allergic illnesses and bronchial asthma. The current treatment is to start by giving analgesics, which can however have similar negative effects. In many cases it is sufficient to drop Aconite ear drops (which have been slightly warmed in the hand) into the ear several times a day. However, this must not be done if there is any damage to the eardrum. Ear infections require close supervision by an experienced doctor, and no treatment should be carried out without medical supervision. As a first aid measure before consulting a doctor you can put a drop of the oil onto some gauze dressing and put this into the ear canal. This will not cause any harm in the case of a damaged eardrum.

The Arnica comp./Apis and Arnica comp./Formica ointments already mentioned in Chapter 7 on the birch also contain Aconitum. The ointment which contains extracts of honey bee (Apis) is recommended for acute pain in the muscle and around the tendon insertion, and that containing ant (Formica) for chronic conditions.

Finally, Wala also makes the (usually prescription-only) concentrated oil extract Aconitum e tubere W 5% oleum, which is recommended for using as an oil dispersion bath. I have tended to use it for local application, by dabbing a little of the oil onto the appropriate nerve endings for severe pain caused by infection of the paranasal sinuses or *trigeminal neuralgia*, a treatment which often leads to a sudden decrease in the pain. Similar effects can be achieved for what can be very unpleasant *neuralgia after shingles* (Herpes zoster). However, due to the poisonous nature of the oil, it is not recommended for self-treatment.

CHAPTER 27

Chicory

When by the wayside you notice masses of sky-blue stars lighting up in the morning of a dry day in late summer, then a real feeling of happiness comes over you. While such a wealth of flowers might be rather overpowering in May, the mood around chicory is marked by a quiet cheerfulness. The plant does not appear at all vigorous. You need to go looking for the leaves. The larger ones are all near the ground, while further up there is almost nothing but dry stems and little pointed leaves. You may come across a chicory plant in the evening when the flowers from that day have wilted and fallen off. Looking at it, you could doubt for a moment whether this undergrowth, almost as tall as a man, is still alive. This many-branched form immediately reminds a physician of nerve fibres.

Everything seems to consist of lines and branchings. But then you notice little buds at the ends of the shoots and in the forks. Every morning, some of these open. They bloom for a day and on hot days wilt by noon. But until then – and even on cloudy days – you have the feeling of seeing a bit of heaven when you look at them from the distance. From close by you can see that the linear principle dominates even the flowers.

Like many medicinal plants described here, chicory also belongs to the daisy family. However, unlike the sunflower, for example, with its fleshy receptacle and large numbers of seeds in the centre of the flower surrounded by a ring of yellow ray florets, the flower heads of the chicory consist entirely of ray florets, which point outwards like blue radii. At the end of each petal are five points, indicating that this petal is made from five narrow radiating individual petals that have merged.

It is scarcely credible that, in mid to late summer, during flowering

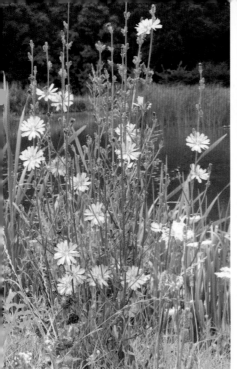

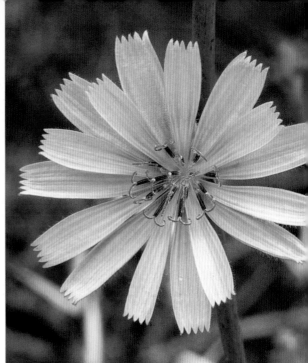

The chicory is reduced to such linear forms that at first all you notice are the flowers.

The flower of chicory.

time, up to 2,000 flowers can appear on this plant. If you rub the stem between your finger and thumb you can feel how dry and hard it is. It is not surprising that it contains large amounts of silica (which, in the mineral world is found, for instance, in quartz with its transparent crystalline, sharp-edged appearance). If you break off a piece of the plant, after a while you can see a little latex, a milky fluid, seeping out from the site of the injury. This is reminiscent of the dandelion, though the latter rapidly secretes a large quantity of white milk.

Latex is often found in plants that can work on the liver and gall bladder. Another indication of this in the chicory is its taste. If you chew on a stem or even on a root it tastes quite bitter, though not nearly as bitter as something like the yellow gentian. It is a pleasant, awakening, digestion-stimulating bitterness that we encounter here (there is additionally a slightly 'alkaline' background taste which comes from the alkaline salts).

The aromatic bitter taste is the reason why chicory also turns up in our lives far from the roadsides. Chicory (or endive) appears on our tables as a salad or steamed vegetable. It is obtained by digging up chicory roots in the winter and keeping them in a warm place in order to make the plant 'shoot'. It then produces fat leaf buds up to 20 cm (8 in) in length in which the leaves of a chicory plant are crowded together. This can be eaten as a bitter-tasting, appetite and digestive stimulating salad or as a steamed vegetable.

Chicory forms a transition from a food to a medicinal plant – or at least to a valuable dietetic food. After a *diarrhoeal illness* or in cases of an

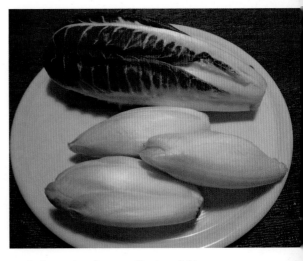

Radicchio and endive are offspring of chicory used for culinary purposes.

inflammatory intestinal disease, many foods cannot be tolerated and cause stomach ache. Steamed chicory (or radicchio, which is likewise obtained from the root of a red-leaved type of chicory) can then be valuable and gentle on the stomach and form a transitional stage to a more comprehensive diet. When the digestion has become stronger, the 'predigestion' by heating or steaming can gradually be left out and raw food enjoyed again. The rather bitter endive salad, for example, can then be important as it also aids digestive functioning. This salad was bred from a close relative of the chicory *(Cichorium endivia).*

Chicory helps to strengthen and regulate the digestion in a gentle manner. It can stimulate both the production and release of digestive secretions from the stomach, gall bladder and pancreas and the synthesis of new substances in the liver. This is also the way that composite preparations (in which chicory is combined with other plants and substances in a potentised form) work, as is the case in homeopathy but above all in anthroposophical medicine. Chicory can assist the attempt to increase the breakdown and synthesis of food material in order to cure diseases in which 'foreign material' (in this case the food) is not properly dealt with, leading to symptoms in the skin or kidneys, for example. In anthroposophical medicine in particular, chicory is not only processed in the form in which it occurs in nature. Its activity can also be directed by growing it on soils that contain specific metals in a dynamised form. A completely original development in anthroposophical pharmacy is represented by the medicines in which a plant such as chicory only functions as a inspirational 'model' for an elaborate new creation in the laboratory (see also page 280).

Perhaps there are still other things 'by the wayside' that would benefit from being taken up and developed further, as has been done with chicory in a variety of ways.

Chicory (*Cichorium intybus*)

In Italy, Greece and some other countries, the chicory leaves are sometimes collected for salad or eaten steamed like spinach, and the cultivated forms of chicory and radicchio are often used as a salad or vegetable. They have a stimulating effect on the appetite and are usually tolerated well during and after *gastrointestinal problems* when steamed.

In hard times the roots were dried and roasted at home in order to make them into a kind of coffee substitute. There are several products that contain roasted chicory root, such as cereal coffee or New Orleans coffee (a mixture of Arabic coffee and roasted chicory root), for example.

Potentised chicory

In anthroposophical pharmacy Cichorium is used both as a single remedy and also in compositions. Wala produce globules from a rhythmised charge made from the whole plant under the name of Cichorium e planta tota, 5% in D3 and D6 and with the same name as ampoules in D4. Weleda supply both alcoholic drops of a mother tincture under the name of Cichorium, ethanol. Decoctum (Mother Tincture) and a rhythmised aqueous preparation Cichorium Rh D3 and D6 drops.

These remedies stimulate the digestive process in the stomach and duodenum. This is where the food is broken down and 'overcome'. If this does not take place fully it can cause inflammatory processes which may play a part in such things as *eczema* to *neurodermatitis, bronchial asthma* and also in *inflammatory intestinal diseases* such as *colitis ulcerosa* and *kidney disease*. I use Cichorium/Pancreas comp. more frequently than the single remedy. This contains an organ preparation from the pancreas, which supports the functioning of the gland that produces the strongest digestive enzyme. The other components are Cichorium and antimony (stibium) which display similar delicate radiating forms. Both of them enhance the forces of organisation and form in us. I generally prescribe 5–10 globules before meals. The effect is often also noticeable in a gradual improvement in food hypersensitivities.

Cichorium and vegetablised metals

Cichorium Plumbo cultum means 'chicory grown with lead'; in other words, the plants have been grown on soil fertilised with lead. This sounds appalling, as lead can be a deadly poison. However, in normal potentising the concentration of a substance decreases geometrically (while, to use Hahnemann's phrase, its 'spiritual content' increases), until it can no longer be detected quantitatively. So there is no measurable amount of lead in this special chicory preparation. However, it is not only the pharmacist who sees to this but also the plant (see page 292). As has already been described for other plants, the lead compounds are first prepared and potentised and then they are used to treat the soil on which the chicory is to be grown. This chicory is made into compost. Chicory is grown on the compost and these plants are also composted and used to grow new chicory, which is then processed into the final medicine. This, like a 'normal' chicory plant, no longer contains detectable levels of lead, but the 'lead forces' are active in a special 'vegetablised' way. Cichorium Plumbo cultum is available as alcoholic drops in D2 and D3 and as aqueous Rh D3 drops (Weleda).

How can lead be beneficial as a medicine? One aspect is that lead can impart permanence. We are familiar with this from red lead paint for protecting iron objects exposed to wind and weather against rust. Red lead is itself 'rusted' or oxidised lead which prevents iron from oxidising.

If these 'shielding' effects of lead are combined with the structuring action of chicory, this can help people to be less dependent on effects from the outside world. It has frequently been observed that Cichorium Plumbo cultum can help people with extreme *sensitivity to odour* to be less affected by the smells in their surroundings. This remedy can also often produce an improvement in people with *'multiple chemical sensitivity'* who experience negative effects on their health due to low levels of chemical contamination in their environment which have no effect on other people (as yet). Similar observations have been made for *food hypersensitivities*. Other forms of dependency such as *addictive tendencies* (smoking, watching television, gambling, etc.) have also been alleviated by this remedy according to the reports of a number of physicians.

Chicory is also used to 'vegetablise' tin. The method used resembles that described above for lead. One preparation of this kind is Cichorium Stanno cultum (*stannum* is Latin for tin). Weleda manufacture alcoholic drops of this in D2 and D3, aqueous Rh D3 drops and D2 and D3 ampoules. It has been reported that this remedy has been of service in assisting depression with liver symptoms (for example digestive disorders when eating fatty foods). It may also be of relevance for liver diseases and diseases of the nervous system, but there is insufficient evidence so far to be able to make a conclusive judgement about this.

Chicory as a 'mineral model'

It was indicated earlier that in anthroposophical pharmacy new medicinal creations are produced inspired by plant models (page 278). One example of this is chicory and the remedy Solutio Alkali comp., which is produced by Weleda. This remedy does not contain any chicory as such, but the study of this plant provided the crucial stimulus, the 'model' for this remedy.

The ashes of chicory contain alkaline salts and silica. The plant is characterised by bitter substances and its latex contains substances similar to resin. To manufacture Solutio Alkali comp., minerals are processed representing natural alkaline salts, quartz and the bitter-tasting resinous myrrh, which acts to 'combine' or 'glue together' the individual substances.

The 'original' chicory itself promotes digestion. The Solutio Alkali comp. manufactured on this model apparently increases the effect in such a way that the remedy produced by Weleda in Switzerland is able to help patients who have lost a large part of their intestine due to operations. The Austrian paediatrician Dr Reinhard Schwarz reported that a child who only had 20% of his small intestine after an operation and was starving due to the resulting severe 'short bowel syndrome' recovered significantly thanks to this remedy.[1]

The remedy can also work well for *psychological problems* arising because a person has not managed to achieve what they set out to do.

There is only a small amount of experience with remedies like this, but it seems likely that a great deal more can be expected in this area.

CHAPTER 28

Stinging Nettle

Anyone who has come into contact with the stinging nettle as a child (and who hasn't?) may not have found it very pleasant, but will have learned to respect this plant. There are not many plants with such efficient defences. And its poison is not something insidious which only makes itself felt hours later, but has an immediate and unmistakable message: do not trifle with me!

In late autumn its evenly serrated leaves have mostly disappeared, but its now dark stem still stands upright as though it wants to say 'this is my place, don't come too close!' It will stay like this throughout the winter – a sign of the almost 'iron' strength this plant contains.

The gardener can make use of the powerful defensive side of this plant by soaking the fresh leaves for a day and using the water infused with the effect of the nettle to spray on plants that have been attacked by pests, or on those that he wants to protect. A completely different side of the plant is put to use if he leaves the nettles lying in the water for a few days. The leaves decompose surprisingly quickly and a dark, strong and rather sulfurous-smelling slurry is produced which is an excellent fertiliser. However, the nettle is not only nourishing for plants. The most common and beautiful of our butterflies have lived on nettle leaves as caterpillars; for example, the peacock butterfly, small tortoiseshell and red admiral. The nettle is also a delicacy for cattle. A farmer told me recently that ill cows and goats who refuse touch any feed almost always start eating happily if you put nettle hay in front of them.

The nettle can be a tasty food supplement for us as well. Turkish bureks filled with steamed nettle taste better than with any other filling. Nettle sprouts can also form a delicious addition to spring salads

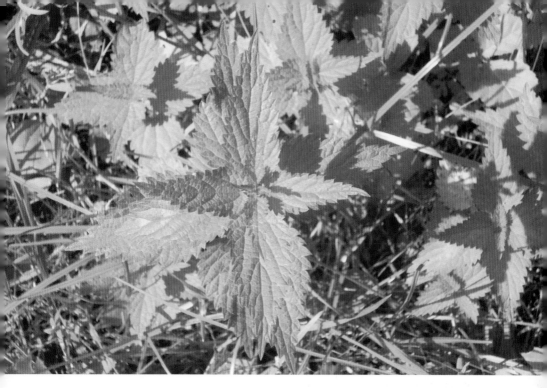

The pairs of opposite leaves are arranged to form crosses, one above the other.

and contribute to good health not least due to their amazing level of iron (analyses show that this plant contains almost twenty times the iron found in such things as pork escalope; its protein content is also unusually high and exceeds that of soya beans). The secret in the preparation lies in the fine stinging hairs on the leaves, which consist of glass-like silica and behave like sharp needles. These hairs break off when they are chopped up and rolled with a rolling pin, so that the nettles lose their painful side. Heating them also helps to 'disarm' them.

The nettle is not only nutritious itself, but it also indicates nutrient-rich and especially nitrogen-rich soil. If there is a patch of nettles in a particular place, it is quite likely that, long ago, this was the rubbish dump or even the toilet of a long vanished house or castle. The plant now re-establishes order in the soil by removing the excess nutrients.

To see one of the plant's particularly striking features, you need to observe it carefully in summer. Sit down in front of a nettle patch on a still, hot day and watch the flowers. You will suddenly notice a little 'explosion', which emits a yellow cloud. Soon after, more of these events can be detected and you might even hear an accompanying crackling sound. If you look closely, you will see that the flowers look

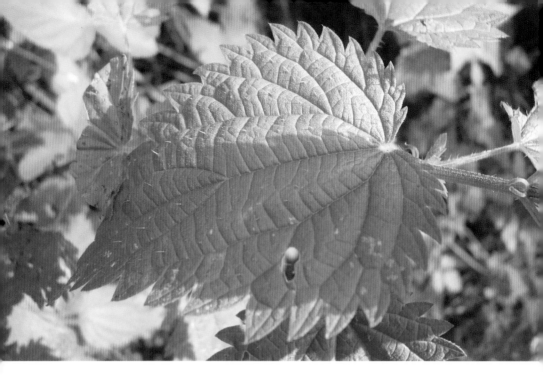

The stinging hairs can be clearly seen on the leaves.

like little clenched fists. The 'fingers' are the filaments, which suddenly stretch out and fling the pollen into the air. This does not happen in all plants, and you can observe that there are two different types of flower, which occur only on one or other plant. Male and female flowers are borne on different plants, so that one makes pollen while the other produces fruits. These fruits taste a bit nutty and are said to have an invigorating effect.

However, not everyone will enjoy observing these pollen explosions. As this pollen is a powerful allergen, people who suffer from hay fever can also react 'explosively' to it with violent sneezing fits.

The fibres from the stems can be used to make high-quality cloth, but first and foremost the stinging nettle is a major medicinal plant with an amazing range of effects. In line with the homeopathic principle that symptoms of disease can be healed by a substance which produces the same symptoms in healthy individuals, it is clear that preparations made from nettles can be beneficial for burning *itchy skin conditions* (for example *nettle rash*) and also for *burns*. But nettle can also have a beneficial effect on inflammation deeper inside the body. It has been used since olden times for *joint inflammation*. As a small child I watched amazed as an old woman treated her legs with a bunch of

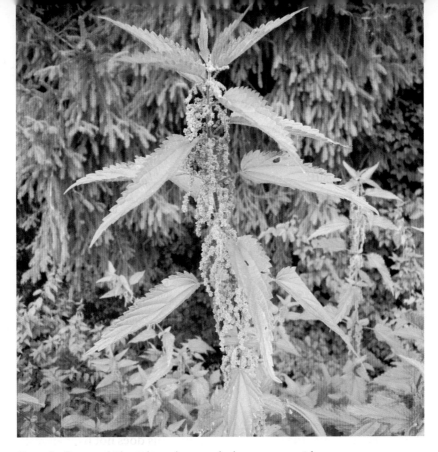

Even the flowers which are borne between the leaves are greenish.

nettles she had pulled up. When she noticed me, she explained that it helped her rheumatic pains. Less hardened souls take internal stinging nettle preparations, which also demonstrate anti-inflammatory effects in laboratory tests. Studies have confirmed that preparations made from nettle leaves significantly reduce the need for analgesics in rheumatism patients. In addition, the stinging nettle can help to check the sometimes rapidly advancing cartilage degradation in *inflammatory rheumatic disorders.*

The nettle roots have a very different effect: they can counteract problems in minor to moderate *enlargement of the prostate* in older men. One of the findings is that the increasing change with age from testosterone to oestrogenic hormones (which allow the prostate to grow) can be inhibited by extracts from stinging nettle roots. So you could say that the Mars-like action of the 'iron' stinging nettle helps to prolong 'masculinity', even at the level of the hormones. Presumably the traditional use of hair tonics which are made using stinging nettle roots and which are claimed to counteract hair loss in men can also be explained by the effect on the hormonal changes. In any case, medicines which are used for genetically determined *male hair loss* (androgenic alopecia) inhibit the same hormone conversion enzyme (5-α-reductase) as the extract from stinging nettle roots.

The often rapid effect on prostate problems presumably has another reason: thanks to the anti-inflammatory effect of the nettle, the enlarged prostate gland can reduce rapidly, which eases the pressure on the urethra. The urinary stream becomes stronger and there is less interruption to sleep due to the urge to urinate.

Nobody who has studied the stinging nettle will be surprised that it has a strengthening effect and supports our iron metabolism. *Iron deficiency* leads to tiredness and a susceptibility to infections, amongst other things. Both of these can be improved by nettle.

The 'iron' side of the plant can be further enhanced if it is cultivated on soil fertilised with iron as is done in anthroposophical pharmacy. In this form the nettle can promote the formation of blood and the defence against infection.

But its therapeutic effects by no means end here. Besides all those already mentioned, the leaves have a slight germicidal action, which is why they were used as wound dressings during wartime shortages. Many other areas of application could be added to this.

Experimental-scientific phytopharmacology has recently found that extracts of stinging nettle are astonishingly effective against *tuberculosis bacteria*. For 35 years no new tuberculostatic substances had been found and more and more patients suffered from antibiotic resistant mycobacteria.[1] At this stage these laboratory findings cannot be used for patients directly, but there is a tradition of using stinging nettle in tuberculosis in naturopathy (Sebastian Kneipp recommended it for treatment of this condition). So there is hope that this new discovery could be useful in future. Again, we can see the power of this strong plant.

Rudolf Steiner explained in his Agricultural Course for farmers, 'the nettle is a regular jack-of-all-trades which can do an amazing amount.'[2] The nettle stems that remain visible in late autumn and throughout the winter are like exclamation marks after this statement.

Nettle (*Urtica dioica*, stinging nettle, and *Urtica urens*, annual nettle)

Only a few of the many therapeutic effects of this jack-of-all-trades, the nettle, can be described here.

Stinging nettle can easily be collected yourself. For using as a vegetable or for adding to a salad the soft young shoots are best. They are suitable for a spring detox. In addition to appetite stimulating bitter herbs such as yarrow, the nettle is valued in a detox as a good source of vitamins and as a diuretic which therefore 'cleanses' the blood. It is advisable to wear gloves and long-sleeved clothing when collecting it. To avoid stinging your tongue on the salad, wrap the leaves in a dry cloth and roll this a few times with a rolling pin or a glass. This breaks off the fine stinging hairs so they can no longer penetrate the skin.

When collecting nettles for making tea there is really no difference between the common stinging nettle and the annual nettle, although the common one may have more powerful stings. Older plants are also suitable for drying, but these should not be cut too late in the year (July at the latest). You can tie the stems into bundles with the leaves and flowers attached and air dry them. They will then lose their stinging capacity.

Nettle tea

The dried herb can be chopped up small or crushed. The correct proportions are 2 teaspoons of this to 1 cup of boiling water. Leave to infuse for 10 minutes and then, depending on preference, drink the tea as it is or (if the taste is not interesting enough) with the addition of some honey and lemon. Midwives often recommend nettle tea with lemon during pregnancy because it prevents excessive *anaemia*. A slight drop in the level of haemoglobin is normal during pregnancy. What would be a sign of anaemia at any other time is normal during pregnancy and even a certain protection against thrombosis. However, the drop in haemoglobin should not be too marked and nettle tea can help to avoid recourse to mineral iron supplements. It can also assist the body in absorbing and utilising iron well. The tea also has a mildly diuretic effect, thus countering a slight tendency to *fluid retention* (*oedema*), which often

I learned about another way of using nettle from a patient which has frequently proved beneficial. The patient was considerably overweight and suffered from the frequently associated problems of high blood pressure, a tendency to a fatty liver and a high cholesterol level. The patient had tried many ways of losing weight but this was never successful in the long-term. The next time he appeared in my practice for a check-up he looked fit and energetic and had lost a considerable amount of weight. His blood pressure was excellent and his blood lipids and liver function results had normalised. I asked him how these changes had come about and he told me that it had been suggested that he regularly make himself a 'green smoothie' from a small handful each of nettle, dandelion and ground elder (the weed most gardeners fight against doggedly but without success). Adding water, and some kiwi and banana to improve the overall flavour, he made a smooth paste in a kitchen mixer. This drink replaced one meal a day. His condition was maintained by continuing with this herbal drink and, since then, many patients have copied him successfully. I suspect that this success is not due merely to replacing one main meal with the low-calorie and low-fat yet filling drink, but mainly to the effect of the herbs in stimulating the metabolism, and to their valuable contribution to the diet. As well as a positive effect on the feeling of hunger, there was also no longer a deficiency in the important dietary components, which is a feature of the food we otherwise tend to eat. I would not like to draw any conclusions as to whether his regular outings to the garden or elsewhere in his surroundings to collect the necessary herbs also contributed to the loss in weight. However, this certainly would have done the garden good, and studies have shown that there is no activity more beneficial to our long-term health as working in the garden.

occurs in late pregnancy. On the other hand, marked fluid retention must be seen by a doctor as it can be the first sign of pathological changes (for example pre-eclampsia).

Nettle tea can also be useful for *rheumatic conditions*. Besides its action in promoting excretion which may contribute to lowering uric acid levels, nettle tea has a direct anti-inflammatory effect (see below).

Nettle extracts

In phytotherapy, nettle extracts are often administered nowadays as tablets, capsules or sugar-coated tablets. In this form large amounts of the nettle substances act directly on the metabolism and have an anti-inflammatory effect. A distinction must be made between preparations made from nettle leaves and those from roots.

Extracts from nettle leaves are used for their diuretic effect. This can be useful for assisting in cases of *bladder infections* and also for the prevention of kidney gravel in patients who have already had bladder or *kidney stones*. A second area of application for these kinds of leaf extracts is based on the anti-inflammatory 'anti-rheumatic' effect which can be helpful both for *inflammatory rheumatic diseases* and for problems caused by arthrosis. For instance, Rheuma-hek is used for both indications at a recommended dose of 2 capsules twice daily. These preparations are generally tolerated well, however, sensitive patients may occasionally experience gastro-intestinal symptoms or – in the case of sensitivity to nettle – allergic reactions.

Remedies made from nettle root extracts are primarily recommended to relieve the symptoms of slight to moderate *enlargement of the prostate* (grade 1 to 2). This can help the urinary stream to become stronger again, an excessive urge to urinate can decline, as can the necessity to pass water frequently in the night. However, in the case of prostate problems, a proper diagnosis is needed before any self-treatment as a benign age-related enlargement of the prostate can cause very similar symptoms to a slight inflammation or even – much less frequently – the start of a carcinoma. Well-known remedies made from nettle roots are, for example, Natu-prosta, Prostaforton and Bazoton.

At the interface between phytotherapy and anthroposophical medicine is the preparation Menodoron (Weleda), which has proved

289

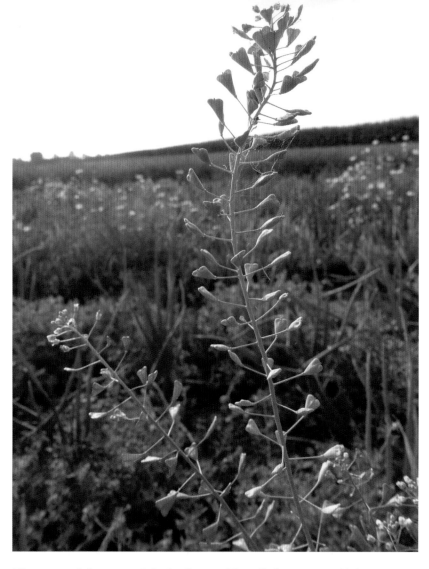

The very regularly structured shepherd's purse (Capsella bursa-pastoris) *has a styptic effect and is used to regulate menstruation in the composite remedy Menodoron.*

beneficial for varied menstrual disorders. If it is used for a sufficiently long time (at least 3 months), then this remedy can frequently be of help both for *disturbances to the menstrual cycle* (too short or too long intervals between periods) and also for heavy or *painful menses.* Other remedies are better for menstrual cramps on their own, but a tendency to this is often successfully treated by Menodoron. The remedy contains numerous medicinal plants in quite high concentrations, amongst them rather unusually stinging nettle flowers. This may be due to the fact that flowers normally act particularly on the organs of the abdomen and pelvis.

Menodoron should help to stabilise the organ's activity in terms of its rhythmical regulation. Besides nettle flowers, such things as yarrow flowers and shepherd's purse flowers are used, the latter displaying a more beautiful rhythmical flowering structure in its form than almost any other native plant.

Potentised nettle

The use of nettle in homeopathy and anthroposophical medicine is very similar to that in phytotherapy. The mother tincture and low potencies of *Urtica urens* (and *Urtica dioica)* are recommended to *stimulate urination* and for *rheumatic complaints* and also for *nettle rash* (*Urticaria*). Ceres produce a good mother tincture, for example. They claim that the remedy can also be beneficial for psychological symptoms if you wish to strengthen the 'iron forces' and promote the patient's self-assertiveness. The recommended dose is a few drops several times daily (for example 3–5 drops 3 times daily). The single remedy is available as Urtica dioica (from the whole plant, that is leaves and roots) as ampoules (D3 and D6) and globules (also D3 and D6) from Wala which also manufactures Urtica urens (from the leaves) as ampoules in D6 and as globules in D2, D4 and D6.

However, Urtica is more frequently used in a composition with other therapeutic substances. In cases of *nettle rash* (*Urticaria*), which causes itchy skin symptoms (including the formation of weals which resemble those which occur after coming into contact with stinging nettle), good results have been achieved in our practice using Urtica comp. (Wala). In addition to potentised nettle, it also contains potencies of tin and oyster shell lime (conchae or calcium carbonicum Hahnemanni). Both remedies act to limit the fluid processes which have overflowed their boundaries and help to quickly remove the unpleasant weals. Acute symptoms of Urticaria can be the result of an oversensitivity to particular foods or medicines which need to be identified and eliminated. However, it is also possible that these kind of skin reactions are due to (virus) infections or to chronic *overgrowth of yeasts* (*Candida*) *in the gut* or to *chronic infections* (for example of the *nasal sinuses*). While Urtica comp. (at a normal dose of 5–10 globules 3 times daily) may help in such cases to finally clear up the problem, a detailed investigation and elimination of the cause may be necessary.

Another remedy from the anthroposophical pharmacy which is suitable for treating *prostate enlargement* and the accompanying problems is Berberis/Urtica urens, in which nettle is combined with barberry (Berberis vulgaris). Barberry exhibits a 'contracting' effect, which promotes shaping and formation. Globules (5–10, 3 times daily) and ampoules (1 ampoule subcutaneously 1–3 times a week) of this combination are available from Wala and ampoules, drops and tablets from Weleda. The preparations from both companies are also suitable for treating disorganised benign growth processes in the uterus in the form of myomas. A more specific treatment for this is the combination of Berberis/Uterus comp. (ampoules and globules, Wala), a remedy containing a series of other potentised substances which intensify the effect and target it to the female genital region. In a similar way the remedy Berberis/Prostata comp. (ampoules and globules, Wala), which also contains nettle, targets the effect more intensively to the prostate.

Soil enriched with metals or vegetabilised minerals

The relationship between iron and nettle was described earlier (page 286) so it is not surprising that anthroposophical pharmacy also works with nettle which has been grown on soil fertilised with iron. Making a fertiliser of this kind requires a time-consuming multi-stage process. This involves dissolving a mineral compound of the metal (in the case of iron this is pyrite which also contains sulfur) in a strong acid, which releases oxygen, and then condensing it again into a solid in a distillation process. This is followed by another acid treatment, this time using sulfuric acid, so that the sulfur is linked in a different way than it was in the original solid mineral – this time in a mobile soluble form. Next, a 'carbon dioxide producing' acid, red wine vinegar, is used to dissolve the substance and finally a nitrogen compound is used. In this way the metal is combined with the important non-metallic elements of oxygen, sulfur, carbon and nitrogen which, together with hydrogen (an essential component of all acids) are also the key components of protein and are of crucial importance for plant growth.

In the Agriculture Course, Rudolf Steiner spoke at length about these elements (his descriptions there are quite vivid and graphic, but do require some basic knowledge of anthroposophy and are best understood when discussed with others). The last part of the process for preparing the fertiliser involves treatment with warmth.[3] This complicated process dissolves the mineral formed eons ago which has been lying motionless in the depths of the earth and sets the metal contained in it on a path which finally connects it to the plant. Every plant does this to a certain degree when it excretes acids from its roots to release minerals into the soil, making them available in living form. The connection of the dissolved and therefore activated metal with the plant material can be viewed as a kind of potentising. It is comparable to what pharmacists do with their pestle and mortar when they take a mineral or metal and, by grinding it with lactose, crush it increasingly finely so that its surface and efficacy are increased enormously. If you intentionally allow the plant to act as the 'potentiser', then this can produce particularly effective therapeutic substances. As part of this 'potentising process' the plants grown on the soil fertilised with metal are harvested, composted and themselves then used as fertiliser for the next plant generation which is again treated in the same manner. It is only the third plant generation which is used for preparing the remedy.

Nettle fertilised with iron

Weleda makes a preparation of this kind under the name of Urtica dioica Ferro culta. This remedy can be used for slight iron deficiency but can also help in cases of serious *anaemia* when additional iron has to be given, as the herbal preparation then stimulates the processing of the iron into living blood in the body. Urtica dioica Ferro culta is also suitable when you still feel run-down after an illness before full recovery. This remedy can also help to improve the iron forces if there is a tendency to *low blood pressure* and *susceptibility to infection*. The usual dose (depending on age and the severity of the condition) is 5–15 drops of the D2, 3 times daily before meals.

A description of a very efficacious nettle preparation for iron deficiency is also given in Chapter 25 on the yellow gentian.

External use of nettle

Nettle is used as an alcoholic extract in remedies for *burns and scalds*. Combudoron (Weleda) consists mainly of a nettle extract and a small amount of arnica essence; Wala's Burn Lotion and Wound and Burns Gel are similar, but also contain some additional potentised substances. Both Combudoron and the Burn Lotion produce a rapid reduction in pain after heat damage to the skin, if baths and compresses are applied with a dilution of Combudoron liquid or Burn Lotion at 1:10 to 1:20 immediately after the injury has occurred. Experience has shown that the healing process is also accelerated.

After the terrible firestorms following the bombing of Dresden in 1945, the anthroposophical doctor Kurt Magerstädt set up baths with solutions like this where the burn victims could treat their wounds, and it is said that many lives were saved in this way. Combudoron gel or Wound and Burns Gel can be used for small-scale or surface burns and for treating insect bites. It is recommended that Burn Lotion or Combudoron is kept in every household so that first aid can be applied quickly and effectively when a burn occurs. However, seek medical help in all cases of higher degree injuries, in other words those accompanied by blistering or even – in the case of third degree burns – where the skin dies and becomes numb. Revaccination against tetanus should also be considered if necessary.

For large-scale skin damage from *sunburn*, diluted Burn Lotion or Combudoron can also be sprayed onto the skin. One option is to obtain an empty bottle with a spray top from the chemist and fill this with the diluted solution. The reddened skin can be sprayed several times a day, which generally quickly provides relief. In addition, Apis D6 can be taken internally (see Chapter 24 on bees).

Baths with the addition of nettle tincture or oil dispersion baths with Urtica urens 5% W Oleum (Wala) can also be useful for various skin diseases which form blisters. However, treatment of these serious diseases belongs in the hands of a specialist.

Another form of external use is as nettle hair tonic. Many hair tonics which are marketed for using to treat *hair loss in men* contain extracts of nettle root. If you want to remove nettle patches in your garden by digging up the roots, then the opportunity can be used and a hair tonic made from the carefully washed and chopped roots which are put into a container with a good-fitting lid along with 20–30% alcohol and left for at least 14 days before straining off the fluid. If you like, you can scent the extract with a few drops of rosemary, lavender or bay oil to give your hair tonic a personal touch. If you add 5 ml glycerine to 100 ml of the extract it does not have such a drying effect on the scalp as it would otherwise, due to the alcohol content. While this hair tonic will not provide a wonder drug against progressive 'thinning' of the hair, it can be fun to obtain 'added value' from gardening work.

Urtica dioica ex herba W 5% Oleum (Wala) can be used for oil dispersion baths for rheumatic conditions. This has a warming effect and stimulates urination and therefore 'detoxification'. The same indications can be treated with Birken-Rheumaöl (Wala) which, in addition to nettle, contains oily extracts of birch, burdock, arnica and a small amount of an extract made from the red wood ant.

CHAPTER 29

Bilberry and Cranberry

It is always nice to receive a present. On your birthday and at Christmas this might be expected, but it is particularly pleasing when it is a surprise.

This may happen to us when we are strolling through the woods. Anyone who collects mushrooms knows the feeling, when they go on a mushroom hunt in late summer or early autumn and suddenly discover a group of delicious boletus. But for many, gathering mushrooms is too risky – after all, you might pick a poisonous one. And on top of that they still have to be cleaned and fried. But when we find berries, this can arouse an immediate feeling of happiness. Ripe raspberries can scarcely be surpassed, but if we come across a whole patch of bilberries in a sunny clearing in the woods, then there is no stopping us until our teeth and tongue are dyed a deep purple. When we pop the dark, slightly flat-topped spheres into our mouths and slowly squash them with our tongue until the tasty juice escapes from the bursting berries, we may ask ourselves why bilberries do not always taste so good. But the wild berries have actually always been like this! The fact is that the cultivated berries that we get in shops are much larger than the wild bilberries, but their juice is as pale as their flavour is bland. The inside of the 'real' bilberries is purple through and through. This enables them to capture the heat of the sun particularly well. When the sun shines they heat up far beyond the ambient temperature. In his famous multi-volume botanical work, *Illustrierte Flora von Mitteleuropa*, Gustav Hegi says of the bilberry that, on a sunny day once 'inside a basket of bilberries (at 11 o'clock) a temperature of 40°C (104°F) was measured, although the air temperature was far below this'.

Without a doubt the smell of bilberry plants on a sunny day is

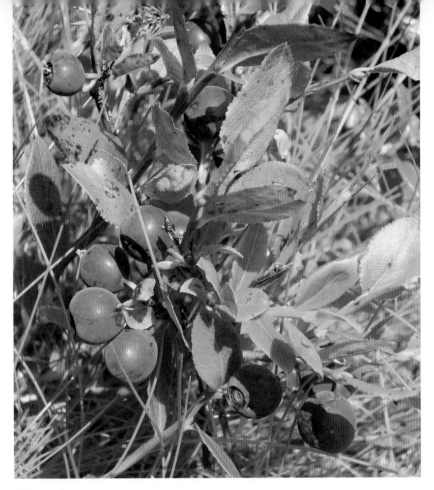

Bilberry plant.

absolutely wonderful. This is not due solely to the berries but also comes from the pine needles which usually cover the ground where bilberries grow. But there is another darker and fuller component of the scent which is reminiscent of earth on which the first raindrops fall after prolonged summer heat. This smell comes from root fungi, the mycorrhizae, which form a dense mat around the roots of these small-leaved plants. The roots never actually touch the earth but are always immersed in a felt of fungus. So in fact we have discovered berries and fungi at the same time.

The bilberry mycorrhizae help to extract minerals from the rocks which the plants then absorb. They weather the stony substrate (this is usually granite and its relatives because bilberries like soil rich in silica) and create humus. However, the humus which is produced in bilberry patches is very acidic, partly due to the thick carpet-like mat of roots

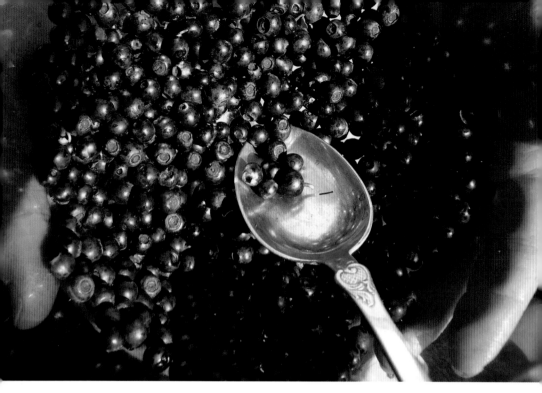

Harvest from a walk in the woods.

and plants. This means that scarcely anything else can grow in a stand of bilberries.

This is one element of the bilberry, which reappears in its phytotherapeutic effect. In the past dried bilberries were an invariable part of any home pharmacy because they are very helpful for *digestive upsets* and *diarrhoeal diseases*. Bilberry not only calms the stomach, but also tastes good (in any case, better than some diarrhoea medicines). Digestive disorders are usually due to a disturbance in the microbial balance of the wall of the intestine. Foreign microbes which do not belong there have spread. While in the past these cases were often treated with bactericidal antibiotics, often resulting in an even greater imbalance, nowadays what are known as probiotics tend to be given. These are medicines and foods containing useful bacteria which are part of our healthy gut flora. If there is enough of them they can drive out the troublemakers – just as the bilberries do on the forest floor. (Incidentally, for this reason cowberries and cranberries which are relatives of the bilberry are able to prevent *bladder infections* as they stop the formation of a dense layer of bacteria on the mucosa of the bladder if we eat these berries or drink their juice).

298

While the alleviation of mild diarrhoea is welcome but not especially noteworthy, in recent years bilberries have achieved publicity in a more serious connection. Cancer cells simply grow without any regard for their surroundings. It is possible that bilberry juice can often induce apoptosis in cancer cells. This is a process of autolysis – whereby the cell dissolves itself in an orderly fashion – which can occur in all healthy cells when they are too old or damaged to fulfil their original functions. A characteristic of cancer cells is that apoptosis (programmed cell death) no longer takes place, which is why they can become dangerous.

The 'bilberry power' can obviously help us to once again be 'master in our own house' and to repulse 'intruders'. It is unlikely that any *cancer* has ever been cured by bilberries alone, but they will probably contribute to cancer prevention and be beneficial in the case of disease.

It is mainly the anthocyanins, the pigments in the bilberries, which are responsible for this effect, so it is good for our health if we accept a gift from the forest now and again – and not simply buy the pale bilberry relatives in the shop. For some time, people were afraid of berries from the forest, assuming they could transmit the fox tapeworm and therefore the serious disease echinococcosis. However, studies have produced no evidence that people who suffer from echinococcosis eat bilberries more frequently than healthy people.[1] It is more likely that breathing in dry dusty earth when ploughing, or keeping dogs and cats which have not been properly wormed, are important factors. The recognised authority on this disease, Professor Klaus Brehm (Associate Professor for medical parasitology at the University of Würzburg, chairman of the informal WHO working group 'Echinococcus basic biology') has diproved the assumption that this illness can be passed on through berries.[2] Anyone who wants to be completely sure just needs to heat up the berries for a short time. They are also a healthy delicacy as compote or jam.

Bilberries (*Vaccinium myrtillus*)

As mentioned, eating bilberries has numerous beneficial effects on health. You can easily collect the berries yourself. The berries can be frozen or turned into juice or jam. The anthocyanins which are ascribed a prophylactic effect against cancer are not affected by this. Recently there has also been evidence that bilberries can *lower cholesterol levels*.

It is less advisable to leave the juicy berries to dry in order to keep them for treating *diarrhoea* because the drying process takes a long time and the berries may spoil. It is therefore better to obtain dried berries from a health food shop.

Bilberry tea

Nowadays bilberry leaves are rarely used to produce tea; they yield a very bitter and astringent tea. The dried berries, however, can be made into a cold extract or into actual tea. The extract obtained is stronger if you first crush the berries in a mortar. Add 3 tablespoons to 250 ml (8 fl oz) of water and either leave to stand for about 8 hours before drinking the extract at intervals during the day, or simmer for about 10 minutes. In both cases you can eat the leftover berries. I find that the cold extract tastes better and is more effective. However, as the cold extract takes longer to prepare, at the start of an illness it can be simpler to start out with the decoction and then continue the treatment with the cold extract.

An extract of blueberries or bilberries like this has a slightly 'constipating' effect in cases of diarrhoeal disease and encourages regeneration of the inflamed mucous membrane of the gut. This treatment appears to be particularly effective for *summer diarrhoeas* and *traveller's diarrhoea*. Bilberries are also said to reduce feelings of *nausea*. Leaving aside the use of bilberry, any diarrhoea accompanied by severe abdominal pain, high fever or a serious effect on general health naturally requires medical attention. More severe diarrhoea which can lead to dehydration and adverse effects on the circulatory system should be treated with electrolyte replacement solutions which can be obtained in any pharmacy.

If the bilberry preparation does not produce an adequate improvement, then the anthroposophical remedy Bolus alba comp. (Wala) often works well. Add 1 heaped teaspoon of the powder to half a glass of water and drink a sip every half hour.

An extract of this kind is also recommended for infections of the *mucosa of the mouth* (for example for *stomatitis aphtosa* in children). It should be used to rinse the mouth several times a day.

Cranberry (*Vaccinium macrocarpon*)

This plant, which is native to North America and a close relative of the blueberry, has a flower that resembles the head of a crane, which is where the name comes from. *Macrocarpon* means 'large-fruited' – and indeed the shiny red fruits of up to 2 cm (1 in) are astonishingly large.

It has already been mentioned that cranberry juice restricts the attachment of bacteria to the wall of the bladder. This applies in particular to E. coli, the most frequent causative agent of bladder infections. However, at 300 ml (10 fl oz) per day – even 250 ml (8 fl oz) twice daily according to one study – the required amount of juice is very high and not every stomach can tolerate this. If the preventative effect fails, this is most probably due to an underdosage.

Current research results indicate that the juice can also help to combat a *Helicobacter pylori infection* of the stomach. Helicobacter pylori is a bacterium which is involved in the formation of *stomach ulcers* and certain forms of stomach cancer. However, I do not have any experience so far of treating this infection with cranberry.

Cranberries contain large amounts of vitamin C – 30 to 40 mg per 100 g (3 ½ oz) – so that they are also useful in this respect. The berries and the juice obtained from them have a 'natural preserving agent' due to their benzoic acid content. Patients suffering from *renal insufficiency* (who need to limit the quantity of fruit and vegetables they eat due to the potassium content) should beware because cranberries contain a large quantity of this mineral. However, for patients who have to take diuretics – for example, to lower blood pressure – the potassium content is actually useful because these drugs can lead to a loss of potassium. Patients suffering from *kidney stones* should find out from their urologist whether they have calcium oxalate stones. In this case the quantity of fruit and vegetables with high amounts of oxalic acid should not be too high (so avoid rhubarb, spinach and cranberries). However, for other kinds of kidney stones (such as apatite, struvite and brushite stones) cranberries should actually have a beneficial effect.

CHAPTER 30

Grapevines

October is the month of late ripening. The grain has long been brought in, most apples have been collected from the trees, but the vintners are still hoping that the last warm rays of the sun will give the grapes a little more sweetness and flavour on these days when morning mists linger. For a long time in spring the dark gnarled fibrous vines looked as though they were dead, until finally light green translucent shoots burst forth from them. The tendrils soon spread out, and hidden beneath them, inconspicuous greenish flowers developed which finally developed into the juicy round grapes. Now in autumn they show staying power – and their quality can go on improving right up to the first frosts.

The grapevine is deeply connected with the earth. It is said to be able to obtain water from a depth of up to 20 metres (65 ft) in order to pass it onto the branches. Even its parts above ground look like roots. Along with the water it carries dissolved minerals to the surface, which may be one reason why the expert palate can taste the location of the vineyard in addition to the grape variety and vintage.

But naturally the mineral-rich fluid brought by the vine is not all that the grapes need for their development. It also requires a meeting of the sun with the leaves, without which no grapes can ripen. The sap is spread over a large area where it is permeated by the light so that a variety of material transformations can take place. First comes the formation of grape sugar, then the production of more than one thousand substances which have been detected in wine. Some of these are only produced during fermentation in the wine cellar. But many are made in the leaf which breathes through tiny closeable pores, absorbing carbon dioxide and light and combining these with the sap from the vine in such a way that plant material is produced.

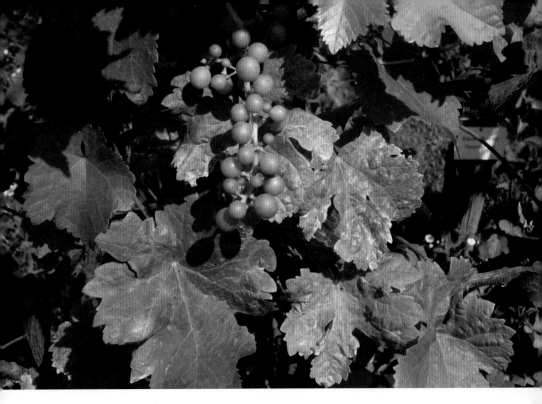

Vine.

Our intestine is somewhat comparable to what the earth is to the plant. We absorb all the food material and all the water that we need from it. However, before the blood, which has been enriched with material from the outside world, is allowed to penetrate into our actual insides, it passes through the liver. There, everything is 'tested' and anything poisonous or foreign broken down as far as possible and transformed into our own substance. Only when our own substance has been produced through complex material transformations does the enriched blood from the liver, an organ lying just below the diaphragm, flow via the short vena cava up into our central organ, the heart, which sits on the diaphragm in the thoracic cavity. In the plant, the organ for transforming and creating substance is the leaf. In us it is the liver. It also has large surfaces, which are of key importance and over which fluid streams are conducted. But, unlike the plant, they are not spread out in the light but lie hidden inside. In the liver, there are actually a great many fluid streams involved in these metabolic processes. There is the stream of blood saturated with substances and carbon dioxide from the portal vein, which collects the blood flowing

303

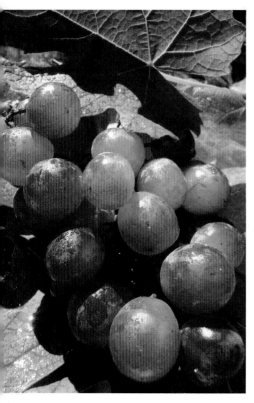

The sweetness in the grapes is made by the light which is absorbed by the leaves.

from the intestine. Some arterial, oxygen-rich blood is added to the liver. Lymph is produced, as is bile. Newly created substances – protein, fat, even dextrose (grape sugar) – go into the blood of the vena cava, which flows directly from the liver into the heart. The liver cells themselves are in a slow moving flow so that anatomists have called it the 'streaming liver'.[1] In principle, every plant leaf is related to the liver, but in the grapevine, with such a juicy fruit, this is true to an even greater degree.

In anthroposophical medicine preparations made from grape leaves have proved successful in the treatment of *liver disorders*. While drinking alcoholic wine in excess damages the liver, grapevine leaves – the part of the plant that produces glucose (the basis of alcohol) – can be a remedy for the liver.

A frequent sign of impaired liver function is an intolerance to fats. Could the knowledge of the medicinal value of vine leaves lie behind its culinary use? Anyway, it may be that Greek cuisine, which is very rich in fats, can be made more digestible by dolmades, stuffed marinated vine leaves. Like almost all liver remedies they also taste slightly bitter and therefore contrast well with their salty sweet filling of rice and raisins – which of course also come from the grapevine.

Healing effects are also attributed to the juice of the grape itself. Red wine in particular – when drunk in small quantities – is reputed to do the blood vessels and heart good. It is also said that it can provide protection against arteriosclerosis which can lead to vascular obstruction and, in cases of heart attack or stroke, cut off the blood supply to large areas of organs in a disastrous manner. It is the blue-red pigments in the grapes, the anthocyanins, which are probably important for the preventative effect in this case. These anthocyanins are present in red grape juice as well as red wine and there is evidence that regularly drinking a little red grape juice can be useful.

So it appears that the grapevine is important for two of our central organs, which are very closely linked anatomically and only separated by the diaphragm. Of course it does not provide any miracle remedy with which to avert an acute crisis. However, it produces effects that could contribute to maintaining health in the longer term.

Then of course there is another completely different reference to the grapevine. In the seven 'I am' sayings in St John's Gospel, Christ speaks about himself using seven images. For example, he describes himself as 'the good shepherd', 'the light of the world', 'the resurrection and the life'. On one occasion, just after the Last Supper at which he offered the wine as his blood, he compares himself to a plant and includes his disciples in this parable: 'I am the true vine and you are the branches.' The branches, tendrils and leaves emerge from the vine, receiving what has come from the depths of the earth, allowing this to be permeated by the light of the sun, and thus creating the basis for the fruit. Everything they absorb is received as a gift from above and below. However, they change it into something new. We can meditate on an image like this for a long time and may eventually notice that something new is created in ourselves.

Grapevine (*Vitis vinifera*)

The grapevine does not play a major part in general naturopathy. It is only in the wine-growing regions of France that tea infusions are made from vine leaves and local applications used for the lower legs for venous congestion. In fact, a therapeutic effect was observed for *leg ulcers* (ulcus cruris) using a combination of local compresses using vine leaves and internal application. This is similar to the more common use of cabbage leaves for this indication.

As already mentioned, small quantities of red wine or red grape juice are said to have a beneficial effect in *preventing arteriosclerosis*. A 'grape cure', where the intake of most foods is limited for a few days while increased quantities of grapes are eaten can be helpful. This is

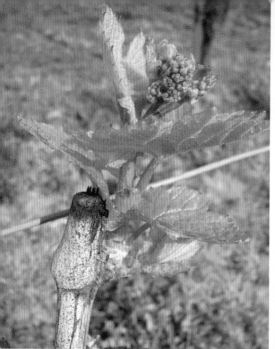 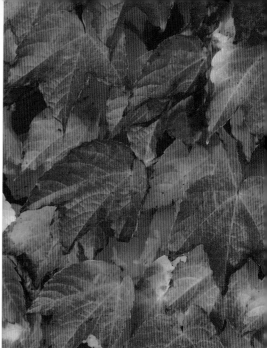

In late spring when the leaves appear on the dead-looking vines, it feels like a resurrection.   *Extracts from red vine leaves are used for varicose veins and leg sores.*

due to the increased intake of potassium and grape pigments which are believed to protect the blood vessels, have an antioxidant effect and even prevent cancer. A requirement, however, is that there is no sugar metabolism disorder, because the grapes contain a great deal of dextrose which leads to a rapid rise in blood sugar.

Grapes in proprietary medicines

A dried extract of the extremely colour-intense grape variety Teinturier du Cher is the active ingredient of Antistax tablets. They help relieve discomfort caused by *venous varicosities*, for example, 'heavy legs', feeling of congestion and calf *muscle cramp* during night. Prof. Christoph Schempp of the University Dermatology Clinic, Freiburg, Germany, recommends this remedy as an adjunct treatment of polymorphous light eruption.

The most frequent use made of the grapevine as a medicine are Hepatodoron (Fragaria/Vitis) tablets from Weleda. They are manufactured from dried vine leaves and strawberry leaves and have a positive effect on the *liver function* (see also Chapter 10 on the strawberry). Hepatodoron (Fragaria/Vitis) can often be beneficial in improving liver function and the quality of life in various types of *liver function disorders* and diseases (for example in *viral hepatitis* and toxic damage caused by medication or alcohol). It often decreases *daytime fatigue* and has a beneficial effect on psychological disturbances (*loss of initiative, mild depression*). However, even without the presence of a 'real' liver disease, there can be 'liver weakness' which can manifest as *sleep disturbance* with a tendency to wake up around 3 am. The Chinese understood this to be the 'optimal functioning time of the liver,' and modern physiology also knows that around this time the liver function that is important in the first half of the night – synthesising substances – gradually declines, and the production of bile and its storage in the gall bladder begins instead. With its help, fats in the digestive tract are made accessible. In this way a maximum amount of important substances for releasing warmth and therefore for daily activity are made available. If you regularly waken up at around 3 am, this can be a sign of a liver weakness. Sleep is often improved by chewing two Hepatodoron (Fragaria/Vitis) tablets before going to bed. Because carbohydrate metabolism is also largely dependent on the liver function, the complementary use of this remedy can help to improve metabolic function in patients with diabetes combined with disturbances to fat metabolism (in what is known as metabolic syndrome).

Taking Hepatodoron (Fragaria/Vitis) can also improve chronic constipation which can likewise be a sign of a deficient liver function. Other disease conditions which depend on the liver (for example some forms of *dry eczema, rosacea*) can respond to the administration of a combination of grape and strawberry leaves in this form. The beneficial effect on *varicose veins* and *leg sores* mentioned above can also be seen in connection with an improvement in liver function. It is of note that 80% of the liver volume is venous blood and a therapeutic effect on the liver often has an effect on the venous system.

Another medicinal preparation made on the same basic combination as Hepatodoron (grape and strawberry leaves) is Vitis comp. tablets (Weleda). These tablets contain a further potentised preparation of calcium and formic acid (Calcarea formicica D2) and potentised antimony (Stibium metallicum praeparatum D5). This stimulates the structural forces in the metabolism. This remedy is used mainly as a complementary treatment for *malignant diseases*.

CHAPTER 31

Bryophyllum

October sees the end of the active period for most of the plants around us. Many annual herbs disappear after having produced the seed into which they have concentrated their essence, in order to unfold again the next year. Many trees, however, exhibit another high point when they glow red or gold in the clear autumn light before going into winter dormancy. The whole plant then displays colours that we normally come across only in flowers. And indeed their colours and scents – which are intended to attract animals, but which also speak to our feelings – arise from decomposition processes, while the green leaf serves only to synthesise substance.

In temperate latitudes the phases of plant growth are determined from outside by the seasons. If these are absent (as in the tropics), plants from temperate latitudes get 'out of rhythm'. For instance, in India I saw a miserable apple tree with branches bearing a couple of flowers, a few ripening apples and some young sprouting leaves, all at the same time.

Many houseplants come from the tropics and survive because of the constant warm conditions in our homes. Some (such as the wealth of orchids which originate around the equator) are notable for their magnificent flowers. Others have particularly beautiful leaves; others have an unusual reproductive behaviour. The latter is the case for the *Bryophyllums*, meaning 'sprouting leaf' in Greek, which is why this old name persists although the family is usually known botanically as *Kalanchoe*. The characteristic feature of these plants is that they can produce complete new little plants for the next generation directly from their leaves without having to flower, pollinate, set seed or have a

The daughter plants sit on the edge of the leaves of the Bryophyllum.

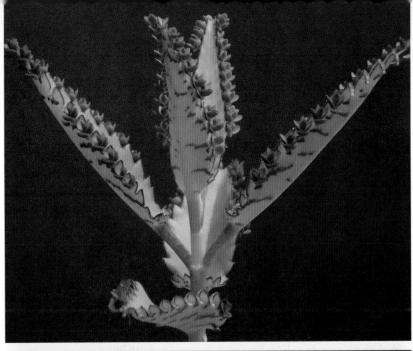

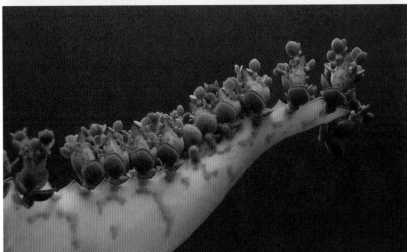

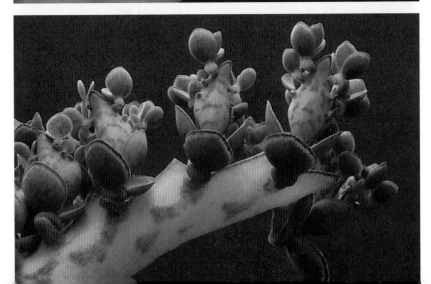

dormant period in between (although they *can* do this). Young plants are produced continuously from the leaves of the mother plant. In one species this happens at the edge of a leaf when it touches the ground, in another case new little plants sprout from the wound of a torn leaf. One particularly pretty species has fleshy leaves which are toothed at the edge, just like our stinging nettles. New plants grow from all the indentations on the edge of the leaf like a string of pearls and sometimes even a 'grandchild generation' can appear.

For Goethe, encountering Bryophyllum was proof of his view that the leaf is the central organ of the plant from which all other parts (including the whole flower) arise. Bryophyllum shows that this applies to the whole plant. This expresses an unusual and almost unrestrained vitality in the plant, which can sometimes become tiresome when the daughter plants fall off and end up growing in places where we do not actually want them.

It is no surprise that such a vigorous and unusual plant can also be a powerful remedy. In the 1980s the anthroposophical gynaecologist Werner Hassauer discovered a relationship between the characteristics of bryophyllum and pregnancy and used extracts of the plant when there was a risk of premature birth and pre-term labour set in.[1] This type of treatment is now standard in anthroposophical hospitals and gynaecological practices in order to lessen *pre-term labour* or overly strong contractions and to improve the nutrition of the developing child in the womb. Several comparative studies have shown that this type of treatment can be just as effective as the use of standard drugs.[2] It was also shown that children born subsequently did better if their mothers had been treated with bryophyllum and the mothers had significantly fewer side effects than with the conventional procedure. Laboratory tests also showed that bryophyllum extracts significantly reduced the tendency of the uterine musculature to contract too strongly.[3] The efficacy of the plant preparation was indicated by patients often becoming mentally relaxed, having improved sleep and showing a degree of drowsiness. Overall it has been found that bryophyllum can relieve an over-excited mental state which expresses itself in nervousness and agitation.[4] A tendency to pre-term labour is often associated with tension and too much stress in the mother-to-be and with the inability to reduce this.

310

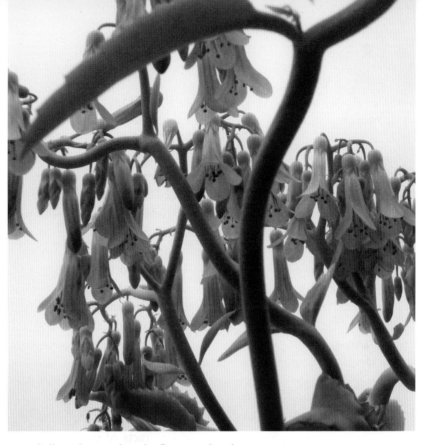

Bryophyllum also reproduces by flowers and seeds.

Other areas of application for this plant have developed over the course of time and it is nowadays also used for various conditions of *excessive agitation.* The juicy bryophyllum, which has the ability to survive long periods of drought, is also applied externally where there is a need to improve the vitality of the skin or to counteract excessive dehydration and irritation due to external stresses (such as frequent washing). Finally, bryophyllum is evidence for another of Goethe's views: that the inner nature of an object or living being can be recognised from its appearance. This means that the pharmacist and physician (at least those with an anthroposophical approach) can recognise the effects of a remedy by becoming closely acquainted with it, for example, by making careful observations of the plant throughout its life-cycle. It is obviously just as important to determine if our discoveries can be verified objectively (including carrying out laboratory tests). In the case of bryophyllum, objective tests impressively bear out our observations.

Bryophyllum

In the plant's tropical home it is used in traditional medicine, whereas in Europe it is used almost exclusively in anthroposophical medicine. Even if you cultivate bryophyllum, it is not suitable for making into remedies yourself, because there are bryophyllum species which can have toxic effects at higher concentrations.

The (already mentioned) effect of bryophyllum on *pre-term labour* has now been confirmed in several studies on human beings. Compared to conventional treatments, it displayed equal efficacy with fewer side effects. Laboratory studies on surgical specimens have also shown that bryophyllum has a relaxing effect on the musculature of the uterus. Relaxing effects of a psychological nature were also observed.

Bryophyllum 50% powder (Weleda), which also improves sleep and has a certain strengthening effect, is often prescribed orally in less serious cases. The usual dosage is 1–2 pinches 3 times daily or a single dose at bedtime. This remedy can sometimes help very thin 'run-down' people to build up their own vitality again.

In more serious cases of *early labour*, obstetrical departments of anthroposophical hospitals often give bryophyllum as a 5% intravenous drip – up to four 10 ml (⅓ oz) ampoules in 1000 ml (35 fl oz) saline – which may be administered throughout the day if necessary. Naturally this kind of application requires expert supervision (usually of a gynaecologist).

Potentised Bryophyllum

Weleda manufactures Bryophyllum D5/Conchae D7 aa as ampoules of 1 ml and 10 ml from a combination of potentised bryophyllum and potentised oyster shell. Time and again this remedy has proved to be very helpful when injected into the vein of an agitated patient during house visits or in the practice. *Extreme agitation and tension* then often ease quickly. The remedy can even be used for psychiatric treatment in suitable cases, where it produces no significant side effects. It can also be helpful for morning sickness. The remedy can also have a beneficial effect on *inflammatory allergic skin conditions* which are clearly related to *psychological tension*. Interestingly, antiallergenic effects have also been demonstrated for bryophyllum in laboratory tests.

Potentised Bryophyllum comp. combines it with silver and a potentised organ preparation of the uterus and is available as globules and ampoules from Wala. In this form it can have a releasing and relaxing effect on *increased irritability,* particularly during menses or in the *menopause.* The remedy can also be helpful for a far less advanced tendency to pre-term labour, for example in cases of professional or private stress and tension. It can be beneficial especially for states of emotional agitation caused by fluctuating hormone levels during menopause and puberty and also for cases of *premenstrual syndrome* when the emotional state is severely affected.

The technique for vegetablising metals has already been described earlier (page 292). For bryophyllum this is done using silver. The Bryophyllum Argento cultum (Weleda) obtained in this way is used for such things as sleep disturbances and shock symptoms. It is especially effective for people whose 'restorative powers' are too weak or who are also suffering from *disorders of the reproductive organs.*

External use of Bryophyllum

Bryophyllum is a succulent plant, meaning one which has thick fleshy leaves and which creates lush green life even in hostile arid environmental conditions. This was a guiding principle in the development of Dr Hauschka Hand Cream, which contains bryophyllum extracts in order to protect hands from *dehydration* due to frequent washing, use of disinfectants, etc. It was accidently observed that this cream can also be useful for other parts of the body where the skin has a tendency to dry out due to stresses such as frequent washing or the effects of the sun.

CHAPTER 32

Ivy

In November the last leaves are blown from the trees, although in October they still had such beautiful glowing colours. Soon the branches are dark and bare. So it is no coincidence that spruces and firs which remain green appear in our houses as Christmas trees – along with a couple of smaller plants which also clearly have no intention of joining in the general period of dormancy. All are mysterious – and legends and customs have grown up around them. The Christmas rose only reveals its magic during the advancing winter, but the clumps of mistletoe become increasingly visible from the start of winter, the more the leaves of their host tree are shed. Their berries gleam bright white until Christmas, bringing delight not least of all to those who kiss under their twigs. The red holly berries, showing between the spiny green shiny leaves, make a colour contrast to this white. The holly is inseparably linked to the common ivy, and not only in the famous Christmas carol and in the charming children's book, *The Story of Holly and Ivy* by Rumer Godden.

These evergreens may catch our attention from time to time as early as November. This is the time when our thoughts turn to the past and we try to draw close to those who have died. The festivals of All Saints and of All Souls, Rememberance Day in Britain and Veterans Day in the United States all fall at this time of year. Many graves are covered by the perennial dark green ivy which often also creeps over gravestones and walls and climbs up trees – giving a romantic appearance of life even in winter. In ancient times, ivy was a symbol of loyalty and everlasting friendship – and indeed it not only appears green all year round, but is so tenacious that it rarely disappears once it has become established.

But at the same time it is not immutable. Have you ever taken a second look and then asked yourself: 'is this actually ivy or not?' You

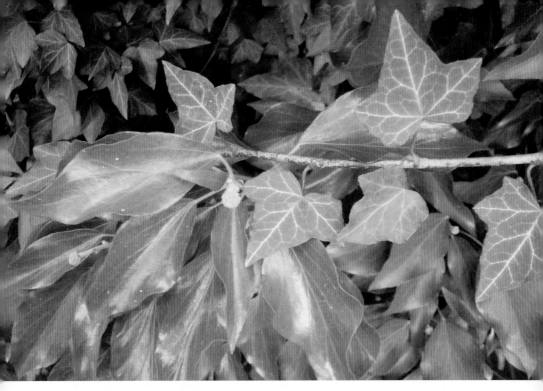

The upper part of the picture shows the original five-pointed leaves. After the blossoms appear, the leaf shape changes (lower part).

know it with its five-pointed leaves which keep close to the ground, appearing from shoots whose aerial roots cling onto the substrate everywhere, be it soil, masonry or bark. But now and again, in places where ivy has grown for decades, it appears quite different: lighter, shinier and ovoid, the leaves only pointed at the end. And, sure enough, there at the end of the shoots are inconspicuous greenish clusters of flowers, still surrounded by flies and wasps in late autumn when nothing else is left in flower. Our question about whether this is ivy is soon answered because, when we search, we can still find its original form. The form we are used to is the one which appears on the ground while the shoots with flowers and transformed leaves have raised themselves up and become free-standing, reaching towards the light, although the plant is otherwise a noted shade species. It appears as though, along with its sexual maturity (which it only achieves after decades of uniform growth), the plant suddenly becomes more independent in every way.

Change of shape, metamorphosis, is something we are familiar with in any case, and this is often connected with conquering a new 'element'. The earth-bound caterpillar confined to its plant transforms

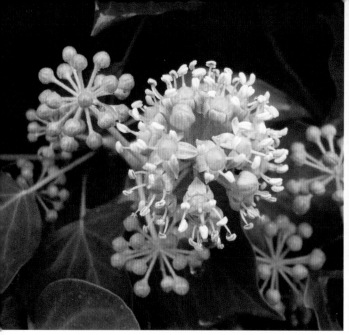
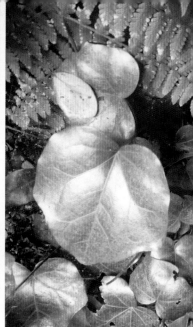

Ivy flower.

itself into the butterfly which can rise unfettered into the light and air; the tadpole grows legs and lungs and climbs out of the water onto the land as a frog (in fairy tales this transformation goes even further and a prince appears). These transformations take place 'upwards' – and this is exactly what we see in ivy. When flowering takes place something completely new is set in motion; the plant's whole form changes. It no longer has to cling on tightly, but gains a relationship to lightness and light and to the animal realm.

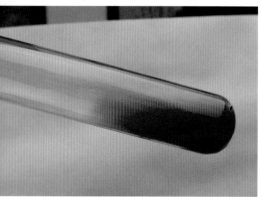

Ivy iodine: for a terrestrial plant, ivy contains an unusually large quantity of iodine. If you heat a crystal of this element it sublimates as a rising purple gas.

Interestingly, something also takes place in terms of its chemical substances: it develops an unusual amount of iodine.[1] This element which is common in the sea – in water – also has a 'propensity to air and light'. It 'sublimates' in chemical terminology; in other words, it easily and directly transforms from a solid into a gaseous state without passing through the liquid state, and as a gas it can be detected by its characteristic smell (and the purple colour of its vapour). However,

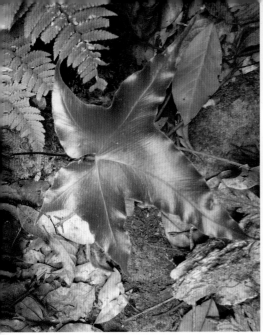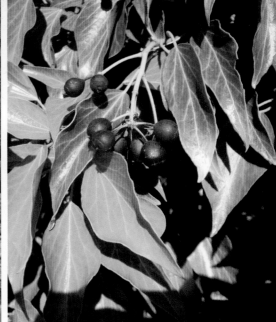

The different leaf shapes of the ivy are clearly visible here on the sub-species Hedera helix canariense.

When the ivy starts to flower it produces shiny pointed ovate leaves which reach towards the light.

it seems that without iodine the transformations mentioned above cannot take place. Interestingly, tadpoles show a similar inability to transform without iodine; if you remove the thyroid gland which produces iodine, they stay as water creatures without any legs or lungs and never turn into frogs.

In our own development we also pass at birth from the water world of our mother's body on to 'land', and then air needs to pass into our lungs which were previously filled with liquid. Thus it is not surprising that an iodine deficiency during pregnancy impairs maturation of the lungs.

If we have an infection of the respiratory tract, appearing to us as a *cold, bronchitis* or *cough*, our respiratory passages and lungs often take half a step backwards. They are no longer dry and filled with pure air but blocked with liquid and rattling mucus. The role of healing is then to 'take a proper step forward' again, to step onto the 'land' and to dry out what has regressed into the liquid element. Ivy is renowned for being able to help with this and a series of cough remedies contain it as the active basis with both a mucolytic and anti-irritant effect. The active ingredients are called 'saponins', soap-like substances (*sapo* is Latin for soap) that create foam if you blow into a solution of them. However, foam is 'a lot of air in a little water' and this indicates exactly

317

the direction in which our infected respiratory tract must develop. Everything about the nature of the ivy indicates that this is the type of transformation with which it is able to assist.

I should just mention that developmental regression can go even further in us, specifically when cancer cells arise which in many respects behave in ways which were normal in the embryo (developing in a bladder of water) but are 'abnormal' beyond the embryonic period. It has been discovered that ivy extracts can be effective in treating cancer cells in the laboratory and this once more allows a comparison with mistletoe with which it shares the room at Christmas. However, this will be dealt with in more detail in Chapter 35.

Ivy (*Hedera helix*)

If you want to collect common ivy leaves for making tea this is best done in late summer, in August or September, shortly before the plant flowers. It is best to use the shiny ovate leaves from the flowering shoots. However, the use of ivy as a tea is not customary for two reasons. Dried ivy leaves have a peculiar musty smell and you have to be careful with the quantity used because too much can cause stomach complaints and may actually aggravate bronchial problems. For these reasons ivy is almost always used as a proprietary medicine. Do not use poison berries of ivy.

Ivy as a medicinal tea

If, despite the above-mentioned deterrents, you still wish to use ivy as a tea, then for an adult use ½ teaspoon of the dried and crushed leaves (not more!) to 1 cup of boiling water and leave to infuse for 5 minutes. This method of application is not recommended for children due to the difficulty of judging the dose.

Ivy in phytotherapeutic proprietary medicines

Ivy combines a mucolytic effect with anti-inflammatory and germicidal ones and an antispasmodic effect in the bronchia. Preparations made from ivy can therefore be helpful both for bronchitis and for a slight *bronchial oversensitivity* with a tendency to spasm and *dry cough.* Proprietary remedies are available as sugar-coated tablets, drops, elixir or effervescent tablets, for example under the names of Prospan, Hedelix, Cefapulmon mono.

A largely experimental aspect of the use of potentised ivy is based on the fact that, like mistletoe and Christmas rose, it is one of the winter flowering plants that Rudolf Steiner stated were suitable for treating *cancers.* There are some initial results for this use of ivy in connection with *thyroid cancer.* In common with ivy, the thyroid contains a great deal of iodine and is the most iodine-rich organ by far. Its 'hunger for iodine' is also the reason that the thyroid is especially at risk after accidents to nuclear power plants where radioactive iodine is released. After the Chernobyl disaster the rate of thyroid cancers rose enormously in Eastern Europe, especially in children, and it is to be feared that this could be similar in areas of Japan exposed to the effect of radioactive iodine. However, the iodine levels in the Japanese were far healthier than those in the Ukraine even before the reactor accident at Fukushima due to their traditional diet of seaweed and fish which contain iodine: so the thyroid was less prone to absorb radioactive iodine. Nevertheless a large part of the radioactive nuclides in Japan were blown out to sea. As described above with tadpoles (page 317) the thyroid and the hormone it produces are also responsible for transformation and maturation processes such as the development of our lungs during the embryonic period or the transformation of the tadpole into a frog. So this is another area where the relationship between ivy and the thyroid appears. To understand whether the use of potentised ivy for thyroid cancer will prove as successful as mistletoe is for other cancers, we must wait until there is more evidence.

CHAPTER 33

Blackthorn

Even the calendar – with All Saints and All Souls days – has November begin with thoughts of death. Nature is naturally linked to the process of dying and at this time of year, darkness is increasing rapidly. It is hard to believe that some fruits are only just becoming ripe and edible. This is the case with blackthorn, which looks like a symbol of death from the plant world during the cold months of the year.

The shrub has black bark and numerous long sharp-pointed thorns, which shoot out from the twigs in all directions and can turn a blackthorn hedge into a thorny thicket more impenetrable than the rose thicket around Sleeping Beauty's castle. It might give you the creeps to learn that a now rare bird with the revealing German name of *Neuntöter* (meaning 'kills nine'), the red-backed shrike, likes to impale its prey – large insects, small birds or even mice – on the thorns of the blackthorn. Old legends often suggest that Christ's crown of thorns was woven from the branches of this plant. Few other plants represent the forces of death better than the blackthorn.

In a legend about this plant, the Creator rushed to the aid of the blackthorn when it was 'unjustly accused' of evil, by showering it with white flowers in spring so that it stood as though wrapped in a white bridal veil. After that, all suspicion of evil was silenced. Every spring since then it is like a miracle when, in barren places like railway embankments, abandoned quarries and other spots exposed to the light, a fragrant veil of white erupts from the stark black of the blackthorn virtually overnight. It almost seems to float above the bushes. The blackthorn thicket is enveloped in a cloud of delicate scent like marzipan. But even this has two sides. The scent comes from a compound produced by the plant called *amygdalin* (from the Greek

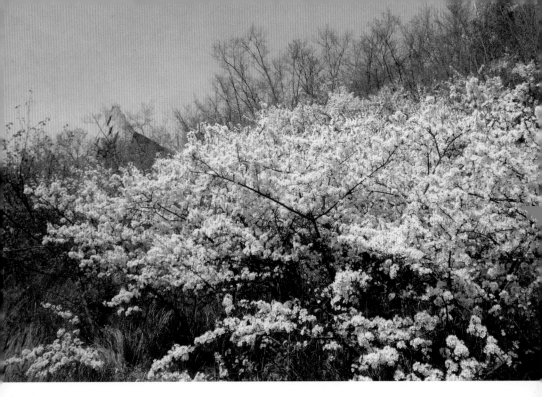

Flowering blackthorn.

word for almond), which contains highly diluted hydrocyanic acid. This has a stimulating effect in small amounts, but hydrocyanic acid is a strong and terrible poison with an asphyxiating action.

So we find a polarity in the blackthorn. It carries the forces of death in it, but at the same time the ability to overcome them. Could this be why it can awaken so impressively and beautifully to new life when most other plants are still dormant, waiting for warmer days? It also reveals amazing vitality in the fact that it can bear its firm fresh fruits into the last months of the year when other fruit has long been harvested, fallen to the ground or rotted. Frost (which finishes off more delicate herbs, wilts leaves and spoils many kinds of fruit) actually helps to ripen the fruits of the blackthorn. The fruits look so enticing as they become an increasingly deep blue in autumn. But anyone who tries one will spit it out again in disgust. Although the fruit looks beautiful it will still be indescribably sour for many weeks. Due to high tannin levels, its juice seems to shrivel up the tongue and leave it numb and leathery for several minutes.

The basic theme appears here again. Tannin, which is found in such large amounts in blackthorn sloes, has been used to tan leather

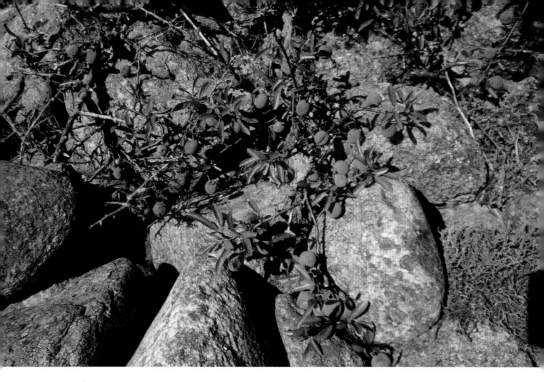

Sloes.

since ancient times. The most living part of the skin, the proteins contained in it, are coagulated by the tannins. They are contracted into microscopically thin threads in which all life is finally extinguished. Yet, at the same time they will remain durable and supple for years in the leather that is produced. An animal skin that is not treated with tannin rots after a few days with an indescribable stench or – if it was dried quickly – becomes hard and brittle. Tannin can do both: mortify and make skin (largely) resistant to bacterial breakdown while at the same time retaining the lifelike suppleness which characterised the skin or fur on the living animal. Fortunately, biting into sloes before they are ripe only makes your tongue temporarily a little 'leathery'!

This experience can point to the first of the therapeutic effects. When mucus membranes become too 'lively' and lacking in form, or if they even start to disintegrate due to inflammation, then extracts from blackthorn and other tannin-rich plants can help to stabilise the form and strength of the mucosa and to activate its healing capacity. This can happen with *inflamed gums.* Another reason for using preparations made from sloes is the 'loosening' of *nasal mucosa* in *colds* or excessive and unstructured growth forces which lead to *mucosal polyps.*

When the first frosts have passed over the sloes, the tannin content falls and sweetness arises. A sour flavour still remains, but the taste is no longer off-putting it becomes refreshing. You can sense that the entire forces of a year have been concentrated in the berries. Few other plants expose their fruits to wind and weather for longer, from the early spring blossoming all the way to being ripe for harvest in late autumn. So it seems only natural that the blackthorn can give new strength to those who have themselves experienced an encounter with the 'forces of death' due to serious illness or personal crises, and who have already recovered from being seriously ill but have not yet returned to full health. In this phase of *convalescence*, of regaining strength, the blackthorn can be an energy-giving support. Blackthorn juices or elixirs made with sugar can be just as helpful as pharmaceutical preparations such as globules, drops or injections.

In anthroposophical pharmacy, blackthorn is often combined with iron. The character of this metal 'fits' particularly well with the plant that produces one of the hardest native woods and whose thorns look like iron spikes. One method of fusing them consists of putting the sloes along with the iron mineral haematite through a rhythmical process of heat and cold, light and darkness, resulting in the preparation Prunuseisen (Wala). In another type of preparation the sloes are processed with the very iron-rich water of a mineral spring into Levico comp. (Wala). Both these processes produce remedies which are used to good effect in anthroposophical medicine for extreme *weakness* or *exhaustion* (or weakness, prostration). The 'spring blackthorn' can also be made into medicines. The flowers and soft shoot tips which burst from the black branches can also be made into invigorating remedies.

What was so black and lifeless throughout the winter not only awakens to new life and strength, but can also impart some of its hidden forces to those who need them. What seemed to be a symbol of death can also contain the hope of resurrection.[1]

Blackthorn (*Prunus spinosa*)

Due to the thorns, collecting the flowering blackthorn in early spring (March to April) is just as difficult as harvesting the ripe fruits in November. The flowers should be thoroughly dried in a well-ventilated place. They should not be stored for too long as they gradually turn brown and quickly lose their original scent. The fruits can be successfully processed into sloe juice in a steam juicer to which usually 20% (sometimes more) sugar is added.

Use in phytotherapy

Phytopharmacological research has not found any strong active ingredients in the flowers, which is why they are no longer of importance in phytotherapy using concentrated substance. Their most common use is as a gentle laxative for *constipation*. After all, Sebastian Kneipp wrote that, 'Blackthorn flowers are the most innocent laxative and should not be absent from any home pharmacy.' Remarkably, however, blackthorn flowers are also recommended 'to prevent and treat *diarrhoea*'. This looks like a contradiction, but with herbal medicines it is often the case that they primarily have a balancing effect on an organ function and can therefore in fact be used when this is out of balance in one direction or the other.

Apart from this, the flowers are also known to have a mild *diuretic* effect. For this purpose they are sometimes mixed with nettle leaves, horsetail and/or bean pod.

The flowers are also sometimes used in tea mixtures for *colds* (for example along with elderflowers and lime flowers) particularly as they have a slightly sudorific effect. This is also the reason that they are used 'for purifying the blood' for example as part of a fasting cure in the spring.

To make pure blackthorn flower tea, add 1 heaped teaspoon of dried flowers to 1 cup of boiling water and leave to infuse for 5–10 minutes. The fruit juice is taken several times a day by the tablespoonful as a tonic (for example after infections).

Homeopathy

Blackthorn is of little importance in homeopathy. Its use is approximately the same as that for traditional folk medicine. Prunus spinosa is given in low potencies (mother tincture to D3) for *stomach complaints* with *bloating* and *constipation* and for stimulating urination in *heart disease.*

Anthroposophical medicine

While blackthorn may play only a minor role in homeopathy and phytotherapy, in anthroposophical medicine it is an important plant, and has proved successful in treating a number of health problems.

Like the above-mentioned home-made sloe juice, Organic Blackthorn Elixir (Weleda) is given for *exhaustion* and for post-treatment *after an infection, a serious illness, after childbirth or after an operation* (1–2 teaspoons 3 times daily). Prunus Essence (Wala), also made from the fruits, is used similarly. In cases of exhaustion due to various causes, add 2–3 tablespoons to a full bath (these kinds of baths have also been known to help in some cases of *muscular disorders*) or use the remedy for compresses (1–2 teaspoons to 125 ml / ½ cup of water). It can also be added to washing water in this concentration. In bedridden patients the strengthening and slightly tanning effect can strengthen the skin and make it more resistant to *bedsores* (*decubitus*). I have the impression that this application also improves the venous return flow from the legs. This effect is even more pronounced in Aesculus/Prunus Essence (Wala), which, besides blackthorn, contains extracts of horse chestnut, borage, oak bark and golden rod. Mild water retention in the legs can also be improved by using compresses and washing with this essence.

The contracting, structuring and invigorating effects of sloe can be beneficial for *swollen nasal mucosa* which is why sloe extracts are included in Nasal Balm (Wala) and Schnupfencreme (catarrh cream, Weleda). The latter also contains *Berberis* which is structure-promoting, and preparations of bryony (*Bryonia*) and coneflower (*Echinacea*) that, like potentised cinnabar, target the action specifically to the acute head cold (which may include inflammation of the sinuses). This remedy contains some other ingredients such as decongestant peppermint and eucalyptus oils. A roughly peppercorn-sized quantity should be put into the nose several times a day.

Wala Nasal Balm has also proved beneficial for *acute head colds,* particularly when accompanied by thick dry secretions. It also contains extracts of sloe and Berberis with some other essential oils and a small amount of Peruvian balsam. Allergies sometimes occur to the last-named substance and also to the lanolin it contains, and in such cases the remedy should not be used. An important substance for the effectiveness of this remedy is the high content of colloidal silica, which promotes formative forces. In cases of *allergic rhinitis,* the nose balm eases breathing, especially if it is used before exposure to pollen (for example, before leaving the house). It has also proved successful as a complementary therapy for *sinusitis.* Finally, it can be helpful in *preventing snoring* in patients in whom snoring is caused by congestion of the nasal mucosa at night. Very young children, who should not have essential oils applied around the nose, can be given Nasal Balm for children, which does not contain oils of this kind.

In cases of a tendency to *nasal polyps* which are characterised by viscous, disordered growth, besides Nasal Balm (Wala), Hayfever Nasal Spray (Gencydo, Weleda) can be effective. This is because polyp formation is often partly caused by allergies. In addition, the plant extracts of lemon and quince have a contracting and formative effect. Help can also be obtained from giving subcutaneous injections once or twice weekly with Prunus spinosa, Fructus Rh D3 (Weleda) along with the organ preparation Tunica mucosa nasi Gl D15 (Wala).

An extract of sloe is also contained in Rosmarinus/Prunus comp. Gel (Wala) which was covered in Chapter 21 on rosemary. During and after menopause, the remedy stimulates the vaginal mucosa and helps to counteract itching and oversensitivity. It is also helpful for itching around the anus.

The blackthorn shoot tips (*summitates* in Latin), which are harvested and processed in spring and contain the buds or flowers and leaves in the process of opening, are almost more important than the fruit. These contain all the spring energy of the plant.

Weleda makes Prunus spinosa, summitates mother tincture and – without alcohol – the same as an Rh preparation in D3 and D6 as drops and D3 and D5 as ampoules. Wala supplies the rhythmically

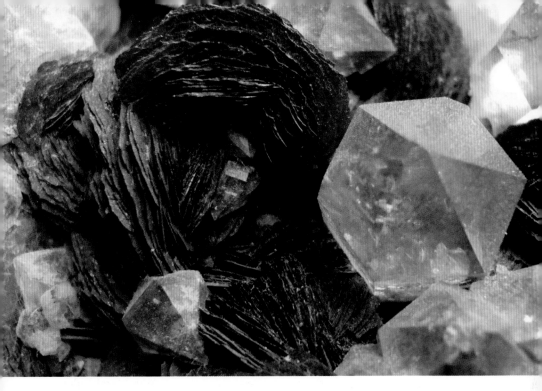

Flower-like crystallized haematite (with quartz crystal).

treated preparation Prunus spinosa e floribus et summitatibus (from flowers and shoot tips) 5%, D2, D3 and D6 as ampoules and D2, D3 and D6 as globules. These remedies often work amazingly well for *cardiac insufficiency* and for conditions of *exhaustion* during and after serious illness. The more serious the situation, the lower the potency chosen in this case. As a rule the dose is 1 injection daily or 5–10 globules 3 times daily.

The blackthorn fruit is used to produce Prunus spinosa, fructus mother tincture and Rh D3 ampoules. If you bear in mind the contracting effect of sloes, then it is not surprising that good results have been obtained from this remedy for polyps in the mucosa of the nasal sinuses, which often consist of loose poorly-structured tissue.

Blackthorn flowers and shoot tips can be combined with haematite. This is the mineral form of ferric oxide, which forms silver-gleaming and sometimes flower-like crystals ('haematite rose' or 'iron rose'). It is produced by Wala under the name Prunuseisen in D6 ampoules and D3 globules. This involves adding the finely powdered mineral to the plant/water mixture. Then for seven days, morning and evening, it is stirred, cooled and taken outdoors. In between, it is warmed in

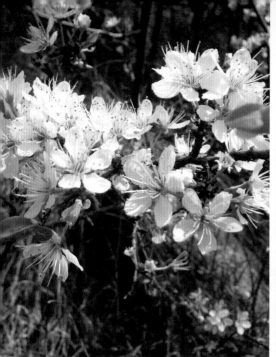
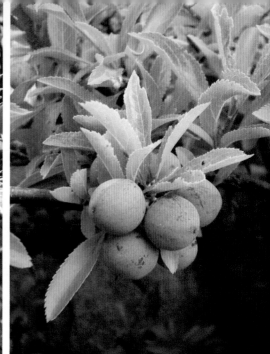

Blackthorn flowers and berries.

darkness. The remedy is made stable and long-lasting through this rhythmical treatment and is connected more strongly to cosmic forces. This medicine has a noticeably strengthening effect and, due to the iron component, is also suitable for treating *anaemia* and *low blood pressure* (hypotension). Prunuseisen is also contained in the composite remedy Levico comp. This remedy has the addition of water from the Levico spring which contains copper, iron, arsenic and sulfuric acid and is famous for its strengthening effects. It also contains St John's Wort *(Hypericum)* in low potency, which stimulates the inner forces of light and counteracts depressive tendencies.

Aurum/Prunus (Wala) which is available as globules and ampoules, has a similar strengthening effect on the 'inner sun forces'. My impression is that Levico comp. is particularly helpful when the inner light appears temporarily clouded by illness or strain while Aurum/ Prunus is indicated by more deep-seated persistent exhaustion, often with a feeling of being cold.

Skorodit Kreislauf injection and globules (Wala) are very specifically targeted to stabilising the circulation. In addition to Prunus spinosa e floribus et summitatibus D5 they also contain the iron mineral scorodite, camphor D3, white hellebore Veratrum D3 and an organ

328

preparation of the pituitary gland. The remedy is very helpful for a tendency towards *blacking out* or *feeling faint* when getting up (postural hypotension), for example in pubescent adolescents and also in women who are anaemic. It also has a strengthening effect on the musculature in neurological diseases (something first pointed out by the neurologist Andreas Rivoir). The usual dose is 5–10 globules 3 times daily. Injections can be more effective for muscular diseases.

If the exhaustion is primarily of an emotional nature, then injections (1–3 times weekly) with Aqua maris D3/Prunus spinosa, Summitates D5 (Weleda) are often very helpful. Aqua maris is seawater which contains numerous trace elements, but primarily common salt which is a famous remedy in homeopathy for depression under its old pharmaceutical name Natrium muriaticum; especially when chronic worry which cannot be discussed is preying on the mind.

Last but not least, the blackthorn flowers are very valuable as an oily extract. They also have a strengthening effect in this form. Malvenöl (Wala) contains oily extracts of blackthorn, mallow, St John's wort, lime flowers and elderflowers. It often has a very stabilising effect for frail patients who are prone to illness and infection when used regularly as a whole-body embrocation in the evening. Good results have also been obtained for delicate children. The same applies to the pure blackthorn oil, which is used as Prunus spinosa e floribus W 5% Oleum (Wala) for oil dispersion baths which are usually administered once or twice a week.

CHAPTER 34

Frankincense

Frankincense does not normally count as a medicine. The word denotes a tree, its resin and the smoke that is produced when you lay it (or a mixture which contains other components) on a glowing piece of charcoal. Smoke is known to quickly lead to controversy, and in the case of incense there are also declared opponents. They believe that it is linked to 'mumbo jumbo' or can even cause nausea. Others, however, find that it adds an additional sensory quality to a spiritual mood, that it evokes Christmas and the Three Kings, memories of childhood – or simply that it smells nice.

However, it can be agreed that frankincense touches our soul, which in ancient languages was often denoted by the same word as the wind or air, and we ourselves can feel that all strong emotions change our breathing.

Although the frankincense tree only grows in a relatively small region in southern Arabia, its resin is used everywhere for ritual acts in which the aim is to turn towards the divine. The highest divinity of the Egyptians was – at least at times – the sun god, and so frankincense was burned at sunrise and sunset. In pre-Islamic Arabia, frankincense was also connected to the cult of the sun god and all the stores of resin had to be kept in his temple. The ancient Jewish Book of Jubilees tells how, after being driven out of paradise, Adam was given a frankincense cutting to take on this journey to earth as a comfort. He burned frankincense mornings and evenings in order to be reminded of the world of his origin.

The link between frankincense and the sun can be found in many other eras and cultures. Even in the Old Testament Jewish ritual, which can certainly not be described simply as sun worship, frankincense

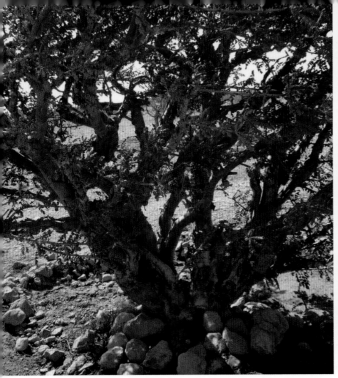

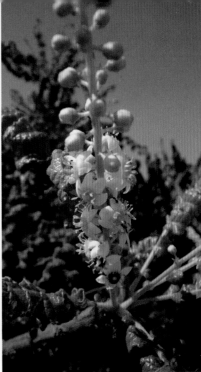

Incense tree in Oman.   *Incense flowers and leaves.*

was burned when the sun appeared above the horizon or disappeared below it.

How can we find this relationship ourselves? Frankincense trees tend to be small and branch early on, and are therefore more like large bushes growing from one point in the ground. Then – almost like an ascending cloud – they spread rapidly upwards. The tree has pinnate leaves, which allow the air to pass through their surface. Even the flowers appear as though they are prepared to spray out. The gesture of lifting itself against gravity into the air, 'to the heavens,' can be clearly seen by looking at the tree.

The branches are covered in a papery, ash-grey bark. If you cut into this deeply enough, then the precious scented resin emerges like blood from a wound and only has to be collected from time to time. This flow lasts up to eight months. When you read botanical textbooks, the reason given for the trees producing resin is always 'to close wounds'. A wound that bleeds for eight months is obviously not very well closed. I therefore asked a botanist friend, Professor Helmut Rehder, who said, 'resins are produced when a plant can perform more photosynthesis (in other words, can absorb the sun's energy) than it needs for producing its own substance.' So resins constitute an 'excess of sun' in the plant, something that also applies to the aromatic essential oils which are contained in frankincense resin, for example.

The water supply of a frankincense tree in the desert is obtained only from dew falling in the night. By contrast, it gets more than enough sun, the effects of which are stored in its resin. Frankincense is therefore a heavenly substance in an earthly guise. When you lay it on the charcoal, it changes into something like its original state and rises up again. If we consider that the human soul also comes from the heavens and will one day return to them, it makes sense that frankincense is a good support when it turns towards this home. This may be the reason why frankincense is part of the burial ritual in many religions.

In many cultures frankincense is also linked to the idea of sacrifice. Botany can give us a clue to this as well. In the tree, resin occurs in special passages formed by tree cells that disintegrate and pour their contents into the space created. Nowadays, it is often claimed that the principle of self-assertion applies to all living beings in nature. Yet here, there is no self-assertion on the part of the cells, but rather a sacrifice allowing something new. In ancient times rituals often used to involve animal blood sacrifices, but were gradually replaced by bloodless sacrifices, like the offering of frankincense.

In later times, substances no longer played the decisive role in ritual sacrifice and offerings. The inner attitude (like offering one's attention, devotion and power of love to the divine) became more important. However, frankincense can still be an expression and a kind of 'bearer' of what is happening in the soul (as it says in Chapter 8 of the Revelation to St John, 'the smoke of the incense rose with the prayers').

Much more could be written about this, but it is now time to discuss the medical aspects. In recent years frankincense has in fact made its way from churches to pharmacies. However, this is usually not Arabic frankincense *(Boswellia sacra)* but mainly its close relative, Indian frankincense *(Boswellia serrata)*. It has long been used in Indian medicine for various *inflammations* and *swelling symptoms* and its use for this purpose is increasing here in Europe. Studies have shown that for *joint inflammation* and serious *inflammatory*

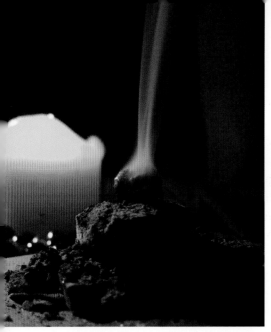
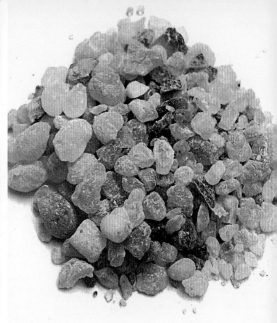

The resin starts to smoke on the glowing charcoal.   *Incense resin.*

intestinal diseases, frankincense preparations can sometimes work as well as conventional medicines.[1] For instance, frankincense can replace cortisone in some cases. This applies to some *brain tumours* with dangerous swelling of the brain. They can be alleviated both by cortisone and by frankincense, and this can lead to improved speech, a reduction in paralysis and greater alertness in particular cases.[2] It goes without saying that for such serious illnesses, the use of concentrated frankincense preparations – which are not yet approved for this purpose in many countries – are only an option under medical supervision (see also pages 334f).

Frankincense is used in yet another way in anthroposophical medicine. In this case it is often processed along with myrrh (the resin of another desert tree which appears completely gnarled and thorny) and gold. Gold, frankincense and myrrh are, of course, the gifts of the three wise men. In a certain sense, these substances accompany the soul as it connects to the body. Where there is a difficulty in establishing this connection, then a remedy made from these substances in potentised form can achieve impressive results (see page 335f). Likewise, the release of the soul from the body at death is also frequently difficult and a remedy of this kind can also be surprisingly helpful in easing this process in the dying person. I have often found that fear and pain decrease and the dying person's real nature can appear lucidly once more. Frankincense seems to be strongly linked to the thresholds of birth and death, where the heavens and earth meet.

Frankincense (*Olibanum*)

A mixture of aromatic resins suitable for burning is often sold under the name of 'frankincense'. True frankincense, however, is a light resin secreted by the frankincense trees *Boswellia sacra* and *Boswellia carterii*. On the other hand, usually the resin of the Indian frankincense tree *Boswellia serrata* is used for medicinal purposes. Due to large differences in quality and potential contaminants, only proprietary medicines from reliable sources are suitable for medicinal use.

Concentrated frankincense

In Germany there is currently no concentrated frankincense preparation licensed for human treatment. However, there has been much research using standardised frankincense preparations from India (for example H15 Gufic), which has been summarised in the German *Ärzteblatt*, for example.[3]

When these types of remedies are used, they are generally imported from abroad on an individual prescription from the attending doctor. Careful supervision by an experienced doctor is necessary for several reasons. The above-mentioned diseases for which the positive effects of frankincense have been documented in studies or for which there is extensive treatment experience are generally of a serious nature. They can themselves lead either to lasting damage or even death, for example, in the case of *brain tumours* with accompanying cerebral swelling. They may also lead to serious complications. This applies, for example, to *chronic inflammatory intestinal diseases* such as *Colitis ulcerosa* and *Crohn's disease* as well as to *inflammatory rheumatic diseases*. In these cases it goes without saying that the treatment must be carefully supervised in order to deal with any dangerous developments which may arise.

In individual cases, frankincense remedies like these have also been very helpful for less dangerous disease symptoms such as *arthritis* pain. However, careful supervision is also required here because frankincense itself can cause difficulties. In sensitive patients it frequently leads to gastro-intestinal problems. When used in high concentrations, frankincense has a detectable effect on metabolic processes. For example, it can prevent the development of special cytokins – substances (for example leukotrienes) which act as 'messengers' in triggering or governing immune responses in the body. However, because these substances have a series of other effects in the whole body, too strong an intervention can produce undesirable consequences. Regular monitoring of the blood count and liver and kidney function is necessary. Just like conventional analgesics, continuous use of concentrated frankincense preparations can cause damage to the kidneys. Changes in the blood count (particularly a decline in the number of white blood cells) may also occur because frankincense in high concentrations has a cytostatic effect, that is, it impedes cell multiplication. This effect can have an undesirable impact on rapidly dividing healthy cells (for example those in the blood-forming marrow), yet it can be useful in treating tumours. It has been shown that frankincense is able to inhibit the growth of *brain tumour* cells in cultures. However, the repeatedly observed improvement in the condition of brain tumour patients being given frankincense has another reason: the 'inflammatory-type' cerebral swelling around the tumour can lead to symptoms such as paralysis, speech disturbances, drowsiness, etc. Like cortisone, frankincense can often bring significant relief by suppressing the oedema. However, a real effect on tumour growth by reducing cell division is probably only possible in cell culture experiments because the concentrations of active ingredients from the frankincense necessary to achieve this cannot be achieved in the brain of a living person. This means that a temporary stabilisation of the situation is produced by these remedies, but over the long term the disease unfortunately usually continues to progress.

Potentised frankincense

Potentised frankincense is occasionally offered with the claim that it helps treat the same diseases in this form as do concentrated preparations. I believe I have seen some indication of this in individual cases when frankincense was prescribed under its pharmaceutical name of Olibanum as powder in a D3 (that is, a preparation which contains 1 mg of frankincense in 1 g of the remedy). However, the medicinal effect was never as strong as that achieved with concentrated preparations. Recently there have even been occasional reports that frankincense can have an inflammatory effect if used in too low a dose.

Aurum comp. Unguentum (Wala) ointment containing frankincense can have some effect on *arthritis of the hand and ankle joints.* Frankincense is used along with gold and myrrh in potentised form in anthroposophical medicine in other situations where it has proved to be a useful remedy. The first to develop and use a remedy of this kind was the physician and curative educator, Karl König. He fled Austria during the period of Nazi rule, founding communities in Britain where people, both with and without recognisable handicaps, lived together. They attempted to support each individual in such a way that he or she could continue to develop and could lead a fulfilling life. The first of these communities, called Camphill, gave its name to the entire movement. Karl König's basic view was that the innermost essence of a person cannot be ill. He believed, however, that there can be physical and emotional circumstances which prevent this essential core of the individual from completely penetrating and forming the body, thus preventing the essential being from coming to expression.

König worked in particular with people suffering from severe autism who were unable to speak. In the search for remedies which could help the souls of such people to 'arrive more fully on the earth', he developed various preparations whose common feature was the use of potentised gold, frankincense and myrrh. König in fact repeatedly found that this was able to successfully stimulate the development of speech and many other abilities. Remedies like these are still important in anthroposophical medical treatment of children with disabilities. But these medicines can also produce undesirably strong effects, which is why it is important to have experienced supervision.

The activity of our innermost essential core, our self or 'I', is visible not only in our speaking and thinking but also in our will and action. This is always linked to changes in our warmth distribution and often to a distinct production of warmth. Using imaging methods such as magnetic resonance imaging, modern brain research demonstrates increased blood flow (and metabolism) in particular regions of the brain. The researchers conclude from this that these regions of the brain are particularly active during the task being carried out by the subject when the images are being made. Because blood flow and metabolism are directly connected to the production of warmth, the brain maps produced in this way also represent 'warmth maps' to a certain degree.

We experience the production of warmth directly and without any technical devices when we carry out vigorous physical activity, but even gentle muscle movements are accompanied by a measurable 'warmth peak'. In this sense, fever can be regarded as an attempt by our self to become 'master in its own house' (the body). This can be experienced directly when invading pathogens are held in check by fever and the immune processes that accompany it. It is also seen when children, in particular, have had experiences with profound emotional effects which they cannot initially cope with and then react by having a high temperature. After the fever, a new stage of emotional and physical maturity can often be observed. The archetypal picture of this is teething fever which can accompany the physical change in the child's mouth and at the end of which the child is ready to 'bite into life' in a new way.

One would expect that a stronger 'presence' of the self, or 'I', in the body can be associated with increased warmth production. It is therefore not surprising that König frequently observed illnesses with a very high fever in his protégés, which appeared soon after the first dose of his gold-frankincense-and-myrrh remedy. Following this, the children almost always developed abilities that no one would have believed them capable of. You almost have the impression that through the fever an obstacle to the full emergence of the self had been 'melted away'. It is probably no coincidence that combustible resins which (as shown previously, see pages 331f) show an excess of 'sun effects' have contributed to results of this kind. But it also appears that, depending on the circumstances, the same substance (in concentrated form) can have an anti-inflammatory effect or (in potentised form) can promote a feverish entry of the self into the body. I have never come across dangerous effects when using such remedies which are made by Wala as Aurum comp. and by Weleda as Olibanum comp. However, Karl König

337

actually experienced some patients developing ear infections and even pneumonia. It is therefore clear that these applications of frankincense also need to be supervised by an experienced practitioner.

The archetype of giving frankincense, myrrh and gold comes from the three kings who went to the infant Jesus, who was likewise entering the earthly world. They worshipped him and, as it were, assisted the soul on its journey into the body.

Nowadays a remedy such as Aurum comp. also has an important place in accompanying the soul out of the body again at the other end of life. In the process of becoming old and dying, this loosening of the soul occurs to an increasing degree. Sometimes, however, the person can become agonisingly 'stuck' on this journey. I have frequently experienced this, especially with people who have had a long battle with an illness and have repeatedly gained a victory over their limitations. They were often successful in not letting something like cancer get them down and regained control over their body. But when the time came to finally let go of the body so that the soul could depart in peace, then the 'habit' of constantly trying to reconnect with the body could become a problem.

I have repeatedly seen similar things, and have also seen that a dying person who appeared to be in anguish once again became lucid and 'present' and stabilised before they then died. This stands in contrast to the disastrous practice of euthanasia, which is sometimes called 'mercy-killing', but nonethless is still an act of killing. When using potentised remedies containing frankincense, I find that they enable the soul to develop and restore a certain freedom. However, their administration does not determine which direction the soul will take, or impose the will of the care-giver over the will of the patient. It therefore appears to me that they can help to provide genuine, morally and humanly appropriate medical support for the dying.

For example, there was one patient who had lived with two types of cancer and numerous metastases for many years, gone through many painful treatments and carried on happily with her work up until only a few weeks before her death. But then the illness which had been successfully combatted for longer than expected finally gained the upper hand and it was predicted that the patient's life could not last much longer. She had been admitted to hospital again because she anticipated that artificial feeding would give her new strength. When the hoped for improvement did not materialise, she was overcome by despair. A continuous, piercing scream escaped the normally self-controlled and amiable woman. Nothing could silence her cries and when I came into the hospital I could hear the wailing several floors away. The patient had ordered the blinds to be let down. She wanted to see and hear nothing and only give expression to the agony in her soul. One ampoule of Aurum comp. transformed the situation. The dying patient quieted down completely, spoke about her life a little, expressed her thanks and said goodbye. She died very peacefully the following night. The nurses and doctors involved were totally amazed at the sudden change. Of course, the administration of the finely dissolved gold, frankincense and myrrh which can usher in life had not lead to her death. But the remedy had helped her to regain freedom when she had become stuck, and it became possible for the dying person to be able to continue on her journey.

CHAPTER 35

Mistletoe

Winter is generally not the time for looking at plants. But it is then that we encounter mistletoe; it appears at most Christmas markets and we can also see it particularly well on the trees after the leaves have fallen. For just a moment we might wonder whether it is a bird's nest or a squirrel's drey. But then the twigs would be greyish-brown, whereas these are a bright green. On some round bunches we even spot gleaming white berries, which ripen in the middle of winter. A few weeks later, when snow lies underfoot, the mistletoe opens its inconspicuous flowers. Everything about misteltoe seems to be different to other plants. So it is no surprise that things happen around it that could not otherwise take place – and kisses are exchanged beneath it unabashed. This, and the mysterious atmosphere surronding this plant can be seen in the beautiful poem 'Mistletoe' by Walter de la Mare:

Mistletoe

Sitting under the mistletoe
(Pale-green, fairy mistletoe),
One last candle burning low,
All the sleepy dancers gone,
Just one candle burning on,
Shadows lurking everywhere:
Someone came, and kissed me there.

The main phase of the mistletoe's activity begins in winter when its host has shed its leaves.

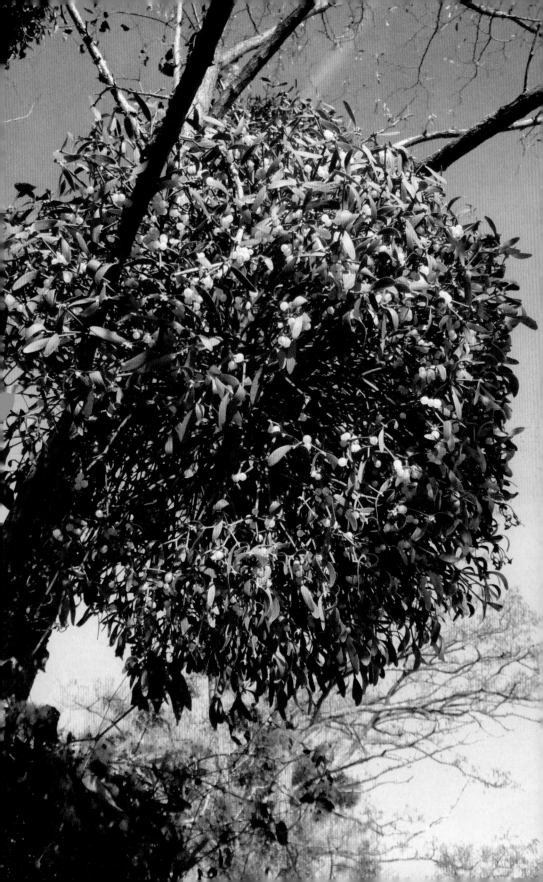

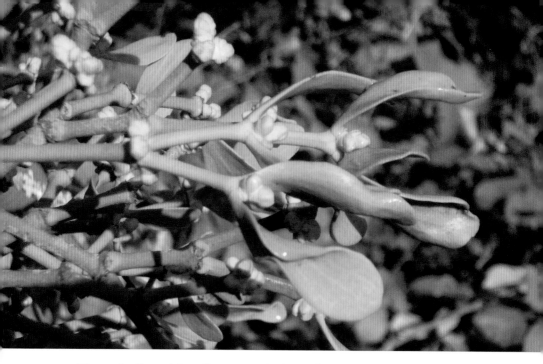

The small yellow mistletoe flowers are quite inconspicuous.

Tired I was; my head would go
Nodding under the mistletoe
(Pale-green, fairy mistletoe),
No footsteps came, no voice, but only,
Just as I sat there, sleepy, lonely,
Stooped in the still and shadowy air,
Lips unseen – and kissed me there.

Mistletoe has always been considered special. Readers of Asterix comic books know that mistletoe berries complete the legendary magic potion for invincibility. They also know that the plant has to be cut with a golden sickle. Somehow it always seems to require special treatment. When dealing with this plant, you constantly encounter aspects of this special nature.

Let us start at the beginning. The life of a 'normal' plant begins when a seed starts to germinate after a period of dormancy in the ground. But in the case of mistletoe, the berry has to be eaten by a bird such as a jay or a mistle thrush. This would be the end of many seeds, but not of mistletoe seeds. Inside the berries are several greenish embryos which – unlike normal seeds – must not dry out and therefore do not

342

undergo any proper dormant phase. Their passage through the belly of a bird is a little reminiscent of the theme of Jonah in the Old Testament who had to spend some time in the belly of a whale before he was ready to carry out his mission. Mistletoe never touches the earth; it is carried through the air by a bird. The mistletoe embryos may then land on a branch along with the bird droppings. They can only thrive on the right kind of branch. Mistletoe never grows on certain trees (for example, beech), and on others it is uncommon (for example, oak). The embryo of pine mistletoe can never grow on a deciduous tree and vice versa. Moreover, not all trees of the same species are suitable for growing mistletoe. Mistletoe is commoner in cities than in the country and it becomes more abundant with increasing air pollution. Trees growing on buried water courses are also said to carry more mistletoe. When everything else is right, then light needs to fall on the seeds so that they germinate. While normal plants now produce two cotyledons, the mistletoe seed first produces a snake-like tube, the haustorium, which it uses to attach itself to the bark of its host. The haustorium penetrates the bark and goes deep inside the branch, where it extends 'roots' into the tree's sap-conducting vessels. The mistletoe itself never takes water or mineral nutriments from the ground. This activity is left to the host tree, which therefore has to sacrifice some of the liquid it has obtained (and also some of the substances it has produced).

But what happens in winter when the tree's flow of sap has ceased? Then the mistletoe secretes special sugary substances into the tree's vascular bundle, which act as an anti-freeze agent. It forces a flow of sap in the vessels leading to the mistletoe in order to meet its needs while the other vessels, which only supply the tree, remain dormant.

Once the haustorium and its runners have been formed, the mistletoe also produces leaves. Most plants transform the shape of their leaves depending on their position in the plant. However, all the leaves of the mistletoe look alike. In fact, they look very much like cotyledons, which are rudimentary, embryonic leaves. Not only is the form of the leaves undifferentiated but, in addition, the upper and lower surfaces of the leaves have the same structure; something not found in other plants. By its nature, a plant grows toward the sky and directs its roots toward the centre of the earth. Mistletoe is different in this regard, too. It only grows upwards for the first couple of years, and it then produces regular V-shaped branches. During this time it actually looks like a little tree. When the first flower primordia appear in the third year, the form starts to change completely. For exactly 28 days (in other words, the length of one moon cycle), the individual shoots start to make slow nodding movements, a discovery made by Rolf Dorka and Thomas Goebel using time-lapse photography.[1] They shape themselves into a bush-like sphere, thus assuming a form that the mistletoe retains for the rest of its life. Unlike other plants, it no longer bothers about where the sun or the centre of the earth are. Its centre is completely within itself. Likewise, it no longer seems to pay attention to the seasons and develops its own particular emancipated rhythm.

Even Norse-Germanic mythology mentions the fact that mistletoe is subject to its own laws. It was the only living thing that did not swear an oath not to harm the god of light, Baldur. This made it possible for the scheming Loki to trick blind Hodur into unintentionally killing Baldur with an arrow carved from mistletoe.

Many of the characteristics of mistletoe are in fact akin to those of a tumour. The cell growth in a tumour is also disconnected from its surroundings. Normally, the processes of growth and regeneration are limited. Tissues and organs only grow to a size and shape that serves the entire organism. It can be observed right down to molecular details that a tumour is 'blind' to the signals from the environment. Moreover, it initially grows in the form of a sphere. Tumour cells generally do not have the dormancy periods common to other cells. And a growing tumour has to make a connection to the human vascular system like the mistletoe on its tree. Tumour cells also show signs of being primitive and undifferentiated like the mistletoe. Mistletoe therefore presents a 'natural image' of a tumour in a sense. On the tree it can even spread beneath the bark and give rise to new bunches of mistletoe at distant locations, reminiscent of the formation of the metastases of cancerous tumours.

At the start of the twentieth century Rudolf Steiner recommended developing a remedy from mistletoe for treating cancer. Since then, various methods for manufacturing a remedy of this kind have been tested, in which the particular characteristics and effects of the plant have been enhanced or further developed in various ways. No other plant has a more extensive scientific literature.

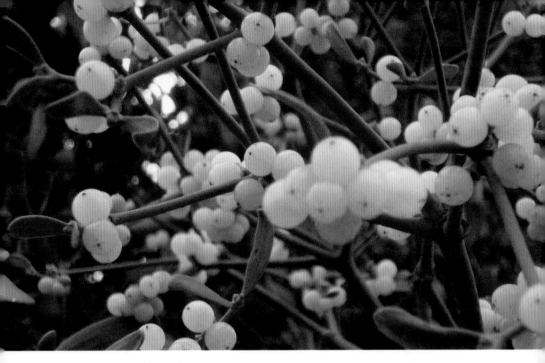

The mucilaginous mistletoe berries ripen in wintertime.

A current book on the topic lists over 3,800 articles on research results obtained from mistletoe.[2] Many studies have demonstrated efficacy in treating tumours. It has been shown that mistletoe extracts can alleviate the side effects of chemotherapy, and in some experiments they were shown to actually increase its efficacy.

In recent years, great success has been achieved in cancer treatment by developing medicines to inhibit the formation of blood vessels (angiogenesis). Growing tumours need this angiogenesis in order to supply themselves with nutrients and oxygen – just as the mistletoe needs to connect to the vessels of the host tree. Interestingly, besides stimulating the immune system and directly destroying tumours, mistletoe also has the effect of inhibiting angiogenesis.[3]

The administration of mistletoe to human beings is done in a number of different ways. Concentrated mistletoe extract can be injected directly into tumours and metastases. This can result in the tumour becoming inflamed and completely – or at least partially – killed. In some hospitals this is practised with impressive results. However, mistletoe can also be injected in smaller doses to stimulate the immune system and improve the patient's overall condition.

Although a great many studies on mistletoe and its application have been published, there is still much more to investigate. Nonetheless, it is without a doubt one of the most interesting, unusual and, one could even say, 'self-willed' plants. It is likewise a powerful remedy for a very serious and prevalent disease.

Mistletoe (*Viscum album*)

Mistletoe is not especially suitable for collecting yourself. To begin with, it is hard to reach it where it grows, high up in trees. The thick, mucilaginous parts of the plant do not dry easily and can easily mould if not treated properly. If you want to use mistletoe as tea you should therefore buy it in a pharmacy. The mistletoe extracts used for treating tumours must be manufactured by skilled pharmacists using special methods and equipment. (see pages 353f).

Mistletoe tea

In folk medicine, mistletoe has the reputation of being helpful in cases of *high blood pressure* or *arteriosclerosis*. This effect is not generally accepted since, up until now, it cannot be attributed to any known substance found in mistletoe. However, I have sometimes had the impression that it can have a relaxing effect and slightly reduce blood pressure when drunk as a tea made by cold extraction. A case of seriously high blood pressure cannot be treated in this manner. But it can be tried if there is only a tendency to raised blood pressure. (Of course, the patient's blood pressure should be properly monitored in this case.)

Add 1 heaping teaspoon of the chopped dried plant to 1 cup of cold water in the evening and leave to soak overnight. Strain the liquid and drink the extract cold in the morning.

When mistletoe is used in the form of injections for cancers this often also produces a regulatory effect on blood pressure.

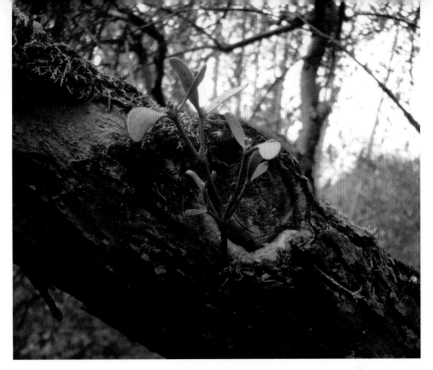

At the start of its development the mistletoe resembles a small upright tree.

Non-oncological use of potentised mistletoe

Mistletoe always grows on trees; it never really comes down to the earth, and it never becomes hardened or fully formed like a 'normal' earthly plant. When used as a medicine, it has a warming effect and it dissolves hardened structures. These characteristics make it easy to understand most of the medicinal applications of mistletoe.

Homeopathy is based on the principle of similarity. According to this principle, if a substance taken in concentrated form produces certain symptoms in people, then this same substance – when given in a highly diluted, potentised form – can be used to heal a patient who presents with these symptoms. The homeopathic use of mistletoe for *dizziness* with a danger of falling and a feeling of floating can be interpreted, in a sense, as a sign of too great a 'similarity to mistletoe', of 'not-being-completely-connected-to-the-earth'. Homeopaths prescribe high potencies of mistletoe for this (for example Viscum album D12 or D30), which are produced by most manufacturers of homeopathic remedies.

However, mistletoe also has a long-standing reputation for treating *epilepsy*. Paracelsus used it for this purpose and many old books on

347

herbal remedies also contain this indication. In recent times the head of the paediatrics ward in the anthroposophical hospital Filderklinik in Germany, René Madeleyn, has reintroduced mistletoe for treating epilepsy on a larger scale.[4] Anthroposophical treatment of epilepsy is based on the insight that epilepsy does not consist only of the actual seizure. Rather, the primary cause is a kind of hardening of the organs, which makes it difficult for the soul and spirit to completely take hold of and permeate the body. The actual convulsion is then only the excessive – and therefore potentially destructive – attempt to permeate the body nonetheless. It stands to reason that a treatment which makes the body 'softer' can prevent seizures. Mistletoe seems to be particularly suitable for achieving this when the convulsions are caused by scars in the brain (from injuries, operations, oxygen deficiency or inflammation). In order to achieve the desired therapeutic effect, anthroposophical physicians often administer gradually increasing doses of mistletoe. This treatment requires experience. As this is such a serious illness it should only be administered under medical supervision. It then often produces good results.[5]

Aside from cancer treatment, mistletoe is used particularly often for *osteoarthritis*. This involves progressive damage of the mucilaginous layer of cartilage which ensures good mobility in all the joints. In the embryonic phase, all the bones which are involved in joints are initially formed as cartilage. This kind of cartilaginous skeleton – which is found in many types of fish – would not allow us to be upright or to move on land as it would become deformed due to the effect of gravity. Large parts of our bones therefore become ossified and calcified. A translucent elastic cartilage normally remains only in the joints, enabling the surfaces of the joints to slide over each other. Increasing age and one-sided movement of, or pressure on, the joints can cause not only damage to the cartilage but also calcified bony growths (exostoses), which cause pain and increasingly restrict movement. Administering mistletoe locally around the joint can have a warming effect and can enhance the circulation and nutrition in that area. This counteracts the stiffening tendency as well as the pain. This treatment re-establishes the joint's 'mistletoe quality' as

Mistletoe does not adapt to its environment but, like a tumour, grows spherically in all directions.

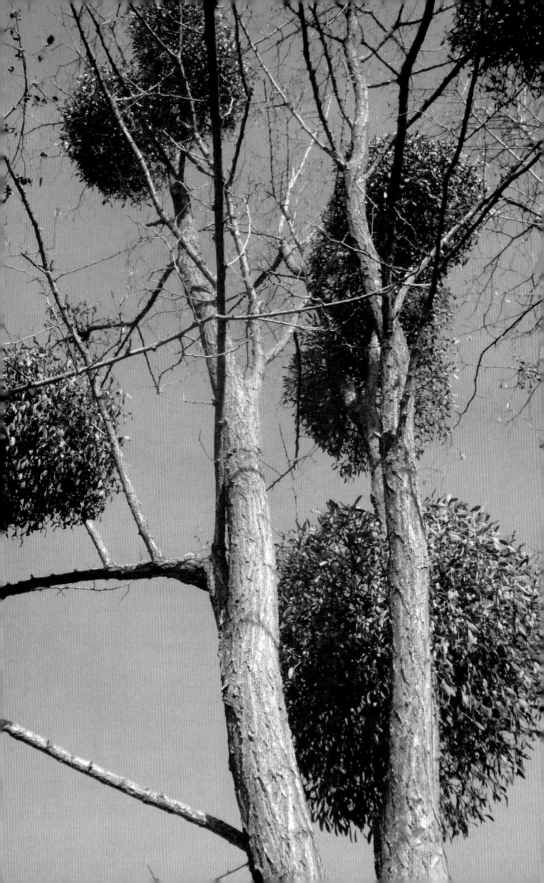

it were, restoring the inside of the joint to a state of 'weightlessness', such as the mistletoe displays on the tree. In this treatment mistletoe is injected intradermally to produce wheals in the skin. This usually results in reddening and warmth production around the injection site in the days following. Sometimes the pain in the joint can increase temporarily, but afterwards there is almost always a shorter or longer-lasting improvement. Normally, mistletoe grown on apple trees, poplars or willows is used for these injections. It is the same as that usually used for cancer treatment. Some of these products are Iscucin, Iscador, AbnobaViscum, Helixor and Vysorel and also Plenosol (although the last is not an anthroposophical medicinal preparation). Mistletoe ampoules which have not been subject to the special manufacturing methods for cancer treatment (see pages 351f) can also be used, such as Viscum Mali e planta tota D6, D4, D3 or D2 (Wala).

Mistletoe can also produce a significant improvement in 'rheumatic-like' muscular complaints such as fibromyalgia syndrome. Good results have been achieved particularly with mistletoe grown on willow. This tree displays a strong connection to movement even in its form. Moreover, it is also closely linked to the movement of fluids which can be disrupted in such illnesses (willow mistletoe is produced under the name of Iscucin Salicis).[6] Fibromyalgia syndrome is characterised by persistent aching pains in the muscles and by pain caused by pressure on a point on an enthesis (the spot where a muscle or tendon attaches to the bone). Patients often suffer from fatigue. Sometimes the mistletoe treatment is combined with other forms of heat treatment (for example hyperthermia, in which externally heating the body produces a condition akin to fever).

Lastly, mistletoe (again, often willow mistletoe) can be very helpful for inflammatory rheumatic diseases, such as rheumatoid arthritis, when used in highly potentised form. The dosage has to be administered very carefully because too high a dose can lead to relapses. However, used carefully by an experienced practitioner, mistletoe can also bring about a significant improvement in the quality of life.[7] Giving too high a dose or increasing the mistletoe treatment too quickly can also have a detrimental effect in other diseases where the immune system is malfunctioning (autoimmune disease) such as multiple sclerosis or some *inflammatory thyroid diseases*. For this reason, the treatment should always take account of the patient's overall situation.

It was mentioned earlier in Chapter 17 on the lime (or linden), that mistletoe in higher potencies can sometimes lead to an impressive improvement in sleep. In addition it often has a significant effect in improving mood, which is why it sometimes forms part of the treatment for depression.

Mistletoe for cancer treatment

In current medical practice, the attempt will be made to surgically remove any cancerous tumour by operation, or to destroy it by radiation whenever possible. Nowadays, chemotherapy is sometimes administered before an operation in order to shrink a tumour which is otherwise impossible to remove, or which cannot be removed without causing significant damage. Subsequently the tumour can be entirely removed with a smaller operation. In some cases chemotherapy is recommended after removal of the tumour in order to reduce the risk of the tumour recurring or producing metastases elsewhere in the body. If there are already metastases, these can sometimes be removed surgically. In other cases, palliative chemotherapy is recommended which – although it cannot cure the cancer – may reduce the symptoms and delay the advancement of the disease. This covers the main options available from conventional cancer treatment.

Many patients and doctors feel that this approach, which solely focuses on and deals with the tumour, is insufficient for regaining real health. Various measures from psychotherapy through physical training and appropriate diet to art therapy and vocational rehabilitation are also offered today. These aim to rally the patient's own forces, overcome the effects of the illness and, if possible, gain enough strength to surmount the conditions which have contributed to the occurrence of such a serious disease. Complementary medical therapy extends and complements conventional medical practices and expands the possibilities both for treating and for understanding illness. It makes use of medicines, and mistletoe in particular, in treating cancer. In fact, mistletoe therapy is the most widely used complementary medicinal therapy of all.

The starting point for this was an indication by Rudolf Steiner. He said that remedies made from mistletoe should eventually have such a powerful effect that they would lead to a complete cure for cancer – when possible, even without the surgeon's scalpel.

At present this aim has only been achieved in a few isolated – but impressive – cases.[8] Recently a randomised clinical study took place with about 220 patients with locally advanced or metastastatic pancreatic cancer, which is one of the most malignant types of cancer. The patients who had mistletoe therapy showed a remarkable improvement in quality of life and a highly significant and clinically relevant longer overall survival rate compared with those without such therapy.[9] Mistletoe therapy has become an invaluable adjunct therapy at all of the above-mentioned stages of cancer treatment. It is applied in very different ways, depending on the situation.

In cases where patients declined localised treatment such as surgery or radiotherapy, injecting concentrated mistletoe preparations into the tumour and its immediate surroundings often achieved a significant reduction of the tumour or even its disappearance. This was normally preceded by a phase of inflammation triggered by the mistletoe, often accompanied by a marked fever. For treatment of cancer of the pancreas, which is often inoperable and progresses particularly rapidly, mistletoe achieved at least as good results in terms of patient survival rates as did the standard chemotherapy treatment.[10] In the case of liver metastases, this type of injection with concentrated mistletoe preparations in addition to (or in place of) the normal treatment for metastases has become a successful routine treatment in some specialised hospitals.[11]

Mistletoe preparations can also have a direct effect on tumour cells if they are injected into accumulations of water containing malignant cells in the pleural cavity or the abdominal cavity. This often leads to a long-term 'drying up' of the discharge and thus to an improvement in the condition of the patient.[12] In some cases of bladder cancer one option is to introduce mistletoe preparations into the bladder using a catheter.[13] This use of very high doses of mistletoe, which generally leads to a strong localised inflammatory reaction and fever, is used occasionally. However, it is much more common to administer smaller amounts of mistletoe by subcutaneous injection. These can reduce the side effects of normal treatments such as chemotherapy and radiotherapy and stabilise the patient's health.[14] Finally, mistletoe is also given to stabilise the immune system and with the aim of reducing the risk of a recurrence of the disease after successful cancer treatment. It has in fact been shown that this type of stabilising mistletoe treatment improves the health of the patient and gives them a better chance of long-term freedom from illness compared to patients who have not had any additional treatment.[15] It is only in recent years that the experience of many (former) cancer patients, who complain of increased tiredness and a significant reduction in their fitness, has been taken seriously. This disorder, known as *cancer fatigue syndrome*, has now been partly attributed to the treatment (particularly to chemotherapy and radiation), but can in part be due to the cancer itself. It has become apparent that patients who are treated with mistletoe suffer less from this debilitating syndrome. However, movement and art therapies also have a beneficial effect in this respect.

Different mistletoe preparations

Mistletoe therapy has been developed for almost a century as part of anthroposophical medicine. Starting from Rudolf Steiner's findings and indications, various routes were taken to develop effective cancer medicines from the raw plant. This resulted in preparations such as Iscador, Iscucin, Helixor, AbnobaViscum and Vysorel. All the mistletoe preparations supplied by anthroposophical pharmaceutical manufacturers combine the juice from mistletoe plants harvested in midsummer and around midwinter. The mistletoe is found in very different situations at these times. On a deciduous tree, for example, it is completely shaded by the crown of the tree in the summer and completely exposed to the light in the winter. Likewise, it is found in differing phases of its own development. For example, it will be full of berries in the depths of winter, or fully in the growth phase in summer. At opposite times of the year it contains differing amounts of various substances, which, while they all produce an anti-tumour action, do this in different ways. For instance, in summer more viscotoxins are produced that work to kill cancer cells directly. In winter, it contains more lectins that work indirectly via the immune system. By combining the juices from plants harvested at different times of the year, the 'totality' of the mistletoe can be better represented than if it was only harvested and processed at one point in time.

Various elaborate and sophisticated techniques are used to produce diverse types of mistletoe preparations. Their intended purpose is to increase and enhance the effect of the mistletoe beyond what the plant produces naturally. Extracting the substances from the mistletoe and preserving the extracts is done in different ways. For example, a fermentation process is used to make Iscador, the plants are frozen for producing AbnobaViscum and they are freeze-dried for Iscucin. This gives each of these preparations typical qualities. Although all the mistletoe preparations can be used for the whole spectrum of indications, according to experienced mistletoe therapists particular preparations are especially suitable for specific treatment situations.

Since mistletoe therapy has become established and due to the impact of sometimes surprising successes in treatment, increasingly intensive research around this plant been undertaken over the last few decades. This has focused especially on individual constituents of the plant. As a result, part of the effect of mistletoe has been attributed to what are known as lectins. These are proteins which react with sugar molecules occurring on immune cells and also on cancer cells in the body. Some of the effects of mistletoe preparations that influence the immune system can be explained in this way.

However, the effect of mistletoe cannot be reduced to one substance or group of substances. Mistletoe contains numerous substances that affect the immune system or destroy cancer cells. But none of these individual substances can explain the overall effect of the remedies obtained from the whole plant. For this reason, established mistletoe preparations (in which only the lectins have been standardised) have come in for a lot of criticism. Another point is that the dosage of some of these remedies is calculated on the patient's body weight (similar to that of conventional oncologic treatments), not on the patient's individual reaction. Some authors argue that such dosages are only calculated on the basis of experiments on a few mice, and are not validated by experience on human beings whose immune system is too individual to influence by uniform medication.

Tailoring the treatment to the individual

Cancer appears in patients with a wide variety of different conditions which need to be improved and healed. So it is not surprising that mistletoe is used in a variety of ways.

The concentration of the mistletoe can be varied. High mistletoe concentrations are normally used with the aim of achieving a localised effect on a tumour. Improving the patient's health during chemotherapy or radiotherapy is usually achieved with moderately high doses of mistletoe, as is strengthening the immune system. A reduction in pain and the establishment of emotional stability in cases of advanced illness can often best be achieved with highly diluted – higher potencies of – mistletoe. Most experienced mistletoe therapists do not simply give a standard dose of mistletoe but rather adapt the therapy to the individual responsiveness and situation of the patient. One indication of a correct dose can be a change in body temperature. Even if there is no intent to produce a significant fever, the attempt is usually made to produce a certain increase in the average body temperature and to strengthen the rhythmical rise and fall of body temperature between morning and evening. Another indication is that the general health of the patient should improve when the individual mistletoe dose is optimised. A small (roughly coin-sized) reddening of the skin around the injection site is aimed for in specific cases. Some therapists measure immunological test parameters as a target criterion.

The method of administration can be modified. Mistletoe is normally injected subcutaneously. This is the usual form of application for a therapy to complement conventional tumour treatments, such as chemotherapy or radiotherapy, and also after complete removal of cancerous tumours. It was mentioned that an application as close to the tumour as possible is recommended when treatment is aimed directly at the destruction of cancer cells. Some experienced mistletoe therapists also obtain good results by administering mistletoe through an intravenous infusion as an adjunct therapy during chemotherapy or in the case of advanced symptoms including metastases. These more intensive forms of treatment may result not only in greater efficacy, but also in a greater possibility of side effects. For example, allergies can be more serious, which is why this kind of treatment should only be carried out in an environment where any side effects can be dealt with properly if necessary.

A basic way of individualising mistletoe treatment is evident from observing nature. As already mentioned, mistletoe grows on very different host trees. Mistletoe growing in the crown of a deciduous tree (which is in full sunshine in winter) is different from that growing in a conifer. Also the sap content differs in different trees at various times of the year. So mistletoe plants growing on deciduous trees and on conifers are in fact different in terms of their constituents and also their effects.[16] As a general rule it can be said that mistletoe growing on deciduous trees tends to promote inflammatory responses, which can cause tumours to decrease in size. On the other hand, mistletoe from coniferous trees tends to improve the patient's health and to strengthen the immune system. Particular qualities are accentuated, depending on the specific type of tree acting as host to the mistletoe. For example, amongst the conifers, pines tend to be characterised by light and structure, while the dark and more uniform spruce is characterised by warmth qualities. During decades of experience in using mistletoe, indications have emerged about the particular efficacy of mistletoe from specific trees for specific kinds of tumours. For example, *malignant melanomas* appear to respond particularly to almond mistletoe, *basal-cell carcinomas* of the skin, in contrast, to birch mistletoe. However, different types of constitutional or emotional characteristics (including the gender of the patient) can also be important for the selection of one or the other host tree species.

In view of the various aspects touched on here it is clear that mistletoe therapy can be administered in a routine manner in straightforward treatment situations, for example for what is known as 'adjuvant' therapy to stabilise the patient after complete tumour removal. Nonetheless, it can also be adapted very individually to the needs of the patient. There are even situations where it is beneficial to use preparations manufactured by different methods, to use mistletoe from different host trees in alternation, or to alter the specifics of the therapy depending on the progress of the disease. True mastery in using the mistletoe can then go beyond routine treatment protocols and can develop a true and proper healing art.

CHAPTER 36

Christmas Rose

Christmas roses have become rare in the wild, where they are most often seen in beech and spruce forests on limestone. However, closer to human habitation, we may see them looking out innocently from a patch of melting snow and we cannot tear ourselves away from the miracle of such beauty bursting forth from a frosty, lifeless world. Although some people know that mistletoe also flowers in winter, it does so in inaccessible places high up in the trees. Moreover, its tiny yellowish flowers are not really very impressive: you have to know about them to recognise them as flowers at all. Be that as it may, mistletoe (at least on account of its white berries) is also a well-known Christmas decoration.

New birth in a world that has outwardly died away can scarcely be more clearly felt than through a marvel of flowering such as this. To the poet Eduard Mörike, who found a Christmas rose in the middle of winter over a grave, it became a symbol of resurrection.[1]

> Daughter of the forest, relative of the lily,
> I have looked for you for so long, unknown,
> And it is in a foreign churchyard, bleak and wintery,
> That I have found you, O beauty, for the first time.
>
> Whose caring hand it is that has allowed you to bloom
> I don't know. Nor do I know whose grave you are
>   protecting.
> If it is a boy's, he has found salvation,
> If it is a girl's, her fate was lovely...

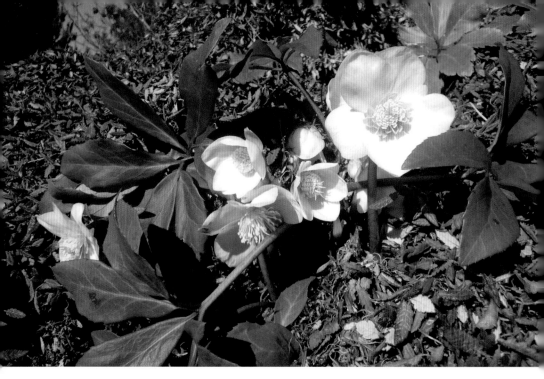

Christmas rose often grows wild in the undergrowth of broad-leaved woodland.

How sensitively the poet captures the nature of the flower is apparent from the initially bewildering lines below:

> You are beautiful. You are a child of the moon, not the sun.
> What for other flowers brings joy would be deadly for you.
> Your chaste body, all frost and scent, is nourished by
> The balsam sweet air of heavenly cold.

Of course Christmas is the time when in the northern hemisphere the sun is above the horizon for the shortest time and the full moon for the longest, where the path of the full moon is as high in the sky as the sun is at midsummer. But more is hidden in this phrase, 'child of the moon'. The moon is the most visible 'transformation artist' in the sky. Every day it looks different and appears in a new place amongst the constellations. The Christmas rose is also a powerful 'transformation artist'. What we perceive as white petals are actually the sepals, which are normally green and inconspicuous beneath the petals. The petals in other flowers normally catch our eye because of their size and colour. However, in the Christmas rose, the actual botanical petals

358

only appear on a second careful look. They are almost covered by the many yellow stamens. The actual petals have become greenish tubes, known as nectaries. As the year progresses, what appeared to be 'petals' at Christmas start to 'recall' their origin as sepals and turn increasingly green in colour until they finally look like leaves in spring. What touched our hearts so strongly as a white shining petal now appears overgrown by the plant's vigour.

From the timing of flowering all the way to the details of its botany, everything about the Christmas rose is a little odd or even abnormal. Another word to describe someone who is abnormal is 'lunatic' from *luna,* the Latin word for the moon, meaning literally 'like the moon'. Thus preparations made from the Christmas rose have been used for centuries for *psychiatric disorders*. This was certainly always a delicate matter as the Christmas rose is poisonous. However, in potentised form (as it is used in homeopathy and anthroposophical medicine), it can be very helpful. For the medicine of ancient times and the Middle Ages in which the relationships between organs and celestial phenomena were perfectly obvious, the brain was the organ with the clearest relationship to the moon. The brain indeed mirrors all the processes in the body and the sense perceptions of the outer world as the moon reflects the sun's light.

In fact, potentised Christmas rose, in the hand of an experienced practitioner, can be beneficial for some *brain diseases*. It can alleviate brain tumour symptoms which threaten the function and order of the brain: excessive and uncontrolled vital functions in the brain, pathological fluid retention and pathological growth, can thus be reduced. This helps patients bring clarity to their thoughts and actions. Good results are also repeatedly made with Christmas rose preparations for *dementia*. The plant can contribute by allowing the emotions to 'blossom' once again when they have been as 'overgrown' and overcome by pathological metabolic processes as the Christmas rose flower which turns green.

Modern substance research has also found specific evidence. For example, ecdysone, a substance of which the Nobel prize-winner Adolf Butenandt managed to extract a few milligrammes from 500 kg of silk moth larvae in the 1950s, has been found in the plant. In insects, ecdysone provides the trigger for moulting and transformation of the larva and therefore contributes to the amazing metamorphosis of the worm-like caterpillar into the magnificent butterfly. Why the Christmas rose needs the transformation hormone ecdysone is not totally clear. It has been suggested that it could protect against insect pests which, if they eat Christmas rose, will emerge from their pupae too soon and therefore die. The fact that this plant can manipulate the insects' processes of metamorphosis can be seen as further proof of what a master of transformation it is. When ecdysone is ingested by higher animals and people it is reputed to inhibit tumours and promote nerve regeneration – in other words, this constituent of the Christmas rose actually works in areas that have been seen as being 'characterised by the moon' – and so we have here a present-day confirmation of old knowledge and poetical insight.*

Christmas rose (*Helleborus niger*)

Due to its poisonous nature the Christmas rose is no longer used in conventional phytotherapy. On the other hand, it is used with increasing frequency in potentised form. Samuel Hahnemann, the founder of homeopathy, dealt in detail with the Christmas rose in his thesis to become a faculty member at Leipzig university. Nowadays it is only used in potentised from in homeopathy and anthroposophical medicine.

Collecting or preparing Christmas rose yourself is not an option. It is also not suitable for self-treatment because it is primarily beneficial for serious illnesses for which individualised expert supervision is essential. However, it is a very attractive garden plant, which gives

---

* The well-known French novelist Christian Signol addresses the Christmas rose in a different way in his novel *Une année de neige*. The little grandson of a couple living a simple life in the Pyrenees falls ill with a life-threatening leukaemia. Chemotherapy is able to reduce the suffering but not cure it. In a moment of semiconsciousness, the grandfather (who is knowledgeable about plants), lets slip the suggestion that the rare Christmas rose which can be found flowering in the snow could bring healing or at least relieve the powerful feelings of cold which repeatedly overcome the boy when his illness worsens. Henceforth the Christmas rose becomes a symbol of hope for recovery and when, towards the end of the book after a long search, the grandfather finally finds the plant in the mountains and gives it to the grandson, he is then indeed cured – whether this is due to the plant's own powers or to the emotion which it releases, the author leaves open.

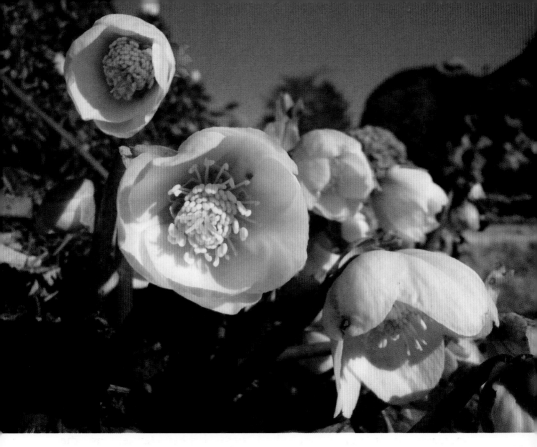

Christmas rose also appears in the mountains.

pleasure with its impressive flowers at a time when scarcely any other plants show signs of life.

Potentised Christmas rose

As the uses of this plant in anthroposophical medicine include those applied in classical homeopathy, no clear distinction will be made between the two therapeutic approaches here. However, their methods for producing the medicines differ. In homeopathy an alcoholic extract is prepared from the dried rhizome of the Christmas rose and this is then potentised, whereas anthroposophical pharmacy uses the whole plant.

Wala harvests whole flowering plants in winter and processes equal amounts of the above-ground (flower and leaf) and below-ground (rhizome) parts. The pulp made from the chopped plant and the juice obtained from it are cooled down morning and evening, stirred and exposed to the light, and in between are kept in the dark at 37°C (99°F). This process is an attempt to increase the vitality of the juice and bring the substance 'closer' to the human being. The plant extract can be kept without a preservative (alcohol) due to the fermentation process which sets in. The pressed residue is burnt and the ashes added to the juice in order to include part of the mineral components of the plant in the medicine. This basic substance is used to produce Helleborus niger e planta tota globules (Wala) in D6 and D12 and ampoules in D3, D6, D12 and D30.

The anthroposophical medical company Helixor harvests the Christmas rose – like the mistletoe – at opposite seasons in the middle of winter and summer. In winter only the flowers with stems are harvested, in summer the leaves and rhizome. The plant parts are frozen and finally an aqueous extract is made over two hours, from the flowers on the one hand and the leaves and rhizome on the other. Similar to the mistletoe (from which Helixor also makes a medicine) the summer and winter juices are combined in a special mixing process in a special apparatus. A vortex is formed in the winter (i.e. flower) juice and the summer (i.e. leaf/root) juice is slowly dripped into it. Helixor only makes ampoules (which can however be drunk) under the name of Helleborus niger in the potency levels D3, D4, D5, D6, D12, D20 and D30.

Just as in mistletoe we distinguish a non-oncological treatment from the cancer therapy, this distinction also needs to be made for the Christmas rose. Both winter-flowering plants were recommended by Rudolf Steiner for cancer treatment. In contrast to the mistletoe which 'flees the earth', Steiner said that the Christmas rose which is deeply connected to the earth is more suitable 'for the male constitution' (which, however, does not mean giving it only to men). It has now indeed been demonstrated that the juice of the Christmas rose like that of mistletoe can destroy tumour cells in surprisingly low concentrations.

The whole character of the action of the mistletoe is a dissolving and warming one, as can be seen from its effectiveness for arthrosis for example. When it produces fever this tends to dim the patient's consciousness. The Christmas rose, in contrast, tends to have a cooling, ordering and clarifying effect. This can be clearly seen in its non-oncological areas of application.

As mentioned earlier in this chapter, in a number of instances there have been some very good experiences in treating *dementia* and conditions similar to dementia (for example after *brain injuries* or *brain haemorrhages,* after *radiation treatment to the head,* etc.) in which, besides a deterioration in memory, poor concentration and disrupted orientation, there is also an impression of mental dullness. It appears that Helleborus can be particularly helpful for heavily built patients in whom the metabolism predominates. It can also improve *epilepsy* if the characteristics mentioned are present.

It has been reported that *premature babies* and children who have suffered an *oxygen deficiency at birth* have shown an unexpectedly good (mental and physical) development when given Helleborus in higher potencies (D12, D30).[2]

The paediatrician Georg Soldner repeatedly found that Helleborus often produced a major improvement or even a cure in children suffering from a *kidney disease* (nephrotic syndrome) which often gives rise to water retention in the tissue (oedema) and a deterioration in the ability to concentrate.[3] This disease is normally treated with cortisone and Helleborus has also worked in cases with insufficient response to cortisone. *Fluid retention* and *swelling* (for example of the testicles) in general are often improved by Helleborus. Mörike saw the Christmas rose as a 'daughter of the moon'. In this context we can see in the tides how the fluids of the earth are connected to the moon, which is interesting in relation to swelling and fluid retention in tissues improved by using Christmas rose. Incidentally, it is noticeable that many symptoms which are normally treated with cortisone respond well to Helleborus. Chemically, cortisone is a steroid; as is the active substance ecdysone mentioned above, which is contained in Christmas rose.

Helleborus was already used in ancient times for *psychiatric illnesses* (to which the dementia disorders mentioned belong). In recent times it has been discovered that depressive states with anxiety, accompanied by physical signs (somatisation) and particularly if there is also the impression of a certain dullness, can often be improved very quickly using Helleborus.[4] This applies all the more if the patient easily loses his temper (compare the ordering 'cooling' effect). Quite often, patients who suffered from a repressed or 'buried' trauma from a long time in the past responded particularly well to this treatment.

The use of Christmas rose for cancer has (like mistletoe) developed out of anthroposophical medicine and has no forerunner in folk medicine or homeopathy.

A certain polarity has become apparent in the therapeutic use of mistletoe and Christmas rose for treating different types of cancer (just as the occurrence of the plants, one in the tree tops, the other on the ground, are opposites). Mistletoe acts particularly on 'hard' and 'slow' tumours (such as cancer of the colon). It is more effective in 'cool' patients: most cancer patients had not had a fever for a long time and tended to have a low body temperature. Helleborus acts more on rapidly progressing cancerous diseases which tend to disintegration (such as *lymphomas* and different types of *leukaemia,* often accompanied by sweating and raised temperature). Tumours which metastasize early (and in this sense are also 'disintegrating', 'centrifugal') such as malignant melanoma or some bronchial carcinomas, can likewise provide an indication for the use of Christmas rose. Brain tumours, which are often accompanied by a loss of mental clarity as described above, can also be a reason for using Christmas rose. As mentioned earlier, its shining white flowers – completely atypically for a flower – become 'dulled' to green in the course of time and start to increase in size. This may suggest that the plant is 'being smothered by growth forces'.

The basic characteristics described here can only provide an indication, which should help to develop an initial understanding of the use of this plant.

A conference on Helleborus in March 2010 reported extraordinarily good progress at times in some seriously ill patients, which was clearly due to the use of Christmas rose.[5] There have also been isolated good outcomes for *prostate cancer* using Helleborus treatment. Nevertheless, research on and testing of the use of Christmas rose is ongoing, and there are as yet fewer definite findings than for mistletoe. This can only be touched on here: in the case of illness which points to this type of treatment, advice should definitely be sought from an experienced therapist and no attempt made at self treatment. Incidentally, an alternating treatment using Christmas rose and mistletoe has repeatedly proved worthwhile.

CHAPTER 37

Ginger and Horseradish

One November a few years ago I went to Indonesia for a few days to join in a family celebration. We were greeted by a sultry-hot, colourful scent-filled tropical world. It was a flood of sense-impressions. We were surrounded by sights, sounds, smells and tastes: unbelievably heavy traffic, animal sounds, sounds of strange music, gleaming flowers, large colourful fluttering butterflies, strongly spiced food. The Indonesian islands were produced by volcanoes and every year they have several earthquakes. In many places hot sulfurous fumes rise from the earth and now and again volcanoes erupt and reform the landscape – the earth here is so powerful, violent and active. It is not surprising that geographers refer to this group of islands as part of a 'ring of fire'.

On our return to Europe, we landed early in the morning as it was slowly getting light. The trees which had still held on to a few coloured leaves when we left were dark and bare and covered in hoarfrost. A uniform grey sky hung over everything. Suddenly we noticed that, despite the long flight, we felt wide awake, that we were alert and centred. There was no longer anything to draw our attention away to an outer world teeming with life – here we could decide for ourselves what we wanted to do and what we wanted to think about. That had been almost impossible where we had just come from. The calm to which we returned felt good.

However, as winter goes on the grey and cold begin to be hard. Our energy dwindles and a little warmth would be good so that we do not catch yet another cold.

How much more our predecessors must have felt this when there was no central heating available and no switch that they only needed to flick in order to make up for the disappearance of the sun in winter.

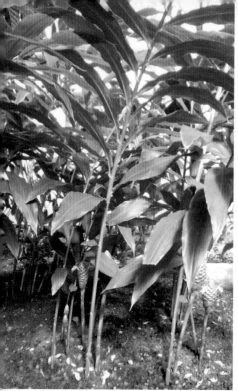
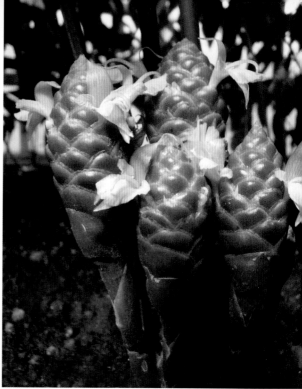

Ginger leaves have a rhythmical structure.

Ginger flowers close above the surface of the ground.

Perhaps it was this need for the sun's qualities which lay behind the fantastic prices paid for hot spices and the perilous journeys our forefathers made to the far-off East in order to obtain them. One of the journeys (which aimed to reach India) led to the discovery of America from where we finally got chilli.

One of the oldest, similarly hot-tasting spices from the tropics is ginger. It is said to have come to Europe from Asia as far back as the ninth century and since then has never been absent for long from kitchens and medicine cabinets. As a matter of fact, almost all spices can be used as medicines, and ginger in particular produces an especially wide range of effects. The rhizome, which we can readily buy as an elongated, branched tuber, is almost the only part used (although the leaf can also be used to make a hot-tasting filling for pastry). When finely grated the root lends a hot exotic taste to many dishes. But as a strong warming drink it can also ward off a *cold* which is just starting.

Stem ginger, which can be obtained by preserving pieces of young ginger tuber in syrup, is equally delicious. It stimulates the digestion but can also relieve nausea. Many sailors chew ginger because it

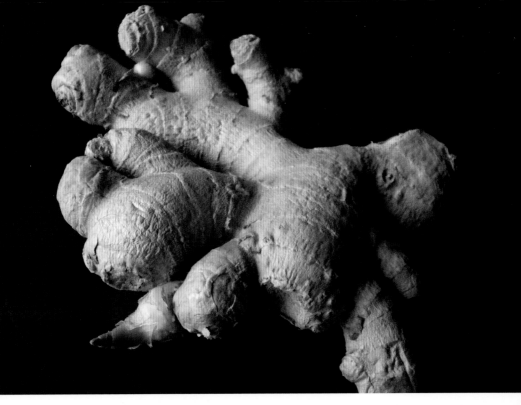

Ginger rhizome with sprouting bud.

prevents the unpleasant effects of rocking waves. It is in fact a good remedy for *motion sickness* and sometimes can even ease the *nausea caused by chemotherapy.*

Ginger also has a warming effect when used externally. Applied to the back as a ginger compress it leads to a deep warming and relaxing effect which lasts for hours and can be beneficial for *lumbago* but is also helpful in many cases of *slipped disc* as part of a treatment programme. It can also bring about an improvement in some *psychological disorders* and – again as part of a comprehensive treatment programme – can help some patients with *depression* to regain a more positive perception of their body and a stronger basic attitude when they appear as though 'frozen' and paralysed.

The ginger rhizome therefore turns out to be a great conveyor of warmth. Almost all the relatives of the ginger have magnificent deeply coloured flowers. In contrast, the flower of the real ginger is less conspicuous, smaller and only pale yellow. It does not store the force of the sun in the flower, where it could be seen, but rather beneath the earth, where it can be felt.

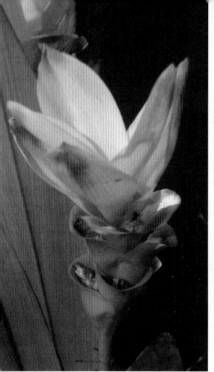
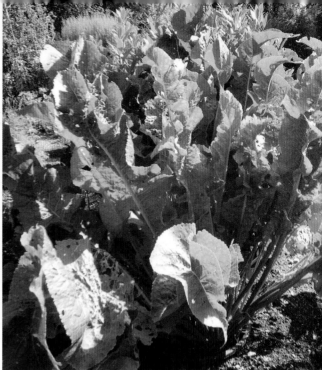

Many species of turmeric have more colourful flowers than the related ginger.

Horseradish plant.

Something similar applies to a plant native to southern-eastern Europe and western Asia which, like ginger, conveys warmth. The cabbage family contains typical plants which grow in a temperate climate. Their flowers are made of four, usually yellow, petals arranged in cross form, which is why they are known as 'crucifers'. They all contain sulfur, that flammable element which is also emitted by volcanoes. The sulfur content can easily be detected from the unpleasant cooking smell but in some plants this is intensified to a burning fiery power. This is the case in mustard seeds and also in the root of horseradish. Unlike its yellow-flowering relatives, this plant has delicate white flowers – but what power appears in the root! In ancient times it was valued so highly that the Oracle at Delphi pronounced the plant to be worth its weight in gold. To treat a *cold with headache*, if you grate horseradish root and put the pulp on the area over the sinuses in the upper jaw or forehead, then the 'swollen' nose will usually clear quickly and the pain be relieved. However, it produces such a burning feeling on the skin that you will soon remove the application, no matter how thankful you may be for the power it provided to withstand the cold.

Ginger (*Zingiber officinale*)

Ginger cultivation began in South Asia, and it is now also grown in East Africa and the Caribbean. It is sold either as a branched tuber (resembling a set of antlers) ground as a spice – or in higher quality, for medical purposes. For therapeutic use it is worth taking relatively fresh powder because the important essential oils gradually disappear during storage. In any case the powder should be stored in an airtight container in a cool dark place.

Internal use

Ginger is hardly ever used in proprietary medicines, but generally used therapeutically in a similar way to its culinary use. Unlike some other plants, therapy and consumption as a food are often similar.

For *travel sickness* and other forms of *nausea* and for *vomiting* (for example during chemotherapy), small pieces of ginger can be chewed and kept in the mouth for an extended period. Anyone who prefers can also eat candied ginger (for example stem ginger) in which the pieces of ginger have been soaked for some time in a sugar solution. Ginger is often used in the form described for morning sickness. There is no adequate scientific basis for this procedure and it is sometimes objected that there is no proof of the safety of ginger during pregnancy. However, this applies to almost all other foods and spices (and also most medicines which are used in this kind of situation). In any specific case you need to decide for yourself whether you wish to use this treatment option, which many midwives consider to be an important part of their therapy. I should just like to add that ginger is not suitable in cases of acute viral diarrhoea with vomiting because it can irritate the mucus membranes which are already inflamed.

At the start of a *cold* and anytime if you feel chilled, a lemon and ginger drink with honey can be beneficial. It has a warming effect and stimulates the mucus membrane secretions, thus liquefying the mucus. Whether the various anti-bacterial and anti-viral properties of ginger are also involved has not been definitely established. In any case, many people find a drink like this of real benefit. Cut 5 thin slices from a piece of peeled ginger and, depending on taste, add 1 or 2 slices

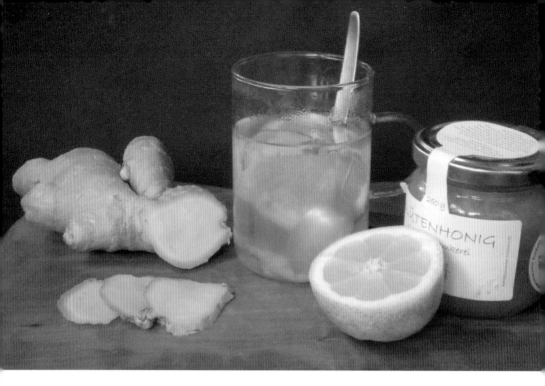

Ginger, lemon, honey and hot water – all that is required for a drink to soothe a cold.

of organic lemon in a glass or cup. Then fill up the glass with boiling water and leave to infuse for at least 5 minutes. Add about 1 teaspoon of honey if desired.

External use of ginger

As mentioned earlier, Ginger can be exceptionally beneficial for *lumbago* and other back disorders which involve *muscle tension* (see page 367). Arthritic pain can be similarly alleviated, as has recently been shown in a New Zealand dissertation.[1] Ginger compresses have also been used successfully for *fibromyalgia* (muscular rheumatism) and depression. Finally, in *chronic bronchitis* or persistent cough, ginger can lead to a deep warming of the chest, relaxation and promotion of healing when applied to the thoracic area.

A ginger back compress is the most suitable for home treatment. The patient should first be allowed to go to the toilet due to the slight diuretic effect of the application. Then make sure that the patient's feet are warm. If they are not, then a hot footbath or hot water bottle on the feet is recommended while the next preparations are made.

The compress requires: 1 heaped tablespoon of powdered ginger, 1 small bowl, 1 pair of rubber gloves if wished, 1 (soft) cotton cloth which covers the area to be treated when folded in two (this is generally the lower back), 1 or 2 dry hand towels, 1 facecloth and at least 1 woollen cloth. A large plastic bag can also be used to protect the bed from becoming damp.

First pour enough boiling water onto the ginger so as to make a paste and leave covered (so that the essential oils do not evaporate) for at least 5 minutes. Because the paste swells and cools during this time, add more boiling water to make a relatively thin paste or slurry in which to soak the (soft cotton) cloth. Then wring out the cloth so that it is relatively dry and no longer drips (it is easier to bear the heat using rubber gloves). Lay the damp cloth (sufficiently cooled) on the area to be treated. Lay a dry towel over this followed by a woollen cloth and wrap the patient firmly so that everything lies tightly against the back. The patient then lies on their back. The cloths tend to lose contact with the skin, especially if the patient has a marked hollow back. This means first that the ginger infusion no longer works on the skin and second that cold air can get in which then achieves the opposite of the desired effect. This can be prevented by folding a hand towel in such a way that it presses the compress gently against the back when the patient lies on it.

The patient should then lie like this for 20–30 minutes. To begin with, they do not feel anything, but after a while a slow, gradually increasing and almost always very pleasant warming effect sets in. Very rarely will a ginger compress cause skin irritation, in which case the compress should be removed if it is felt to be unpleasant.

After a sufficient period the compress is taken off and any crumbs of ginger left adhering to the skin removed with a facecloth. Wrap the patient in the woollen cloth again and leave them to rest for 20 minutes.

These compresses are usually done once daily in acute cases and less often for chronic symptoms.

Another external application for ginger is an oil dispersion bath with Ingwer-Oliven-Öl (Demeter) (Dr Heberer Naturheilmittel). This kind of bath generally has a warming effect for pain in the back, muscles and joints and it stimulates the metabolism. It has a more general effect than the local action of a compress which is especially

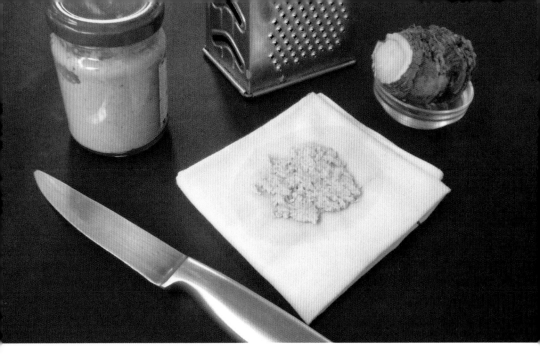

The items for making a horseradish compress.

used on the painful area.

Horseradish (*Cochlearia armoracia*)

Although horseradish is easy to grow in kitchen and vegetable gardens it takes a lot of space and spreads quickly, so it is better to plant it in a separate bed and harvest the roots frequently. As a culinary plant, it can lend spiciness and taste to white sauces when grated finely. It is also excellent as an addition (especially with grated apple, some yoghurt and a touch of garlic) to salads of raw beetroot, which tend to taste rather earthy on their own.

External use

Horseradish proves to be particularly useful in cases of illness. Finely grated (or out of a jar) and eaten on bread, its spiciness usually clears a *blocked nose*. However, it is particularly effective (as described earlier, page 368) when you put horseradish paste on a handkerchief and lay this on the forehead, the neck or the cheekbones. With the last-mentioned case, keep your eyes shut tight, as the rising vapours irritate them.

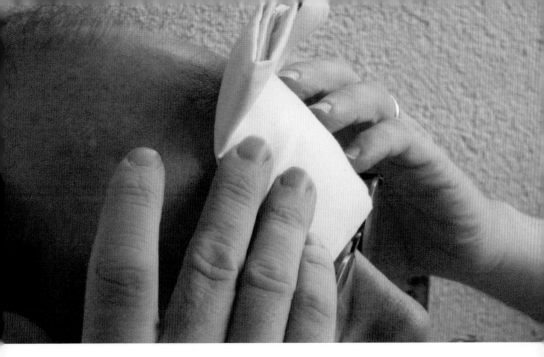

A horseradish compress usually brings quick relief from the symptoms of sinusitis.

The skin rapidly turns red and a strong burning sensation means that hardly anyone can endure this form of application for more than a few minutes. With very delicate and sensitive skin it is better to avoid this direct use on the skin completely. It is then better to use Cochlearia armoracia 10% ointment (Weleda) which is made from horseradish and only leads to a gentle warming of the areas of skin to which it is applied. Both types of application are very good for a bad head cold but also as a complementary application for *inflammation of the paranasal sinuses*.

Anthroposophical medicine has discovered that roots have a particularly strong effect on the nerve-sense system and this is reflected in the beneficial effect of horseradish root on the head described above. Oil dispersion baths using horseradish oil 5% in olive oil (Dr Heberer Naturheilmittel) appear to have an even more immediate effect on diseases of the nervous system which cause paralysis and rigidity. It is reported that such baths lead to a distinct stimulation and internal and external improvement in mobility in patients who have suffered a stroke or have contracted *Parkinson's* or *Alzheimer's* disease.

Internal use

Taken internally (approximately 1 teaspoon eaten on bread at repeated intervals), the antibiotic-like effect can be used. Like many other members of the Cruciferae (for example mustard), horseradish contains glucosinolates from which the spicy-hot, germicidal oil, allyl isothiocyanate, is produced. As they are excreted via the urine they can also help in cases of *mild infections of the urinary tract and bladder.* They are thought to be particularly beneficial in treating coliform bacteria, which are the most common inflammatory pathogens of this region. One proprietary medicine made from horseradish and garden nasturtium is Angocin Anti-Infect N, which should be taken at a dose of 3–4 sugar-coated tablets several times per day. But in this case, self-treatment also requires good self-observation. If there is no clear improvement within two days, if fever sets in or pain in the back indicates that the kidneys are involved, then medical help must be sought immediately. The same applies to a worsening of the general health, increase in pain or blood in the urine. Patients with known restriction in urination (for example due to an enlarged prostate) would be better to avoid self-treatment completely. In those with a sensitive stomach, horseradish in higher doses can lead to upper abdominal pain. However, overall it is truly valuable, and a genuine home remedy.

CHAPTER 38

Gold

Nature gives us substances that can help us when we are ill. In addition to plants and animals (bees were described as an example), minerals and metals can also be processed into effective medicines. A description of gold will be given here as an example of how substances from inorganic nature can improve our health. Gold is one of the metals which are key medicinal substances with a broad range of applications, especially in anthroposophical medicine.

In the New Testament, gold is first mentioned when the three wise men from the East give their gifts to the infant Jesus. Somehow it seems by its very nature to belong to Christmas. How many things on the Christmas tree (and also in the shop windows before Christmas) have a golden gleam, and how much is decorated in gold?

Why is it that we compare and surround the most precious things with gold? Is this only due to its material value and rarity? If that were the case, would it not be more appropriate to use platinum or uranium? Perhaps our high regard for gold goes deeper than this.

The very first metals used by human beings were in fact gold and meteoric iron. The latter falls from the sky from time to time – at first it appears as a shining meteor and if it is large enough not to burn out completely in the atmosphere, then a lump of cosmic material may reach the ground. This is sometimes composed of 'meteoric iron'; a type of cosmic stainless steel made of iron, nickel, cobalt and a few other elements. In a field or in the jungle a 'cosmic gift' like this would hardly be noticed, it would simply weather and gradually mingle with the normal substance of the earth. However, if a meteorite like this falls in the desert, on a glacier, or in an Arctic snowfield, then it easily attracts the attention of an observer. This is why there are some very

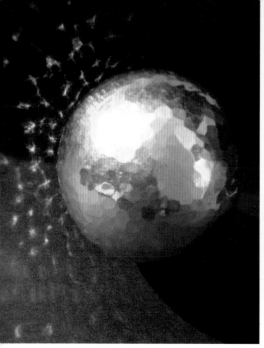

Gold ball.

Gold foil can be so thin that the sun shines through with an emerald green colour. The sun there appears to be surrounded by a halo which resembles the corona (visible during an eclipse of the sun).

old Inuit knives made from meteoric iron, made thousands of years before people were able to smelt iron.

One of the very few other metals which can simply be found in the earth without the need to master complicated smelting processes is gold. It can be found as nuggets, fine flakes in river sand or as a lode in a quartz vein.

The resistance of this metal to all weathering is the reason that it is always found sparkling and gleaming while other metals, which can also be found as a metal, tarnish like silver or gradually dissolve like copper. Its resistance to all external influences is certainly part of the symbolic power of gold and may be one reason why it is made into wedding rings.

It has only recently been discovered that meteoric iron and gold have further things in common. Meteorites also contain traces of gold and it is now assumed that all the gold in the upper layers of the earth (in other words, the gold that can actually be mined) originally reached us through meteors from the cosmos, of which there have been a surprisingly large number in the course of the long evolution of the earth (the surface of the moon which has not weathered gives us some clue about the number of meteorite impacts).

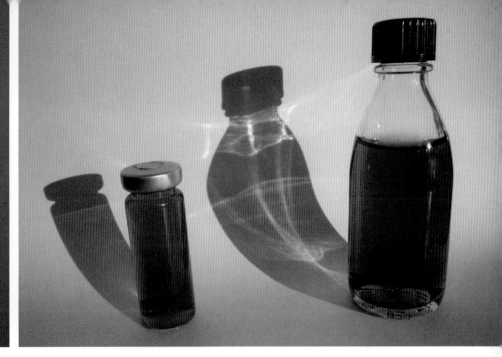

Two samples of colloidal purple gold.

Meteorites and gold therefore connect us to the cosmos. Even the Ancient Egyptians appear to have had an idea that gold has something to do with the cosmos. They depicted it using the same symbol as the sun: a circle with a point in its centre. This is the old astronomical sign for the sun, still used in astrology today. What is expressed by this? The point in the middle is a place of maximum contraction and concentration; the circle, on the other hand, symbolises the periphery or the surrounding space which still has a connection to the point. This is an ingenious way of representing the nature of the sun, which, though being a point in the sky, also fills the whole world with its shining warming effect.

The symbol similarly describes gold. Gold is so dense that it weighs almost 20 times as much as the same volume of water, and nearly twice as much as lead. Using the imagery of atomic theory, physicists say that this is because the atoms in the gold are highly 'condensed' and it is said that the electron shells are 'contracted'. In this picture, these electrons should be whizzing around the nucleus with almost the speed of light and are therefore faster than almost all material that we know. Of course, no one has seen this. However, even at this level of scientific theory, it would appear that in gold, elements of the greatest contraction and a similarity to light exist side by side. Moreover we can also experience this directly, because gold is actually translucent. Gold can be rolled or beaten into such a thin foil that a strong light can penetrate, it becoming emerald green in colour, as can be seen on the photograph on page 376.

The heaviness of gold is matched by the lightness of a gold foil like this. A breath of wind can send it whirling through the room; and the Maya produced birds and butterflies from gold that could float in the air! Using chemical and physical tricks, gold is pulverised into small particles that can be dispersed in water (into what is known as a colloid). The gold is then so fine and 'light' that the particles never precipitate to the bottom of the container, however long you wait. The colour of a gold colloid can be purple, red or rose-pink, depending on the particle size, and is reminiscent of the colours of the dawn. In Ancient Greek this was called *aurora*, so it is no coincidence that the scientific name for gold is 'aurum'. Once again we come across the similarity between the sun and gold.

Gold therefore possesses the capability for great concentration and the lightest expansion to equal degrees. In our own bodies we find this in our circulation. Blood has its centre in the heart. But it is active when it expands far out into the periphery of the body, permeating our organs to the very furthest corner, nourishing and warming. It is then concentrated again into the heart. It is provided with a new impetus there, and then it flows out once more. We can sense why gold crushed by pharmacists into ever smaller particles, potentised and 'expanded' can have a beneficial role in cases of *heart and circulatory diseases*. However, we can also sense why it can be used in anthroposophical psychiatry when an insurmountable lack of light and heaviness are felt in a state of depression and, likewise, when there is an excess of bubbling lightness in a case of *mania*. Perhaps this might even cast light on the gift of the magi when the fullness of the heavens appeared on earth as the little infant in Bethlehem.

Gold (*Aurum metallicum*)

Metals occupy a special position in therapy. It is obvious that they are not involved in phytotherapy: only in anthroposophical pharmacy are they combined with plants via fertilising and composting. Decades after investigating this process in anthroposophic pharmacy, Dr Melvyn Lintern published an article in *Nature Communications* (Oct. 2013), where he showed that eucapyptus trees incorporate gold nanoparticles in their leaves, which they dissolve from deep layers in the earth. This is astonishing, because normally gold can only be dissolved by highly corrosive chemicals like aqua regia. What the plant is able to do calls to mind the pharmaceutical process of potentising. The metal is fused with the plants more in terms of its forces than its substance, as described in the process of soil enriched with metals (see page 292).

In what follows we will expand on the relationship of gold and the sun. Every leaf growing in the open is unthinkable without sunlight to combine with the earthly substance in it. Thus, in every medicinal plant there is a sun aspect, and therefore in the broader sense, also a gold aspect. Naturally gold belongs to inorganic nature, but human beings nevertheless have a long-cherished feeling that metals are something special in comparison with the rest of the mineral world. A mineral is characterised by its solid nature. If it occurs in a particularly pure form, it appears as crystal showing an angular, geometric nature. Metals too can form crystals, but they still display characteristics of the fluid element. A metal – and this applies particularly to gold – can be melted, bent and given new forms. The precious metals – and here again this applies particularly to gold – display a tendency to remain pure, forming no (or scarcely any) compounds with other 'earthly elements'. Gold therefore does not rust and always remains shiny with a metallic reflectiveness. The internal 'vitality' and mobility of the metals is also expressed in the fact that they are conductive to a greater or lesser degree. This applies to electricity and heat as well as to sound; which is why bells are made from metal.

In ancient times, when the world was generally experienced in its wholeness and when heavenly and earthly were felt to be directly related to one another, metals were viewed as being intrinsically connected to the seven classical planets. For example, beautiful copper was connected with shining Venus, and dark lead with dull, slow-moving Saturn. To this day, poets connect silver with the moon.

The justification for the relationship between the sun and gold can perhaps be felt directly. For a modern scientifically inclined mind, we can look at this reciprocal relationship step by step. We do not experience the movement of any other heavenly body so directly as the sun, which rises and sets every day. Yet, at the same time, we think of it as the centre of our solar system around which all the planets including the earth (and us) revolve. However, the solar system is also involved in the movements of the entire universe. Our view of the sun is simultaneously both of active movement and of a still centre (reminiscent of the old symbol of sun and gold). Similarly, gold is simultaneously extremely mobile, or malleable (for instance, as delicate gold thread or flexible gold leaf) and shows an unchanging immobility in withstanding all attacks by normal chemistry.

Likewise, from ancient times our organs were seen in relationship to the effects of the planets and metals, and thus there is a long-standing connection between the sun, gold and our heart. The shining, warming effect of the sun is reflected in our heart in as much as there is no organ in us which can constantly produce a greater amount of warmth (by weight) while at rest. The heart is our centre of warmth and our life is dependent on both the shining of the sun and on the beating of our hearts.

No one doubts that the heart is the centre of our circulation. The blood flows together here from all over the body. It is a principle of blood to be in movement: if it stops for only a few minutes then coagulation processes set in, which are eventually no longer compatible with life. The blood flows everywhere, but with each heartbeat there is a brief moment when the blood in the heart comes to rest before receiving a new impulse to flow from the contraction of the heart.

In the central organ of our life we therefore also find the polarities of forming a centre and stillness, and the greatest dynamism and radiating power. These are similar qualities to those we have found in the sun on the one hand and in gold on the other. This can explain why gold is a key remedy for heart disease in anthroposophical medicine.

Homeopathy develops its knowledge of remedies from observing what are known as proving symptoms; in other words, from symptoms which appear when a healthy person takes a potentised remedy over a period of time. In addition, understanding is built up from experiences which arise from therapeutic use. In this way, knowledge of gold as a remedy has arisen –independently of the observations which have already been made here – which fits well into the picture outlined.

One of the most prominent contemporary homeopaths, George Vithoulkas, received the Right Livelihood Award (also referred to as the Alternative Nobel Prize) in 1996 for his homeopathic work. He described people who are helped by gold as follows.[1] 'Aurum patients are closed people. They do not find it easy to explain their deepest feelings... the person remains closed in their connection to the environment... They prefer to remain alone.' This clearly shows a connection to the chemical resistance of gold, which can also be seen as the lack of a tendency to form connections. However, behind the appearance of correctness and inviolability there is another side. 'Aurum patients [are] characteristically sensitive to every form of criticism... they "take it to heart" (a favourite expression of Aurum patients)'. Eventually the attitude to life can darken into depression. Interestingly, a picture of the sun also appears here in homeopathy – even though it is a negative picture of it being extinguished. Vithoulkas expresses this as follows: 'Everything becomes darker and darker until not even a single ray of light appears to get through. For these patients it is as though the sun were completely extinguished: there is no reason to carry on with life.' Homeopathy in fact uses Aurum as a key remedy for risk of suicide, which naturally does not mean that in such cases it is adequate just to prescribe a remedy. Every patient in whom a risk of this kind is recognised must undergo a careful and expert examination in order to avert it. Besides any necessary drug treatment and ensuring that the environment is safe, it is always essential to forge a link to the affected person's inner life, which strengthens the will to live again. This can be very difficult in a person whose nature shows very strong traits of 'gold pathology'.

It is not surprising that Vithoulkas came to the conclusion that, for the patients mentioned 'their material position... is very important... [they] accord gold (money) a very high importance.' The organ relationship outlined is also found in homeopathy. 'Interestingly, a relationship between the emotional level and heart disease appears to exist... in the case of aurum, every little anxiety about health is focussed on the heart... aurum is an important remedy if repression [here the homeopath means both emotional processes and the removal of disease symptoms without them really being overcome] has begun to affect the heart.'

Naturally these comments only represent part of the picture. A range of further aspects could be added on the level of the organs, such as a tendency to full-bloodedness and high blood pressure (like an 'excess of gold quality', while the depression described can be seen as 'too little').

Based on the example of gold it may be said that the homeopath's observations and the anthroposophical doctors' and scientists' inner work, study and effort to understand the nature of gold both give rise to a very similar picture in the end. One element in the manufacture of remedies from gold is unique to anthroposophical pharmacy. Usually it either processes gold found in a natural state – for example as nuggets – (Aurum naturale) which always contains traces of other precious metals (particularly silver and copper), or carries out a special preparation stage (Aurum metallicum praeparatum). This involves melted gold being heated to its boiling point in a flask at a temperature of over 3000°C (over 5000°F) and the vapour then being made to precipitate as a 'mirror' on a cold quartz glass wall. This mirror is then scraped off and the distilled gold thus obtained is processed further into a medicine. In this process gold is brought into a gaseous state, in which it was originally present in a cosmos still characterised by immense heat. The gold is thus brought close to its original state but at the same time – in a similar way to the manufacture of distilled water – purified so that any 'impressions' are removed. This purification can also be seen as removing all the human emotions associated with gold, and cleansing its tainted history.

Pure Aurum metallicum praeparatum is available from Weleda as a trituration in D6, D10, D12, D15, D20 and D30, in drop form in D10,

D12, D15, D20 and D30, as ampoules in D6, D10, D12, D15, D20 and D30 and as ointment in D4. There are whole books on metal therapy in anthroposophical medicine, so the remarks here can only provide a selection.[2] Metal therapy is a highly developed therapeutic art, so the following notes are not indications for self-treatment. Rather they are offered to promote understanding of some types of treatment and to give an idea of the great variety of therapeutic applications. In addition, only part of the extensive range of anthroposophical remedies containing potentised gold can be mentioned here.

In cases of *depression*, when there is a need to stimulate 'more lightness' in the inner gold forces, higher potencies (D12 to D30) have proved successful. Depression can have a wide range of causes and accordingly require the strengthening or influencing of quite different organs. One sign that the use of gold is specially indicated is if depression sets in after a heart attack or as a consequence of an illness. This applies especially to people for whom their position and claim to leadership are especially important. A biographical indication for the use of gold remedies can be the lack of a father or the separation of the parents, especially between the ages of 7 and 14. In this period of development the main aim is to absorb 'sun forces' and transform them into one's own abilities. A stable relationship to the parents and the father in particular are especially important for this.

If the soul is not heavy and immobile (as in a depression) but rather excessively dynamic, elated and volatile to the point of an incipient manic disorder, then lower aurum potencies can help to restore stability. For similar reasons, one can use aurum D10 (a relatively low potency) for support in cases of anaesthesia and operations. The drugs used here cause the body and the soul to temporarily 'separate' from one another. Afterwards, the soul needs to connect to the body again in the right way. Sometimes this 'separation' leads to temporary *confusion* (*postoperative delirium*), which can be treated or prevented by this type of remedy. Another medicine containing gold for *support during anaesthesia* is Aurum/Valeriana comp. (Wala) which, besides potentised aurum, also contains potencies of camphor, cactus, strophanthus and valerian, which help the circulation and have an emotionally relaxing effect. I usually prescribe 10 globules of this remedy 3 times daily, from 3 days before until 3 days after the operation. For *fear of flying* and also for *stage fright* and test anxiety or exam nerves, 5 globules can be taken hourly in the acute situation.

Everyone will have noticed that their emotional state can influence the activity of the heart. These kinds of changes in cardiac activity are normally experienced for a limited time, when there is cause for joy, fright or sorrow. However, if they occur repeatedly and with no apparent reason, then Aurum/Lavandula comp. ointment (Weleda) applied to the area around the heart can often produce considerable relief. It can also help to stop sleep being disturbed by palpitations. The ointment can also often help a tendency to *anxiety*. In addition to potentised gold, this remedy also contains essential oil of rose and lavender (see also Chapter 22). A stronger effect can be achieved by using an 'ointment cloth' on which the ointment has been applied in a thin layer and laying this on the heart region. What is known as a rhythmic einreibung of the heart with this ointment, something carried out by specially trained therapists (often nurses or physiotherapists) is particularly effective. For other states of anxiety related to the heart and non-organic heart complaints, Aurum/ Stibium/Hyoscyamus (Wala) can often be a great help. The related remedy, Strophanthus comp. (Wala), (which also contains potentised gold and antimony) was described in detail in Chapter 1 (page 23).

The administration (as an adjunct therapy) of remedies which contain potentised gold can often also have an astonishingly good effect in cases of serious *heart disease* and *congenital heart defects*. Remedies of this kind are for example Cor/Aurum I and II (Wala) in which potentised gold is combined with an organ preparation from the heart (Latin *cor*). In Cor/Aurum I, the organ preparation is used in a low potency, in Cor/Aurum II in a higher one. The high Cor potency is indicated for inflammatory heart disease, the lower one for degenerative conditions (for example *circulatory disorders*). In conjunction with other heart remedies (see for example Chapter 8 on the cowslip and Chapter 18 on the thistle) I have found these remedies to produce lasting stabilisation for serious heart conditions (often with patients who are almost a hundred years old).[3] On the other hand, the paediatrician Georg Soldner has found a measurable improvement in the ECGs of some of his young patients using this remedy. This improvement was seen, for example, when the rhythm of the child's heartbeat was impaired by certain drugs which were given as part of a standard medical treatment (for leukaemia) and a dangerous retardation in the impulse transmission in the heart muscle had arisen.

In Chapter 33 on the blackthorn we mentioned in relation to Aurum/Prunus that gold can be helpful for some *exhaustion conditions*. While this is primarily for exhaustion after (infectious) diseases, a very successful remedy for 'nervous' exhaustion arising in stressful and overtaxing circumstances (for example in single mothers) is Aurum/Apis regina comp. (Wala). Here, rather than metallic gold, a potentised form of a slightly soluble gold salt – Aurum chloratum, which is formed by treating gold with aqua regia – is used. This also contains St John's wort (Hypericum) which itself has a strong relationship to the sun and gold, oat (Avena) which is prescribed in potentised form for promoting sleep and as a tonic for nervous tension, Acidum phosphoricum (a proven remedy for exhaustion), Apis regina (a preparation to which queen bee royal jelly is added) and Ignatia (the seeds of a liana) in potentised form. I tend to prescribe 7 globules of this 3 times daily. As even school children are often under such pressure nowadays that they react by developing *psychosomatic headaches*, it should be mentioned that this remedy can often provide effective relief (particularly around the ninth year of life).

Neurodoron or Kalium phosphoricum comp. (Weleda) has similar effects in some respects, comprising potentised gold and potassium phosphoricum (also used homeopathically for anxiety and exhaustion due to mental stress) and Ferrum-Quartz (Bidor, Weleda), a preparation which is also used for treating *migraines*. The usual does is 1 tablet 3 times daily.

From the range of anthroposophical medicines containing gold, two should finally be mentioned which appear to cover a completely different range of indications. Chapter 14 on horsetail dealt with the group of Disci preparations which can be very helpful for various types of *spinal problems*. Of these Disci comp. cum Auro (Wala) has proved very successful when pain arises from the thoracic vertebrae, often radiating to the front of the chest in such a way that patients fear they have something wrong with their heart. It can also frequently be established that such patients are stuck in circumstances where the 'forces of gravity' dominate and there is a 'lack of buoyancy'. In my experience in these circumstances it is best if the doctor (or another suitably trained therapist) injects an ampoule of the remedy (which is also available as globules) intradermally, into the skin on both sides of the spine in the central thoracic region. The pain often decreases only a few minutes later.

Finally a further remedy which acts on the musculoskeletal system should be mentioned: Cartilago comp. (Wala) which contains potentised gold in the higher D15 potency in addition to birch *(Betula)*, ant *(Formica)*, tin *(Stannum)* and an organ preparation of joint cartilage *(Cartilago articularis)*. This is a proven basic remedy for the treatment of *arthroses.* You may wonder why gold is important for this disease in which the cartilage first becomes rough and then increasingly shrinks. One viewpoint about this is that every reduction in movement weighs down the soul and is often accompanied by mild depression. When the emotions are negatively affected, even small changes in the joints can lead to severe pain and, conversely, even major changes in the joints can often be accompanied by surprisingly little pain if the patient feels emotionally stable. We saw another viewpoint in the description of gold; this metal is connected both with the aspect of heaviness and with overcoming it. This is exactly what is involved with joints (particularly in the lower extremities). The body's load weighs down on them, but they contain small spaces of buoyancy where the load is transformed into movement. At the point where they threaten to deform due to the influence of too much weight, high potencies of gold can be of help. Long-term oral treatment with Cartilago comp., 10 globules 2–3 times daily has proved successful (injections may be necessary to start with for severe pain). Depending on the situation, other (adjunct) forms of arthritis treatment can be considered, from embrocation (for which there is also a Cartilago comp. ointment) through curative eurythmy and physiotherapy to local injection with mistletoe (see Chapter 35 on the mistletoe) or the application of leeches.

This in no way represents all the range of applications of potentised gold (a further important area of application is described in Chapter 34 on frankincense in relation to Aurum comp.). However, it should now be possible to imagine that metals in particular open the door to a whole therapeutic world, which is just as interesting and useful as that of the medicinal plants.

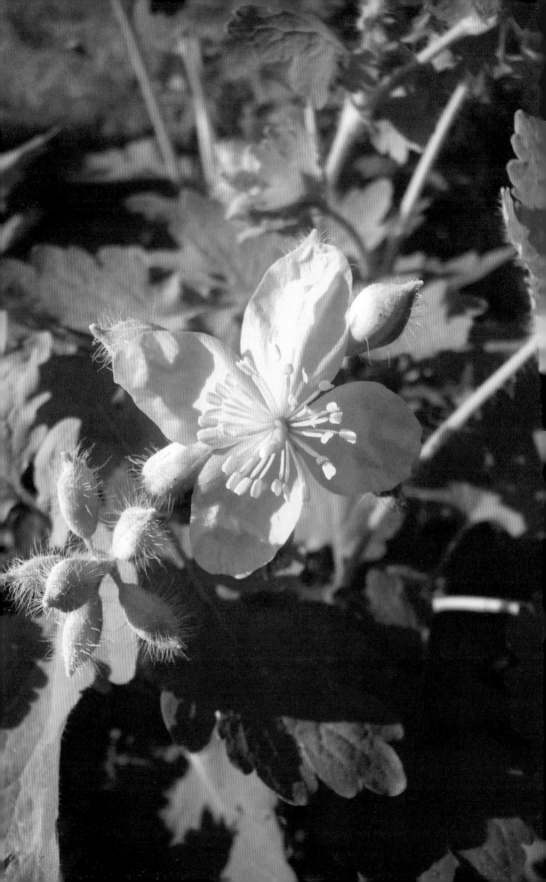

Acknowledgements

Some of my first memories of life include happy discoveries (e.g. daisies) and less happy ones (e.g. nettles) of plants. Long before I went to school I started concocting secret plant potions 'for the spirits in the garden' with my friend Anneli Nenninger-Patzak. Later on, Anneli studied Asian languages and pharmacy and was trained in the traditional herbal medicine of Japan and China. She finally wrote a historically, artistically and scientifically excellent dissertation on a Chinese medicinal plant before opening a pharmacy in our home town. But back then we 'fed' ants with our plant extracts, created 'perfumes' from flowers and tried to 'heal' the small bruises of our playmates by bandaging them with leaves of daisies and plantain. All this and the small laboratory that I set up in our house soon after learning to read certainly required quite some tolerance on the part of my parents, for which I cannot thank them enough. Later, the trust and tolerance of my teachers was of a no lesser order. They allowed me unrestricted access to the school biology, chemistry and physics laboratories whenever I wanted. My old school often enabled me to attend seminars at places like the botanical institute at the University of Munich. All this contributed at various levels to deepening my relationship to, and knowledge of, plants. Our family doctor, Dr Günther H. Werner, who treated our family with herbal teas, homeopathic and anthroposophical medicines, was particularly important for me. He answered my questions and encouraged my thirst for knowledge by providing me with reading material and treating me from early on like a young colleague. I then came across the works of Dr Rudolf Hauschka who, amongst other things, had found ways of increasing the healing properties of plants and making them medicinally beneficial. Early on I tried to reproduce some of his experiments (including at school). When making the rhythmical plant extracts he developed – which require being outside long before sunrise – I had some of my most precious experiences of nature.

Anthroposophy began to open up to me when I started to study Rudolf Steiner's most important basic works along with my school friend Josef P. Schaffer. Right from the beginning of my university days, I attended a working group with other medical students who tried to familiarise themselves with anthroposophical medicine founded by Rudolf Steiner and Ita Wegman. We often met on weekends when we studied a plant together and then prepared a remedy from it. This led to the discovery of some new aspects of these plants which are of relevance to this day when using herbal remedies. I am still in regular contact with almost all the members of this group and, after our medical training, two of them – Andreas Korselt and Georg Soldner – joined me in 1994 in establishing a medical practice in Munich. I have continued regular work on questions relating to our knowledge of nature and the development of our treatment options, especially with Georg Soldner, from which many lectures and – often joint – publications have arisen. Much of this has been included in this book.

Meeting and working with the exceptionally creative doctor, Dr Heinz-Hartmut Vogel, founder of the Medical Seminar at Bad Boll, was very important to both of us. Since the 1980s Georg and I have been involved in the work of this seminar where many important remedies have been initiated and created. Since then I have come into contact with so many doctors and pharmacists who have expanded my knowledge of the healing power of nature that I cannot mention all of them here. My sincere thanks are due to them all and likewise to the many patients who have related their experiences to me and with whom I have been able to experience the effectiveness of herbal remedies. The fact that, even during my medical training, I enjoyed the freedom of using these kind of remedies in the hospital is due to the tolerance and lack of prejudice of my former senior consultants, the specialist for internal medicine and geriatrician Prof. Dr Robert Heinrich and the neurologist Prof. Dr Mario Prosiegel, and to the keen interest and pursuit of a broadening of medicine in my former consultant and friend Dr Mario Paulig.

Mention must be made of a group of doctors who have taken on the task of publishing the *Vademecum of Anthroposophic Medicines*. This project involves anthroposophical doctors from all over the world (currently from 18 countries in Europe, North and South America

390

and Africa) who report on the medicines which have proved to be the most reliable for them. Many of these remedies are made from plants. As a member of the editorial board of this project I enjoy the privilege of being able to read all these contributions in the original and often of entering into correspondence with the colleagues who have sent them and of being able to discuss them with the other members of the editorial team. This has not only taught me a great deal for the treatment of my own patients but much knowledge gained in this way has been incorporated into this book. One of my colleagues in the editorial team – the Austrian paediatrician Dr Reinhard Schwarz – diligently maintains an overview of the current global status of research and shares his knowledge with the greatest generosity. Much of this has also been included in this book.

It is thanks to the initiative of my publisher Frank Berger that this book has come into being in the first place. The extremely trouble-free and skilful copy editing by Maria Kafitz and Christine Christ was equally important. My wife Anne Sommer-Solheim has contributed most of the photos in this book and her artistic eye and support have been of vital help. It is always a pleasure to work on the photos and text with her. She was also the first reader to give creative criticism of each section, followed by the Swiss nurse, Ursi Soldner, to whose knowledge of the external application of medicinal plants I was able to refer at any time. Other friends supplied photos which were difficult to obtain, such as the botanist Prof. Dr Helmut Rehder (who also answered my special botanical questions), Gerdi Orterer who travels the length and breadth of the world, and Dr Friedrich Edelhäuser who heads an excellent training for medical students in anthroposophical medicine at the University of Herdecke. Gardening questions were answered in discussion with the gardener and noted landscape architect Peter Kluska and his wife Dr Edith Kluska-Szügyi, and support with agricultural matters came from my brother Tobias Sommer who works as a tree specialist in the Pyrenees in France and for a long time ran a small biodynamic farm high in the mountains. My friend Herbert Urban, with whom even in childhood and adolescence I pondered chemical and philosophical questions and who is now professor of mathematics, has meantime discovered for himself how many apparent 'weeds' can become delicious accompaniments on our table or can simply be eaten on a walk, and has allowed me to share in this knowledge which I am happy to pass on. Finally, botanical and therapeutic information sent to the author by attentive readers of the first German edition has been included.

After the book was very well received in Germany by doctors, therapists, nurses, non-medical practitioners and students of these professions and by people who simply have an interest in medicinal plants, Georg Soldner suggested that it should be translated into English. The publication was made possible by the generosity of the Medizinisches Seminar Bad Boll and the Christophorus Stiftung who have borne the translation costs. The translation itself was carried out by the botanist Lynda Hepburn with the support of Dr William Riggins. Judith Klahre-Parker kindly helped with questions about English names of remedies. The different language perceptions were finally combined by the publisher Christian Maclean and we hope to have produced a book which can be enjoyed by the reader in different parts of the English-speaking world with their different styles and traditions. To all of these and many whom I have not mentioned, who have all contributed to the production of this book, I extend my sincere and lasting thanks.

Markus Sommer

Photo credits

Gerdi Orterer: page 331 left and right.

Weleda archive, Schwäbisch Gmünd: page 20, 148, 229 right.

The following photos are taken from the free encyclopaedia Wikipedia (www. wikipedia.de): Alvesgaspar: page 276 right; birdy: page 333 left; Curtis Clark: page 187 left; LucaLuca: page 150; Nova: page 276 left; Peter Presslein: page 333 right; Peter Schmidt: page 248; Waugsberg: page 246; Stefan Wernli: page 178; Yikrazuul: page 125.

All remaining photographs are from the author or his wife Anne Sommer-Solheim.

Notes

Preface

1. Translated by William Riggins from Eichendorff, *Werke*, Vol. 1, p. 132. Original German is:
   Wünschelrute
   Schläft ein Lied in allen Dingen,
   Die da träumen fort und fort,
   Und die Welt hebt an zu singen,
   Triffst du nur das Zauberwort.
2. From: Schimmel, A., *Rumi. Ich bin Wind und du bist Feuer.* p. 43.
3. For example, in Steiner's basic work *An Outline of Esoteric Science.*
4. Buber, *Die Erzählungen der Chassidim*, p.187.

Chapter 1: Our Inner Garden

1. Livingstone, *Narrative of an Expedition.*
2. Verbal communication to Dr Karl Köller.
3. Schoner W., Scheiner-Bobis G.: Endogenous cardiac glycosides and ther mechanisms of action. *Am J Cardiovasc Drugs* 2007; 7:173–93.

Chapter 2: Bulbs

1. It would not create a great deal of enthusiasm if the patient were to come to the doctor's surgery with an onion bag, because it is not only the patient who is affected by the side effects of the penetrating smell.
2. Benavides, G.A., Squadito, G.L., Mills, R.W. et al., Hydrogen sulfide mediates the vasoactivity of garlic, *Proc Natl. Acad. Sci.* USA 104 (2007) 17977–82.
3. An overview of the effects of hydrogen sulphide which is created in the body from substances in the plants described, is given in Rui Wang, Giftgas mit Heilkraft, *Spektrum der Wissenschaft* 3 (2011) 22–27.

Chapter 3: Yarrow

1. Leeser, Lehrbuch der Homöopathie, Vol. B/II Pflanzliche Arzneistoffe.
2. Khan, A.U., Gilani, A.H., Blood pressure lowering, cardiovascular inhibitory and bronchodilatory effects of Achillea millefolium, Phytother. Res. 25 (2010) 577–83.
3. Weisser, S., Effekt von Leberwickeln auf die exkretorische Leberfunktion – eine randomisierte Cross-over-Studie. Dissertation Freiburg University 2006.

Chapter 4: Dandelion

1. Science daily Oct. 28 2013: Fraunhofer-Gesellschaft: Making rubber from dandalion juice. www.sciencedaily.com/ releases/2013/10/131028114547. httm
2. Steiner, *Agriculture,* lecture of June 13, 1924.

3. Diederich, K., Taraxacum officinale, *Merkurstab* 60 (2007) 566–71; Paepke, D., Taraxacum off. in der Behandlung des Ovarialkarzinoms, (lecture of May 8, 2010 at second congress Ganzheitliche Medizin in Perinatalmedizin und Gynäkologie, at University Hospital Klinikum rechts der Isar, Munich).
4. Diederich, K., Taraxacum officinale, *Merkurstab* 60 (2007) 566–71.
5. Paepke, D., Taraxacum off. in der Behandlung des Ovarialkarzinoms, (lecture of May 8, 2010 at second congress Ganzheitliche Medizin in Perinatalmedizin und Gynäkologie, at University Hospital Klinikum rechts der Isar, Munich).
6. Jachens also wrote several descriptions of the remedy, such as in *Dermatologie*, and in his article 'Die Behandlung von Hautkrankheiten über die Leber' *Merkurstab*, 2004; 57 (4): 248–59.

Chapter 5: Peppermint

1. There is a large number of species of mint which can only be distinguished by an expert. The real peppermint does not occur in nature but is a cultivated form produced by crossing several mint species.
2. For details see www.jungebad.com
3. Madish A., Heydenreich C-J, Wieland V, Hufnagl R, Hotz J., Treatment of functional dyspepsia with a fixed peppermint oil and caraway oil combination preparation as compared to cisapride. A multicenter, reference-controlled double-blind equivalence study. *Arzneim*

Forsch/Drug Research 49 (II) 11, 925–32 (1999); Hoffmann G, Gschossmann J, Bunger L., Wieland V., Heydenreich C.-J., Effects of afixed peppermint oil caraway oil combination (FPCO) on symptoms of functional dyspepsia accentuated by pain or discomfort, *Gastroenterology* 122 (Suppl 1) A-471.

Chapter 6: Daisy

1. See Mommsen, J., Das ausdauernde Gänseblümchen: ein heilkräftiger Immerblüher, *Merkurstab* 61 (2008) 270–83.
2. This is tyrosinase, which is an important enzyme in the process of producing the dark skin pigment melanin.

Chapter 7: Birch

1. Major, H., Untersuchungen zur Wirkungsweise von Birkenblättern *(Betula folium)* und phenolischen Verbindungen, unter besonderer Berücksichtigung der Beeinflussung von Metallopeptidasen, Dissertation, Berlin 2002.
2. Further information is available at www.imlan.de.

Chapter 8: Cowslip

1. A detailed description of this remedy is given in Sommer, M., Plantago Primula cum Hyoscyamo – ein fast vergessenes Arzneimittel gegen Muskelerkrankungen, *Merkurstab* 61 (2009) 65–72.

Chapter 9: Pasque Flower

1. Vithoulkas, *Essenzen Homöopathischer Arzneimittel,* p. 134.

Chapter 10: Wild Strawberry

1. Steiner, *Introducing Anthroposophical Medicine,* lecture of March 30, 1920.
2. Olsson M E, Andersson C S, Oredson S, Beglund R H, Gustavsson K E, Antioxidant levels and inhibition of cancer cell proliferation in vitro by extracts from organically and conventionally cultivated strawberries, *J Agric Food Chem* 2006, 54:1248–55.
3. Mudnic I, Modun D, Brizic I, Vokovic J, Generalic I, et al, Cardiovascular effects of aqueous extracts of wild strawberry (Fragaria vesca L.) leaves, *Phytomecicine* 2009, 16:462–69.

Chapter 11: Greater Celandine

1. Teschke, R., Frenzel, C., Glass, X., Eichhoff, A., 'Greater Celandine hepatotoxicity: a clinical review', *Annals of Hepatology* 2012, 11, 838–48.
2. A detailed study on the issue of potential adverse reactions to medicines was published on Wala remedies containing Chelidonium and came to very reassuring results. Stahnke, G., Mörbt, N., Jäckel, B., Sobeck, U., Meyer, U., Sicherheit und Unbedenklichkeit von Chelidonium ferm-Urtinktur enthaltenden Arzneimitteln *Merkurstab* 2012; 65 (2) 136–42. Undesirable effects appear to be very rare events which, in any case, seem to occur in the case of very concentrated preparations.
3. Servan-Schreiber, *Das Antikrebs-Buch.*
4. This led to the development of Ukrain, a medicine made from a combination of Chelidonium extract and a cytostatic agent for treating cancers. This remedy is highly controversial. On the one hand there is a series of reports on amazing effects in some cancer sufferers, on the other there are no clear research results which substantiate its efficacy but significant misgivings, particularly because of the cytostatic Thiotepa which is used in its manufacture along with the greater celandine. Ukrain is not licensed anywhere in the EU. At the beginning of 2012 it was classified by the German Federal Institute for Drugs as an unsafe drug whose use is liable to prosecution. A current review is available, 'Ukrain – ein Dauerbrenner' in *Tägliche Praxis,* 53, 2012 (3) 633–35.

Chapter 12: Chamomile

1. In Chapter 3 on yarrow it was noted that when making biodynamic compost preparations, medicinal herbs are processed using particular animal organs. Physicians will notice that those plants often have a therapeutic effect on exactly the organ which is used. For instance yarrow, which is a proven remedy for bladder complaints, is filled into a stag bladder, and chamomile flowers are filled into cow intestines.
2. Breg, M., Fickler, C., Das

Kamillendampf-Sitzbad zur
Prävention von Harnwegsinfekten
bei Frauen. Transplant Unit of
Munich University Hospital.

3. Gyllenhaal, C., Merritt, S.L.,
Paterson, S.D., Block, K.L.,
Grouchenour, T., Efficacy and
safety of herbal stimulants in sleep
disorders, *Sleep Med. Rev.* 4 (2000)
229–51; Viola, H., Wasowski, C.,
Levi de Stein, M., et al, Apigenin, a
component of matricaria recutita
flowers is a central benzodiazepine
receptor-ligand with anxiolytic
effects, *Planta Med.* 61 (1995)
251–52.

Chapter 13: Plantain

1. A detailed description of this
remedy is given in Sommer, M.,
Plantago Primula cum Hyoscyamo
– ein fast vergessenes Arzneimittel
gegen Muskelerkrankungen,
Merkurstab 61 (2009) 65–72.

Chapter 14: Horsetail

1. Husemann, *Anthroposophische
Medizin.*
2. A group of pharmacists
systematically examined the degree
to which different preparation
methods released the constituents
of horsetail. See Meyer, U., Staiger,
K., Seitz, A., Rechnen Sie mit der
Kieselsäure: Pharmazeutische
Gesichtspunkte zu einer möglichen
Optimierung der Equisetum-
Therapie, *Merkurstab* 65 (2012)
112–16.

Chapter 15: St John's Wort

1. Schempp, C.M., Wölfle, U., Meyer,
U., Schaette, R., Johanniskraut

(*Hypericum perforatum L.*):
heilkräftige Lichtpflanze der
Sommersonnwende, *Merkurstab*
2011; 64 (6) 596–606.
2. Lomagno, P., Lomagno, R.C.,
Activity of Hypericum perforatum
oil in the treatment of bedsores in
old people, *Fitoterapia* 1979; 50:
201–5.
3. Glaser, *Erfolgreiche
Wundbehandlung.*
4. Schempp, C.M., Müller, K.A.,
Winghofer, B., Schöpf, E., Simon,
J.C., Johanniskraut (*Hypericum
perforatum L.*) eine Pflanze mit
Relevanz für die Dermatologie,
Hautarzt 2002; 53: 316–21.
5. Schempp, C.M., Pelz, K., Wittmer,
A., Schöpf, E., Simon, J.C.,
Antibacterial activity of hyperforin
from St. John's wort against
multiresistant Staphylococcus
aureus and grampositive bacteria,
Lancet 353 (1999) 2129.
6. Reuter, J., Wölfle, U., Weckesser,
St., Schempp, C.M., Which plant
for which skin disease? *Journal of
the German Society of Dermatology* 8
(2010) 788–796.

Chapter 16: Starry Elder

1. Madaus, *Lehrbuch der
Homöopathischen Heilmittel,*
Volume 3.
2. Schaefer, O., 'Holunder,' in *Der
grüne Ton,* p. 98. German original is:
Sitze ich im Dunkelgrün
Träumend an der grauen Rinde
Eingewiegt vom Sommerwinde –
Sehe ich dein helles Blühn
Überall im Dunkelgrün,
Sehe still dein Wunder,
Sterniger Holunder.

Blätter spielen über mir
Fingergleich im Licht und Schatten
Auf den zarten Phloxrabatten,
Und ich ruhe ganz im Hier,
Glut und Mittag über mir,
Lausche Deinem Wunder,
Sterniger Holunder.

Chapter 17: Lime (Linden)

1. Rispens, J.A., Die Linde: Der Baum des Menschen, *Merkurstab* 59 (2006) 423–35.
2. Further information in Sommer, M., Soldner, G., Therapeutische Erfahrungen mit der Lindenmistel, *Merkurstab* 59 (2006) 435–37.

Chapter 19: Coneflower, Echinacea

1. There has been much speculation as to whether there were in fact cases of syphilis in Europe before Columbus. As far as I understand the current state of research on this question, there are now in fact good reasons to believe that the actual strain causing the life-threatening syphilis was imported from South America at the end of the fifteenth century but that related, far less dangerous but similar diseases (which were probably not transmitted sexually) were present before this.
2. Barrett, B., Brown, R., Rakel, D., Mundt, M., et al., Echinacea for treating the common cold. A randomized trial, *Ann. Intern. Med.* 153 (2010) 769–777.
3. Jawad, M., Schoop, R., Suter, A., Klein, P., Eccles, R., Safety and efficacy of *Echinacea purpurea* to prevent common cold epsiodes: A randomized double-blind placebo-

controlled trial. *Evidence-Based Complementary and Alternative Medicine* 2012. Article ID 841315 dx.doi.org/10.1155/2012/841315.

Chapter 20: Lemon balm (Melissa)

1. See Akhondzadeh, S., Noroozian, M., Mohammadi, M., Ohadivia, S., Jamshidi, A.H., Khani, M., *Melissa officinalis* extract in the treatment of Alzheimer's disease: a double blind, randomised, placebo controlled trial, *J. Neurol. Neurosurg. Psychiatry* 74 (2003) 863–66.
2. Ballard, O.C., O'Brien, J.T., Reichelt, K., Perry, D.K., Aromatherapy as a safe treatment for the management of agitation in severe dementia: The results of a double-blind placebo-controlled trial with melissa, *J. Clin. Psychiatr.* 63 (2002) 553–58.
3. Burns, A., Perry, E., Holmes, C., Francis, P., Morris, J., Howes, M.J., Chazot, D., Lees, G., Ballard, C., A double-blind placebo-controlled randomised trial of *Melissa officinalis* oil and donepezil for the treatment of agitation in Alzehimer's disease, *Dement Geriatr Cogn Disord* 2011; 31: 158–64
4. Fung, K.M., Tsang, H.W.H., Chung, R.C.K., A systematic review of the use of aromatherapy in treatment of behavioral problems in dementia, *Geriatr Gerontol Omt* 2012; 12: 372–82.
5. Kurz, A., Psychosoziale Interventionen bei Demenz, *Nervenarzt* 2013; 84: 93–103.
6. See Akhondzadeh, S., Noroozian, M., Mohammadi, M., Ohadivia, S., Jamshidi, A.H., Khani, M., *Melissa*

officinalis extract in the treatment of Alzheimer's disease: a double blind, randomised, placebo controlled trial, *J. Neurol. Neurosurg. Psychiatry* 74 (2003) 863–66.

Chapter 21: Rosemary

1. When rosemary aroma was introduced into the rooms then the subjects' memory improved and their degree of wakefulness increased, while with the aroma of lavender they were more relaxed but their memory declined. See Moss, M., Cook, J., Wesnes, K., Kucket, P., Aromas of rosemary and lavender essential oils differentialy affect cognition and mood in healthy adults, *Int. J. Neurosci.* 113 (2003) 15–38.
2. Steiner, *Introducing Anthroposophical Medicine,* lectures of April 3 and 4, 1920.
3. Bakirel, T., Bakirel, O.U., Selgen, S.G., Yardibi, H., In vivo assessment of antidiabetic and antioxidant activities of rosemary *(Rosmarinus officinalis)* in alloxan-diabetic rabbits, *J. Ethnopharmacol.* 116 (2008) 64–73. In this work it says: 'Rosmarinus *officinalis* extracts exert remarkable antidiabetic effects.'
4. Jimbo, D., Kimura, Y., Taniguchi, M., Inoue, M., Urakami, K., Effect of aromatherapy in patients with Alzheimer's disease, *Psychogeriatrics* 9 (2009) 173–79.
5. Steiner, *Introducing Anthroposophical Medicine,* lectures of April 3 and 4, 1920.

Chapter 22: Rose

1. Translated from German by Lynda Hepburn, from Rumi, *Ghaselen des Dschelâleddîn Rumi.*
2. Translated from German by Lynda Hepburn, from Atabay, *Die schönsten Gedichte.*
3. Translated from German by Lynda Hepburn, from Rumi, *Ghaselen des Dschelâleddîn Rumi.*

Chapter 23: Arnica and Calendula

1. Eckermann, J.P., *Gespräche mit Goethe,* p. 453.
2. Karow, H., Abt, H.-P., Fröhling, M., Ackermann, H., Efficacy of Arnica montana D4 for Healing of Wounds after Hallux Valgus Surgery Compared to Diclofenac, *J. Altern. Compl. Med.* 14 (2008) 17–25.
3. Steiner, *Introducing Anthroposophical Medicine,* lecture of April 3, 1920.
4. In the study, 128 patients were given the commonly used Trolamin gel after each session of radiation and 126 patients were given Calendula ointment. The allocation to groups was random. Grade II and higher radiodermatitis occurred in 41% of patients in the Calendula group and 63% of patients in the standard treatment group. This means there was over a third less radiation reactions which exceeded a simple reddening of the skin and involved at least slight skin damage, weeping and pain. The women in the Calendula group also had significantly less pain and were more satisfied with the

treatment. Pommier, P., Gomez, F., Sunyach, M.P., D'Hombres, A., Carrie, C., Montbaron, X., Phase III randomized trial of *Calendula officinalis* with Trolamine for the prevention of acute dermatitis during irradiation of breast cancer, *J. Clin. Oncol.* 2004: 12 (8) 1447–53.

5. A number of case studies on this are given in Sommer, M. Lokale und systemische Behandlung mit Calendula bei komplizierten Wundheilungsstörungen: eine Kasuistik, *Merkurstab* 1996; 49 (2) 127–30. An interesting description of this medicinal plant is given in the article by Diederich K, Riggers U., Die Calendula, *Merkurstab* 2005; 59 (1) 47–55.

6. See also Sommer, M., Lokale und systemische Behandlung mit Calendula bei komplizierten Wundheilungsstörungen: eine Kasuistik, *Merkurstab* 1996; 49 (2) 127–30.

Chapter 24: What Bees Tell Us

1. Günther, et al., *Urania Tierreich,* Vol. 3, p. 470.

Chapter 25: Yellow Gentian

1. Deshpande, D.A., Wang, C.H.W., McIllmoyle, E., Robinett, K.S., et al., Bitter taste receptors on airway smooth muscle bronchodilate by localized calcium signaling and reverse obstruction, *Nature Med.* 16, 1299–1304 (2010).

Chapter 26: Monkshood

1. Nilius, B., Properties of aconitine-modified Na chanels in single cells of ventricular mouse myocardium,

Gen. Physiol. Biophys. 5 (1986) 473–482; Iurievichius, I.A., Rosenstraukh, L.V., Ishmanova, A.V., Formation of ectopic stimulation in the heart under the action of aconitine, *Kardiologija* 20 (1980) 75–78.

Chapter 27: Chicory

1. Schwarz R., Alkali comp. Kurzdarmsyndrom, in *Vademecum Anthroposophische Medizin,* p. 53.

Chapter 28: Stinging Nettle

1. Singh, R., Hussain, S., Rajish, V., Sharma, P., Anti-mycobacterial screening of five Indian medicinal plants and partial purification of active extracts of *Cassia sophera* and *Urtica dioica. Asian Pacific Jnl. Trop. Med.* (2013) 366–71.

2. Steiner, *Agriculture,* lecture of June 13, 1924.

3. Dr Wolfgang Engel described the manufacture of this fertiliser and the complex background to the process in detail in Vegetabilisierte Metalle Teil I: Grundlagen des pharmazeutischen Verfahrens und Zubereitung der Metall-Dünger, *Merkurstab* 66 (2013) 4–17.

Chapter 29: Bilberries

1. Kern, P., Ammon, A., Kron, M., et al., Risk factors of alveolar echinococcosis in humans, *Emerg. Inf. Dis.* 9 (2003) 343–49.

2. Heidelbeeren, Bärlauch und Hund: Wo der Fuchsbandwurm wirklich lauert. *Bild der Wissenschaft,* May 30, 2007.

Chapter 30: Grapevines

1. Zajicek, G., Oren, R., Weinreb, M. jr., The streaming liver, *Liver* 6 (1985) 293–300.

Chapter 31: Bryophyllum

1. Hassauer, W., Schreiber, K., Von der Decken, D., Ein neuer Weg in der tokolytischen Therapie, *Erfahrungsheilkunde* 34 (1985) 683–87.
2. Daub, *Vorzeitige Wehentätigkeit*. Vilaghi, I., Decreasing the rate of premature delivery with phytotherapy: results from general practice, *Ther. Umsch.* 59 (2002) 696–701.
3. Planegger, N., Rist, L., Zimmermann, R., von Mandach, U., Intravenous tocolysis with Bryophyllum pinnatum is better tolerated than beta-agonist application, *Eur. J. Obstet. Gynecol. Reprod. Biol.* 124 (2006) 168–72.
4. It has been shown using rodents that Bryophyllum increases the length of sleep (Pal, S., Sen, T., Chadhurim, A.K., Neuropsychopharmacological profile of the methanolic fraction of Bryophyllum pinnatum leaf extract, *J. Pharm. Pharmacol.* 51 (1999) 313–18), and a calming and muscle relaxing effect has also been demonstrated experimentally (Yemitan, O.K., Salahdeen, H.M., Neurosedative and muscle relexant activities of aqueous extract of *Bryophyllum pinnatum*, *Fitoterapia* 76 (2005) 187–93).

Chapter 32: Ivy

1. Mezger, *Gesichtete Homöopathische Arzneimittellehre,* Vol. 1; Stephenson, *Hahnemannian provings.*

Chapter 33: Blackthorn

1. The paper by Ulrich Meyer gives an excellent overview of the blackthorn, its effects and its many uses throughout history: Die Schlehe: Heilpflanze für Zeitgenossen, *Merkurstab* 2011, 64 (2) 100–114. In a further paper Meyer deals with hydrocyanic acid which, as has already been mentioned above, is to be found in blackthorn: 'Dem Stoff sich verschreiben, heißt Seelen zerreiben'. Zur historischen Signatur und toxikologischen Problematik reiner Blausäure, *Merkurstab* 2011, 64 (3) 123–32.

Chapter 34: Frankincense

1. An overview is given by Ammon, H.P.T., Salai-Guggal-(Indischer Weihrauch-) Gummiharz aus *Boswellia serrata, Dtsch. Ärztebl.* 95 (1998) 30–31.
2. A current review of brain tumours also recommends considering the use of incense: Schneider, T., Marri, C., Scherlach, C., et al., Die Gliome des Erwachsenen, *Dtsch. Ärztebl.* 107 (2010) 799–808.
3. Ammon, H.P.T., Salai-Guggal-(Indischer Weihrauch-) Gummiharz aus *Boswellia serrata, Dtsch. Ärztebl.* 95 (1998) 30–31; and Schneider, T., Marri, C., Scherlach, C., et al., 'Die Gliome des Erwachsenen, *Dtsch. Ärztebl.* 107 (2010) 799–808.

Chapter 35: Mistletoe

1. Göbel, Th., Dorka, R., Zur Raumgestalt und zur Zeitgestalt der Weißberigen Mistel (*Viscum album L.*) *Tycho de Brahe Jahrbuch für Goetheanismus* 1986, 167–94.

2. Kienle & Kiene, *Die Mistel in der Onkologie.*

3. Britsch, M., Heidecke, H., Meyer, U., Angiogenesehemmung durch Iscucine: Ergebnisse aktueller Untersuchungen, *Merkurstab* 63 (2010) 218–22.

4. See Madeleyn, R., Gesichtspunkte zur Epilepsie und deren Behandlungsmöglichkeit bei Kindern, *Merkurstab* 43 (1990) 369–84.

5. See also Soldner & Stellmann, *Individal Paediatrics.*

6. Wilkens, J., Sommer, M., Soldner, G., et al., Die Behandlung des Fibromyalgie-Syndroms mit Weidenmistel-Extrakten, *Merkurstab* 58 (2005) 264–71.

7. Simon, L., Chronisches Gelenkrheuma/Chronische Polyarthritis, in Glöckler, *Anthroposophische Arzneitherapie,* Vol. 1, 31.1–12.

8. Orange, M., Fonseca, M., Lace, A., von Laue, B., Geider, S., Durable tumour responses following primary high-dose induction with mistletoe extracts: Two case reports. *Eur. J. Integr. Med.* 2010, 1 (4) 227. Orange, M., Lace. A., Fonseca, M., von Laue H.B., Geider, S., Kienle, G.S., Durable Regression of Primary Cutaneous B-cell Lymphoma following Fever-inducing Mistletoe Treatment: Two Case Reports. *Global Adv. in Health & Med.* 2012 1(1) 16–23. Seifert, G., Tautz, C., Seeger, K., Henze, G., Laengler, A., Therapeutic use of mistletoe for CD30+ cutaneous lymphoproliferative disorder/lymphomatoid papulosis, *J. Eur. Acad. Dermatol. Venereol.* 2007 Apr, 21 (4) 558–60. Werthmann, P.G., Strater, G., Friesland, H., Kienle, G.S., Durable response of cutaneous squamous cell carcinoma following high-dose peri-lesional injections of Viscum album extracts: A case report. *Phytomedicine* 2013 Feb 15; 20 (3–4) 324–27. Mabed, M., El-Helw, L., Sharma, S., Phase II study of viscum fraxini-2 in patients with advanced hepatocellular carcinoma. *British Journal of Cancer* 2004 (90) 65–69. Mahfouz, M.M., Ghaleb, H.A., Hamza, M.R., Fares, L., Moussa, L., Moustafua, A., El-Za Wawy, A., Kourashy, L., Mobarak, L., Saed, S., Fouad, F., Tony, O., Tohamy, A., Multicenter open labeled clinical study in advanced breast cancer patients. A preliminary report. *Journal of the Egyptian Nat Cancer Inst* 1999 11 (3) 221–27.

9. Tröger, W., Galun, D., Reif, M., Schumann, A., Stankić, N,, Milićević, M., Viscum album [L.] extract therapy in patients with locally advanced or metastatic pancreatic cancer: A randomised clinical trial on overall survival. *Eur. J. Cancer* 49 (2013) 19: 3788–97.

10. Personal communication from Dr. H. Matthes, Head Physician, Gastroenterology, Havelhöhe Community Hospital, Berlin. A small retrospective study with 39 patients has shown that intratumoral application of mistletoe extracts in combination

with conventional chemotherapy in patients with advanced, unresectable pancreatic carcinoma was safe and associated with an remarkably long time of survival. The efficacy should be evaluated in a randomised controlled trial. (Schad F, Axtner J, Buchwald D, Happe A, Popp St, Kröz M, Matthes H, *Integr Cancer Ther* Dec 19, 2013 DOI: 10.1177/153735413513637)

11. Wilkens, *Mistletoe Therapy for Cancer.*

12. Werner, H., Mahfouz, M.M., Fares, L., Fouad, F., Ghaleb, H.A., Hamza, R., Kourashy, L., Mobarak, A.L., Moustafa, A., Saed, S., Zaky, O., Zawawny, A., Fischer, S., Scheer, R., Scheffler, A., Zur Therapie des malignen Pleuraergusses mit einem Mistelpräparat, *Merkurstab* 1999, 52 (5) 298–301. Salzer, G., Popp, W., Die lokale Iscadorbehandlung der Pleurakarzinose, in Jungi & Senn, *Krebs in Alternativmedizin,* Vol. 2, pp. 36–49. Girke, M., Debus, M., Kröz, M., Ascites bei Non-Hodgkin-Lymphom (V.a. splenales Lymphom) Remission nach viermaliger intraperitonealer Viscum-album-Instillation, *Merkurstab* 2012, 65 (3) 257f.

13. Schaefermeyer H., Zur Therapie des Blasenkarzinoms, *Merkurstab* 1996, 49 (3) 229–33. Simões-Wüst, A.P., Hunziker-Basler, N., Zuzak, T.J., Eggenschwiler, J., Rist, L., Viviani, A., Meyer, U., Das Mistelpräparat Iscucin Crataegi: Option für die Instillationstherapie bei Harnblasenkarzinom. *Merkurstab* 2007, 60 (3) 251–55.

14. For example, a randomized clinical study showed that patients with breast, ovarian and bronchial carcinomas tolerated chemotherapy significantly better when they were given mistletoe at the same time (Piao, B.K., Xang, Y.X., Xie, U., Mannsmann, U., Matthes, H., Beuth, J., Lin, H.S., Impact of complementary mistletoe extract treatment on quality of life in breast, ovarian and non-small cell lung cancer patients. A prospective randomized controlled clinical trial, *Anticancer Res.* 23 (2004) 303–9. In vitro studies on cell lines of breast, pancreas, lung and prostate cancer showed that mistletoe extracts which where given simultaneously with standard chemotherapeutic agents (doxorubicin, gemcitabine, docetaxel, mitoxantrone, cisplatin) did not inhibit chemotherapy induced cytostasis and cytotoxicity. In higher concentrations mistletoe extracts showed an additive inhibitory effect. (Weinstein U, Kunz M, Baumgartner St, Interactions of standardized mistletoe (Viscum album L.) extracts with chemotherapeutic drugs regarding cytostatic and cytotoxic effects in vitro. *BMC Complementary and Alternative Medicine* 2014 14:6 DOI: 10.1186/1472-6882-14-6

15. A detailed account of the scientific findings on mistletoe therapy is given in Kienle, & Kiene *Die Mistel in der Onkologie,* and in Kienle, Kiene & Albonico, *Anthroposophische Medizin in der klinischen Forschung.*

16. See also Sommer, M., Soldner, G., Die Mistel und ihre

Wirtsbäume – Differenzierung
zur Optimierung der Therapie,
Merkurstab 54 (2000) 29–48.
Wilkens, J., *Misteltherapie*. Soldner,
G., Sommer, M., Wilkens, J.,
Therapeutische Erfahrungen mit
der Lindenmistel, *Merkurstab* 60
(2006) 435–37. Wilkens, J., Die
Weidenmistel beim Blasenkarzinom,
Merkurstab 60 (2007) 446–49.
Wilkens, J., Die Weisstannennmistel,
Merkurstab 62 (2008) 570–83;
Wilkens, J., Die Mandelmistel,
Merkurstab 63 (2010) 29–45.

Chapter 36: Christmas Rose

1. Mörike, 'Auf eine Christblume,'
   translated by Malcolm Wren,
   copyright © 2006, reprinted with
   kind permission. The German
   original reads:
   Tochter des Walds, du
      Lilienverwandte,
   So lang von mir gesuchte,
      unbekannte,
   Im fremden Kirchhof, öd und
      winterlich,
   Zum ersten Mal, o schöne, find ich
      dich!

   Von welcher Hand gepflegt du hier
      erblühtest,
   Ich weiß es nicht, noch wessen
      Grab du hütest;
   Ist es ein Jüngling, so geschah ihm
      Heil,
   Ist's eine Jungfrau, lieblich fiel ihr
      Teil.
   ...
   Schön bist du, Kind des Mondes,
      nicht der Sonne;
   Dir wäre tödlich andrer Blumen
      Wonne,

   Dich nährt, den keuschen Leib voll
      Reif und Duft,
   Himmlischer Kräfte balsamsüße
      Luft.

2. For example, Wilkens, J., *Helleborus
   niger*: Geschichte, Botanik
   und differentialtherapeutische
   Anwendung einer Heilpflanze,
   Merkurstab 63 (2010) 535–49.

3. Soldner, G., *Helleborus niger* in der
   Pädiatrie, *Merkurstab* 63 (2010)
   508–17; Soldner & Stellmann,
   Individual Paediatrics.

4. Schnürer, Chr., *Helleborus niger*:
   Anwendung in Innerer Medizin
   und Psychosomatik, *Merkurstab*
   63 (2010) 518–25; Soldner, G.,
   Helleborus niger in der Pädiatrie,
   Merkurstab 63 (2010) 508–17.

5. Many verbal descriptions are now
   available as articles in a special
   issue on *Helleborus niger* in the
   journal for anthroposophical
   medicine, *Der Merkurstab,* 63,
   Vol. 6 (2010). Contributions
   worth noting are for example:
   Breitkreuz, Th., Helleborus in
   der Onkologie. Kasuistiken und
   Therapieerfahrungen aus dem
   Gemeinschaftskrankenhaus
   Herdecke 2001–2010, *Merkurstab*
   63 (2010) 526–34; Debus, M.,
   Anwendungsmöglichkeiten von
   Helleborus niger in der Onkologie,
   Merkurstab 63 (2010) 551–57 and
   the articles by Wilkens, Schnürer,
   and Soldner mentioned in Notes 2
   to 4 above.

Chapter 37: Ginger and Horseradish

1. Therkleson, T., The experience of receiving ginger compresses in persons with osteoarthritis: a phenomenological study, Faculty of Nursing. Vol. PhD. Edith Cowan University. Perth, Western Australia 2009.

Chapter 38: Gold

1. This and following quotes are from Vithoulkas, G., *Essenzen Homöopathischer Arzneimittel.*

2. For example, Selawry, *Metallfunktionstypen in Psychologie und Therapie*; Selawry, *Zinn und Zinntherapie*; Selawry, *Silber und Silbertherapie*; Walter, *Die sieben Hauptmetalle.* Individual topics also appear in *Vademecum anthroposophische Arzneimittel,* and Girke, M., *Innere Medizin.*

3. More about the possibilities of anthroposophical medicine for heart disease is given in Bavastro, Fried, & Kümmell, *Herz-Kreislauf-Sprechstunde.*

Useful Organisations

UK & Ireland:
Wala & Weleda www.weleda.co.uk

USA & Canada
Weleda usa.weleda.com

Australia
Weleda www.weleda.com.au

New Zealand
Wala & Weleda www.weleda.co.nz

Weleda (international) www.weleda.com

Bibliography

Atabay, Cyrus (tr.), *Die schönsten Gedichte aus dem klassischen Persien*, Munich 2004.

Bavastro, P., Fried, A., Kümmell, H.Chr., *Herz-Kreislauf-Sprechstunde. Ein umfassender medizinischer Ratgeber*, Stuttgart 2003.

Buber, M., *Die Erzählungen der Chassidim*, Zurich 1992.

Daub, E., *Vorzeitige Wehentätigkeit. Ihre Behandlung mit pflanzlichen Substanzen*, Stuttgart 1998.

Eckermann, J.P., *Gespräche mit Goethe in den letzten Jahren seines Lebens*, Munich 1984.

Eichendorff, J. von, *Werke*, Volume 1, Munich 1981.

Girke, M., *Innere Medizin, Grundlagen und therapeutische Konzepte in der Anthroposophischen Medizin*, Berlin 2012.

Glaser H.. *Erfolgreiche Wundbehandlung: Aus der Praxis anthroposophisch erweiterter Krankenpflege*, Stuttgart 2000.

Glöckler, M. (Ed.), *Anthroposophische Arzneitherapie für Ärzte und Apotheker*, Stuttgart 2005.

Godden, Rumer, *The Story of Holly and Ivy*, London 2001.

Gunther, K., Hannemann, H.-J., Hieke, F., Konigsmann, E., Schumann, H., *Urania Tierreich*, Vol. 3, Leipzig 1994.

Hegi, Gustav, *Illustrierte Flora von Mitteleuropa*, Parey 2000.

Husemann, Friedwart, *Anthroposophische Medizin. Ein Weg zu den heilenden Kräften*, Dornach 2011.

Jachens, Lüder, *Dermatologie: Grundlagen und therapeutische Konzepte der anthroposophischen Medizin*, Berlin 2012.

Jungi, W.F., Senn, H.-J. (eds.) *Krebs in Alternativmedizin*, Berlin/Heidelberg 1990.

Kienle, G.S., Kiene, H., Albonico, H.U., *Anthroposophische Medizin in der klinischen Forschung*, Stuttgart 2006.

Kienle, G.S., Kiene, H., *Die Mistel in der Onkologie*, Stuttgart 2003.

Leeser, O., *Lehrbuch der Homöopathie*, Ulm 1973.

Livingstone, David and Charles, *Narrative of an expedition to the Zambesi and its tributaries and of the discovery of the Lakes Shirwa and Nyassa, 1856–1864*, London 1865.

Madaus, G., *Lehrbuch der Homöopathischen Heilmittel*, Vol. 3, (reprint of 1938 ed.) Hildesheim 1979.

Mezger, Julius, *Gesichtete Homöopathische Arzneimittellehre*,

Vol. 1, Heidelberg 1989.

Mörike, E., *Sämtliche Gedichte in einem Band*, (ed. B. Zeller) Frankfurt 2004.

Rumi, *Ghaselen des Dschelâleddîn Rumi*, (tr. Josef v. Hammer-Purgstall) Stuttgart 1920.

Schaefer, O., *Der grüne Ton. Späte und frühe Gedichte*, Munich 1973.

Schimmel, A., Rumi. *Ich bin Wind und du bist Feuer. Leben und Werk des großen Mystikers*, Cologne 1986.

Selawry, A., *Metallfunktionstypen in Psychologie und Therapie*, Ulm 1983.

—, *Silber und Silbertherapie*, Ulm 1966.

—, *Zinn und Zinntherapie*, Ulm 1963.

Servan-Schreiber, D., *Das Antikrebs-Buch. Was uns schützt: vorbeugen und nachsorgen mit natürlichen Mitteln*, Munich 2010.

Soldner, G., Stellmann, H.M., *Individal Paediatrics: Physical Emotional and Spiritual Aspects of Diagnosis and Counseling*, CRC Press, USA, 2014.

Steiner, Rudolf, *Agriculture*, Bio-Dynamic Farming and Gardening Ass. USA 1993.

—, *An Outline of Esoteric Science*, Anthroposophic Press, USA 1997.

—, *Introducing Anthroposophical Medicine*, Steinerbooks USA 2010.

Stephenson, J., *Hahnemannian provings: A Materia medica and Repertory*, New Delhi, 1998.

Vademecum anthroposophische Arzneimittel, (ed. Gesellschaft Anthroposophischer Ärzte) 3ed Stuttgart 2013.

Walter, H., *Die sieben Hauptmetalle. Ihre Beziehungen zu Welt, Erde und Mensch*, Dornach, 2010.

Wilkens, Johannes, Misteltherapie. *Differenzierte Anwendung der Mistel und ihrer Wirtsbäume*, Stuttgart 2006.

—, *Mistletoe Therapy for Cancer: Prevention, Treatment and Healing*, Floris Books, 2010.

Vithoulkas, G., *Essenzen Homöopathischer Arzneimittel nach G. Vithoulkas*, (tr. J.Faust & G. Hieronymus) Frankfurt 1986.

Plant families

Indices are not usually the most interesting parts of a book. But they unquestionably offer a good opportunity for making discoveries. Below is a list of the medicinal plants mentioned in detail in this book, arranged according to their families. A great many medicinal plants are found here as the only representative of their family (for example ivy for the *Araliaceae* and mistletoe for the *Loranthaceae*). But it is very noticeable that there is a concentration into three families: the daisy family, mint family and buttercup family. Over a quarter of all the therapeutic plants in this book belong to the daisy family (*Compositae*, also called *Asteraceae*). This is very striking, but it has to be admitted that this is also due to the fact that the *Compositae* is a very large plant family.

Plants are in principle assigned to the different families on account of the structure of their flowers. The flower of a member of the *Compositae* is actually a community made up of numerous individual flowers. This can easily be seen with the naked eye in a sunflower, which also belongs to this family. The outer flowers each have a long coloured petal, while the inner part of the flower disc is made up of inconspicuous individual tubular flowers which each have stamens and a pistil and produce their own fruits. At every point where a sunflower seed sits there was previously an individual flower of the sunflower flower community. In principle, all members of the *Compositae* family are made up of a 'composite' of individual flowers like the sunflower. A composite inflorescence like this in a way represents the ability to integrate the individual into an overall structure. Might this ability be connected to the fact that there are so many medicinal plants amongst the members of the daisy family? Ultimately, every illness can be viewed as one part of our body no longer being able to perform what is necessary for the whole (it varies from illness to illness as to whether this is a case of 'too much' organ activity – think of the increased mucus production in a cold – or 'too little' – for example in the case of a thyroid insufficiency). What is unusual is that the members of the daisy family almost never produce any poison (in contrast to those of the buttercup family, for example, which all produce substances which irritate the skin and mucus membranes). These characteristics may be a reason that plants from the daisy family are particularly suitable as 'home remedies', which can gently help to restore health when this has begun to falter.

Far fewer plants in this book come from the mint family (*Labiatae*) but they still comprise almost a tenth of the total. The members of this family are characterised by their complicated horizontally-angled flowers resembling a face, where the petals have united into a tube and often make use of a refined tilting mechanism to ensure that every insect visiting the flower gets dabbed with pollen. Many of these 'gestures' point beyond the sphere of the plant towards that of the animal realm. What is typical of plants is actually the production of surfaces, particularly those of the leaves. When plants form enclosed spaces, this goes beyond the plant nature, strictly speaking. The fast reaction of the stamens when an insect penetrates the flower in search of nectar is also an 'animal-like' gesture. The flower, in turning away from the sky into the horizontal axis, also positions itself in the same plane in which the animal lives. Like very many other flowers, the goal of the *Labiatae* is also to attract insects. Many plants make use of scent to do this. It is a characteristic of the *Labiatae* – and especially those with a medicinal effect – that there is also a large amount of scented essential oil in the leaves. It is perhaps not surprising that these plants particularly affect our mood. They can stimulate (rosemary, for example) or relax (lemon balm or lavender, for example) or they relieve organs such as the stomach that have become 'upset' due to emotional stresses (peppermint, for example).

Just as, in individual plants, we can discover gestures in their appearance that reappear in their medicinal effects, gestures typical of the family can also be found, as illustrated by these examples. An index showing the plants in this book arranged according to their families not only has a scientific purpose, but can also be the basis of our own discoveries.

Ivy family (Araliaceae)
Ivy (*Hedera helix*): page 314.

Incense tree family (Burseraceae)
Frankincense (*Boswellia serrata, Boswellia sacra*): page 330.

Birch family (Betulaceae)
Silver birch (*Betula pendula*): page 70.

Nettle family (Urticaceae)
Stinging nettle (*Urtica dioica, Urtica urens*): page 282.

Orpine family (Crassulaceae)
Bryophyllum (*Kalanchoë* (= *Bryophyllum*) *daigremontiana, Kalanchoë pinnata*): page 308.

Gentian family (Gentianaceae)
Yellow gentian (*Gentiana lutea*): page 256.

Honeysuckle family (Caprifoliaceae)
Elder (*Sambucus nigra*): page 169.

Buttercup family (Ranunculaceae)
Christmas rose (*Helleborus niger*): page 357.
Monkshood (*Aconitum napellus*): page 265.
Pasque flower (*Pulsatilla vulgaris, Pulsatilla pratensis*): page 92.

Heather family (Ericaceae)
Cranberry (*Vaccinium macrocarpon*): page 296
Bilberry (*Vaccinium myrtillus*): page 296.

Dogbane family (Apocynaceae)
Strophanthus (*Strophanthus kombé, Strophanthus gratus*): page 17.

Ginger family (Zingiberaceae)
Ginger (*Zingiber officinale*): page 365.

St John's Wort family (Hypericaceae)
St John's Wort (*Hypericum perforatum*): page 158.

Daisy family (Compositae)
Arnica (*Arnica montana*): page 228.
Artichoke (*Cynara scolymus*): page 183.
Blessed thistle or St Benedict's thistle, holy thistle (*Cnicus benedictus, formerly Carduus benedictus*): page 183.
Daisy (*Bellis perennis*): page 65.
Chamomile (*Matricaria recutita,* formerly *Matricaria chamomilla*): page 127.
Dandelion (*Taraxacum officinale*): page 42.
Milk thistle (*Silybum marianum, formerly: Carduus marianus*): page 183.
Marigold (*Calendula officinalis*): page 228.
Yarrow (*Achillea millefolium*): page 34.
Coneflower (*Echinacea angustifolia, Echinacea purpurea, Echinacea pallida*): page 192.
Chicory (*Cichorium intybus*): page 275.

Cabbage family (Brassicaceae)
Horseradish (*Cochlearia armoracia*): page 365.

Lily family (Liliaceae)
Garden onion (*Allium cepa*): page 26.

Lime family (Tiliaceae)
Lime (*Tilia cordata, Tilia platyphyllos*): page 177.

Mint family (Labiatae)
Lavender (*Lavandula officinalis*)
Melissa/Lemon balm (*Melissa officinalis*): page 201.
Peppermint (*Mentha piperita*): page 58.

Rosemary (*Rosmarinus officinalis*): page 210.
Poppy family (*Papaveraceae*)
Greater celandine (*Chelidonium majus*): page 109.

Primrose family (Primulaceae)
Cowslip/Oxlip (*Primula veris/Primula elatior*): page 82.

Mistletoe family (Loranthaceae)
Mistletoe (*Viscum album*): page 340.

Rose family (Rosaceae)
Rose (*Rosa centifolia, Rosa damascena*): page 219.
Blackthorn (*Prunus spinosa*): page 320.
Wild strawberry (*Fragaria vesca*): page 103.

Horsetail family (Equisetaceae)
Field horsetail (*Equisetum arvense*): page 146.

Plantain family (Plantaginaceae)
Ribwort plantain (*Plantago lanceolata*): page 138.

Grapevine (Vitaceae)
Grapevine (*Vitis vinifera*): page 302.

Index of Healing Plants

Index of Ailments

417

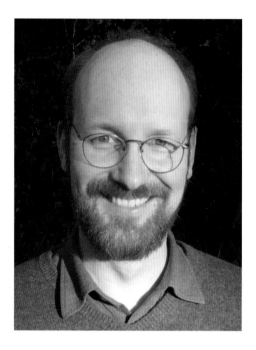

Markus Sommer, born in 1966, studied medicine in Munich and is a general physician there. His experience includes internal medicine, pediatrics, geriatry, neurology, and the practical application of homeopathic and anthroposophical medicine. He is the author of several medical books.